the $800 MILLION PILL

We'll plug along on it for two or three years, and maybe we'll get something permanent—and probably we'll fail.

Martin Arrowsmith

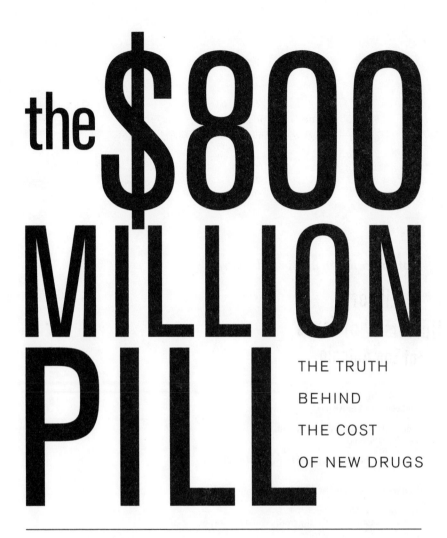

the $800 MILLION PILL

THE TRUTH BEHIND THE COST OF NEW DRUGS

MERRILL GOOZNER

UNIVERSITY OF CALIFORNIA PRESS Berkeley Los Angeles London

For my children and grandchildren

University of California Press
Berkeley and Los Angeles, California

University of California Press, Ltd.
London, England

© 2004 by the Regents of the University of California

Library of Congress Cataloging-in-Publication Data

Goozner, Merrill, 1950–.
  The $800 million pill : the truth behind the cost of
new drugs / Merrill Goozner.
      p. cm.
  Includes bibliographical references and index.
  ISBN 0-520-23945-8 (cloth)
    1. Prescription pricing.   2. Drugs—Prices.
3. Pharmaceutical industry.   4. Consumer education.
I. Title: Eight hundred million dollar pill. II. Title.

RS100.G668 2004
338.4'3'61510973—dc22   2003063422

Manufactured in the United States of America
10 09 08 07 06 05 04
10 9 8 7 6 5 4 3 2 1

The paper used in this publication meets the minimum
requirements of ANSI/NISO Z39.48-1992 (R 1997)
(*Permanence of Paper*). ♾

Contents

Introduction / 1

PART ONE **BIOHYPE**

1 The Longest Search / 13

2 Rare Profits / 39

3 The Source of the New Machine / 61

PART TWO **DIRECTED RESEARCH**

4 A Public-Private Partnership / 85

5 The Divorce / 115

6 Breakthrough! / 137

7 The Failed Crusade? / 164

PART THREE **BIG PHARMA**

8 Me Too! / 209

9 The $800 Million Pill / 231

10 The Future of Drug Innovation / 247

Notes / 261
Bibliography / 281
Acknowledgments / 285
Index / 287

Introduction

In the quarter-century since the dawn of the biotechnology revolution, hundreds of research scientists at the nation's elite medical schools have decamped from their tenured sinecures to join pharmaceutical firms or biotechnology start-ups. Most have set up shop near the institutions that trained them—near Boston, San Francisco, San Diego, or Research Triangle Park in North Carolina. Others have gravitated to the outskirts of Washington, D.C., to be near the National Institutes of Health (NIH), the funding colossus of the biomedical world. Most see themselves as dedicated scientists in the mold of Martin Arrowsmith, the fictional physician in Sinclair Lewis's novel, whose passion to make a mark in the world of research was always leavened by his abiding concern for the health of mankind. But virtually all have lurking somewhere in the corners of their minds another goal. They want to start the next Amgen.

Amgen Inc., however, did not spring from any of the intellectual command posts of the biotechnology revolution. It began in an office park in Thousand Oaks, a skateboard haven about an hour's drive north of Los Angeles, far enough from downtown that local inhabitants sometimes refer to it as Thousand Miles. In that small city of cookie-cutter ranch homes and enclosed shopping malls, a handful of scientists trained at the University of California at Los Angeles and skilled in the new art of recombinant engineering began in 1980 what would eventually become the largest, fastest-growing, and most profitable biotechnology company in the world.

One of the first companies to bring a biotechnology product to market, Amgen has grown to more than eight thousand people working in forty buildings sprawled across its industrial park–like campus. Though Amgen attracted only a handful of top-notch scientists to move there over the years, the company registered nearly $5 billion in sales in 2002 and declared almost a third of that in profit.[1] According to *Forbes Magazine,* investors who plunked down one hundred dollars for stock in the struggling start-up in the mid-1980s would have shares worth more than $1.5 million by 2001, making Amgen one of the business world's most extraordinary growth stories in the decades when such stories were commonplace.

Yet for all of Amgen's spectacular success, virtually all of the company's revenue came from the sale of just two drugs. Both gained approval from the Food and Drug Administration during George H. W. Bush's administration. Both were considered the low-hanging fruit of the biotech revolution, easy targets for the new technology of recombinant engineering. Amgen's big sellers are artificial versions of naturally occurring enzymes that had been identified and isolated well before the company began developing them.

Amgen's first approved drug and its biggest seller is Epogen. It is the recombinant-engineered version of erythropoietin, the enzyme produced in the kidney that signals bone marrow to manufacture red blood cells. The largest patient population in need of erythropoietin is the more than three hundred thousand Americans on dialysis. Their failing kidneys no longer produce it in sufficient quantities to prevent anemia. The federal government picks up the tab for most dialysis patients through the Medicare program, meaning Amgen's financial success has largely come at taxpayer expense. Amgen's other big seller is Neupogen, an artificial version of granulocyte colony-stimulating factor, which tells the bone marrow to produce infection-fighting white blood cells. This drug is a godsend to cancer patients undergoing chemotherapy, whose suppressed bone marrow is in need of extra stimulation.

The health benefits derived from these drugs have come at a hefty price. They are among the most expensive on the market. This is not because the drugs are costly to make. The technology behind recombinant engineering, invented in the mid-1970s, is now rather commonplace and can be conducted by intelligent college students working with lab equipment ordered over the Internet. Nor is the high price justified by the original investment in research and development. Amgen earned the cost of developing these drugs within a year or two of their coming on the market.

Rather, as Amgen's extensive advertising on National Public Radio, in magazines, and in the medical literature puts it, there is only one justification for the high price tags on its drugs. They are needed to pay for the scientists and technicians squirreled away in Thousand Oaks, who are busily searching for the next generation of wonder drugs. It costs more than $800 million to discover a new drug, industry officials have said, drawing their figure from a single, frequently cited study from Tufts University. They have to put a high price on yesterday's discoveries if they are going to conduct the research needed to come up with the next generation of wonder drugs. One set of recent Amgen ads featured a clinician clad in a lab coat peering into a microscope. The caption claimed the company was searching for therapies capable of "dramatically improving people's lives."

Half of Amgen's employees and one of every five dollars earned over the past decade was in fact devoted to what the company called research and development. Yet Amgen's labs were notoriously unproductive in the decade after its first drugs were approved. "It's been a while since a major clinical advance has come out of Thousand Oaks," said Mark Brand, a marketing professor at Johnson and Wales University in Denver who used to be the company's top public relations man. "Their offerings to physicians have not been major league."[2]

In late 2001, after a decade of disappointments, the company's labs finally produced a new drug capable of generating a billion dollars in sales—the financial holy grail of pharmaceutical industry managers and investors. The drug is called Aranesp. The company touted Aranesp as its most significant medical advance since the arrival of its first two drugs. But Aranesp, like Epogen, was for anemia. Was it a dramatic new treatment for the debilitating condition? Company officials said it was. "We believe Aranesp simplifies the treatment of anemia associated with chronic renal failure, with potentially fewer office visits and less disruption to patients' lives," Kevin Sharer, the chief executive officer of Amgen, said.[3]

It is dramatic health claims like Amgen's, and the assertion that only industry can produce those benefits, that justify the high cost of drugs in the United States. North America's pharmaceutical and biotechnology companies have become the primary source of new drugs for physicians looking for new weapons for fighting disease. The hopes of millions of Americans for cures for cancer, Alzheimer's disease, and the other debilitating conditions of aging rest on the tireless efforts going on in the drug industry's labs. But there's a catch. Industry can produce those results only if the American people continue to pay the highest prices in the world for drugs.

This book challenges that assertion by pulling away the curtain that has long shrouded pharmaceutical innovation. It asks two simple questions. Where do new drugs come from? What do they really cost to invent? To answer these questions, I take readers inside the arcane process of drug development for a representative sample of relatively recent discoveries—from their beginnings in academic and government labs to their final approval by the Food and Drug Administration. By viewing the entire process of drug development, I offer an alternative picture to the one painted during the heated debate in Washington over a prescription drug benefit for Medicare, a debate in which politicians and drug industry officials, echoing the Amgen ads, argue that drug prices have to remain high in order to fund innovation.

I first became intrigued by that assertion in 1999 while attending hearings on Capitol Hill devoted to the crisis in Medicare funding. As an economics correspondent for the *Chicago Tribune*, I was tugged in many directions that winter: Alan Greenspan and interest rates; the aftermath of the Asian financial crisis; the budget battles between the Republican Congress and a beleaguered President Bill Clinton. And, of course, there was the story that from the hindsight of our post-Enron world seems almost laughable: Would the president's impeachment trial destroy investor confidence?

But something curious happened to me that busy news year. Whenever I wrote about these stories, I received no mail. No e-mails jammed my computer's inbox. No readers searched out my telephone number. It was as if my dispatches about economic events at the peak of the bubble had disappeared into a black hole. When I mentioned this to my colleagues, they scoffed at my naiveté. Wasn't it obvious? The American public, enjoying the fruits of a raging bull market, was too busy watching the presidential soap opera known as Monica.

Yet when I wrote about the Medicare reform debate—the National Bipartisan Commission on the Future of Medicare was concluding its deliberations about the same time that Kenneth Starr was concluding his—I received a completely different response. Letters to the editor began appearing in the paper. Senior citizens began sending me hand-written notes. Many came on personal stationery, a touching reminder of a fading era when people penned longhand notes to their representatives about matters that deeply concerned them.

The letters all spoke to the issue that bedeviled and eventually stale-mated the Medicare commission. Why, my elderly readers wanted to know, were the prices of drugs so high? Why couldn't the government do something about it? And why couldn't the government provide a pre-scription drug benefit for senior citizens? While 62 percent of Americans take no drugs at all over the course of an average year, three-fourths of the elderly do, and half of them take two or more that require them to follow a daily regimen—usually for chronic conditions like high blood pressure, diabetes, or arthritis. In 2002 the nation's total prescription drug spending soared to more than $160 billion a year and was rising at an 18-percent annual rate. Americans spent more on prescription drugs than on telephones, radios, televisions, and cell phones combined. Well over half of that came out of seniors' pockets. In the richest nation on earth, some elderly Americans were hobbling onto buses to cross into Canada to buy cheaper medicines, while others sawed pills in half or did without basic necessities to get to the end of the month.[4]

There were no significant differences between Republican and Demo-cratic appointees to the commission on the need for adding prescription drugs to Medicare. Everyone agreed that pharmaceuticals had become a key component of modern health care, just as hospital stays and doctor visits had been the main concern when President Lyndon B. Johnson signed Medicare into law in 1965. Yet, with the price of drugs skyrock-eting year after year, millions of seniors were forced to choose between paying for their medicine and paying for the other necessities of life. Leaving Medicare without a drug benefit would turn a program that was designed to provide Americans with medical security in their old age into a mirror image of the nation's health insurance market. A substan-tial minority of the population would be forced to go without.

Yet the appointees to the bipartisan Medicare commission faced a conundrum in trying to add a prescription drug benefit to the system. How could the government afford to add drugs to a program that was already headed for bankruptcy? Although the state of the economy over this decade will determine Medicare's ultimate date with insolvency, the government's actuaries predict the program will begin running chronic deficits just about the time the Baby Boom begins retiring in 2010.

Liberals and progressive Democrats in Congress offered one possible solution to this dilemma. They proposed a Medicare drug program that would act like any other large buyer in the marketplace. Pharmacy benefit managers, who operate drug plans for major corporations, negotiated steep discounts on the prices they pay for drugs. Why couldn't the government do the same? Wielding senior buying power was one way to hold down costs.

Some experts also proposed limiting the choice of drugs that Medicare recipients could buy. In the jargon of the experts, such preapproved drug lists are called formularies. Government agencies like the Veterans Administration and some private-sector benefit managers already use them. Proponents of formularies argued that it makes no sense for the government to pay for lifestyle drugs like, say, Viagra, which is prescribed for erectile dysfunction but is widely used for sexual enhancement. And when there are two drugs on the market for a condition and both work about the same, the government should not pay for the more expensive brand name. Instead, it should reimburse people only if they buy the cheaper generic. A government formulary could sort through the morass of the modern drug marketplace on behalf of senior citizens.

Conservative Democrats and most Republicans on the panel recoiled in horror at these proposals. They took their cue from industry officials such as Alan F. Holmer, the president of the Pharmaceutical Research and Manufacturers Association, the industry's main lobbying group in Washington. Holmer was not one of Washington's more imposing figures. He did not have the golden tan and silver locks of the movie industry's Jack Valenti, nor the technical expertise and insider savvy of PriceWaterhouse's Kenneth Kies, the master architect of corporate tax breaks. Holmer often stumbled over his words when giving testimony and took a long time to formulate his response to questions. Yet he wielded enormous clout on drug issues, and his testimony was always the centerpiece of any hearing devoted to the topic. This was driven in part by the industry's large campaign contributions. According to the Center for Responsive Politics, the pharmaceutical industry raised $26 million for political campaign contributions in the two years before the 2000 election, and in the 2002 cycle it was the tenth largest donor among all industries, up from thirteenth in 2000 and twenty-seventh in 1990. The industry also deployed more than six hundred paid lobbyists on Capitol Hill, more than one for every senator and representative.[5]

But Holmer's influence did not depend solely on this largesse. It also rested on a powerful and compelling argument. The pharmaceutical industry's top official said that without high prices, the innovation that led to new medicine would dry up. It was an argument that invoked fear and consternation among the health-conscious public and their representatives. Americans fervently believe in the power of modern medicine and do not want anything to jeopardize the promising treatments for cancer, heart disease, and Alzheimer's, which the media routinely suggest are just around the corner.

Yet few Americans grasped the argument's startling departure from the norms of modern business practice. Most industries view research and development as something they must do to stay one step ahead of the competition, just as they must reduce the cost of production to maintain profit margins. If they fail to innovate, they risk obsolescence and decline. "If we don't spend our money on research and development, we will die," I've heard more than one chief executive officer say to stockholders at an annual meeting. The drug industry stood this corporate mantra on its head. "If we don't get your money to spend on research and development, you'll die."

The industry was not shy about deploying this argument on Capitol Hill. Testifying before the Senate Finance Committee in May 2000, the industry's top spokesman warned legislators that a disaster would befall the American people if the government tampered with the prescription drug market. Holmer told the committee that adopting a senior citizen drug benefit that imposed any kind of restrictions on price or relied on a formulary would dry up the revenue stream needed for innovation. The U.S. industry was responsible for 370 new drugs and vaccines in the 1990s, half of all pharmaceutical innovation in the world. An industry-sponsored study came out a year later that said the average price tag for developing a new drug had risen to more than $800 million. To raise that kind of money for research, the industry needed every dime it collected from the American people. To limit the price of drugs or to limit the number of drugs that a plan might buy would jeopardize the industry's ability to come up with new breakthroughs. "Government price controls are unacceptable to the industry because they would inevitably harm our ability to bring new medicines to patients," Holmer testified.[6]

Public interest groups, insurance companies, and health care advocates cried foul, claiming the drug companies' reasoning was nothing more than a scare tactic. They wielded studies that tried to poke holes in estimates of the research-and-development costs of a single new drug. They complained bitterly about the industry's wasted search for drugs that mimic those already on the market. They attacked its marketing practices, including the expensive advertising sprees that encouraged patients to ask their doctors for new medicines that were no better than ones just coming off patent. And they pointed to the oversized profits racked up by the industry. Yet most legislators refused to do anything to hold down prescription drug prices when they passed a Medicare bill in November 2003 because they accepted the industry's core assertion that its financial health was the key to innovation.

This book challenges that assertion by delving into the process by which drugs are actually developed. By recounting the history of several of the most significant new drugs of the past two decades, this book shows that the inception of drugs which have truly made a difference in recent years and which will make a difference in the twenty-first century can almost always be found in the vast biomedical research enterprise funded by the federal government. Taxpayer-financed medical research, whether in NIH labs or through government grants to academic and nonprofit medical centers, reached $27 billion in 2003, almost equal to industry spending. But a dollar comparison does not begin to describe the critical nature of the taxpayers' role. Over the years, NIH-funded research played not only the key role in virtually all of the basic scientific breakthroughs that underpin modern medicine but also a central role in the application of those findings to the search for many new therapies. In some cases, government-funded researchers not only conducted the basic research but went on to identify the new drugs and test them in animals and humans, thereby completing the vital tasks required for regulatory approval.

This is not to say that many of the fifty thousand scientists, technicians, and office personnel working in industry labs do not play a crucial role in the successful development of new drugs. Significant advances in medicine require a complex interaction between scientists in the public arena and scientists in industry. The most successful drug companies maintain sophisticated in-house staffs capable of keeping up with the latest breakthroughs in public research. The companies also house scientists who can rapidly synthesize new chemicals that may become new drugs, develop new tools of high-throughput screening and rational drug design, and employ physicians adept at designing and monitoring clinical trials for testing them. But at the same time drug companies and their biotechnology cousins are deploying these skills for the commercialization of important new medicines, a sizable portion of the industry's $30 billion research budget—perhaps as much as half—is spent on drugs that add nothing significant to physicians' armamentarium for fighting disease.

Moreover, big pharmaceutical firms increasingly farm out many critical tasks to highly specialized firms willing to do that work for anyone. There are a growing number of biotech companies, specialty chemical companies, and clinical research firms willing and able to design drugs, screen chemicals, and conduct animal and human studies for researchers who think they have identified a new way to combat a disease. Anyone can take advantage of their services, including research organizations in the public and nonprofit domain.

Yet in the twenty-first century, the breakthroughs that lead to pharmaceutical innovation will take place long before those firms are employed. As the economist Alfonso Gambardella pointed out in *Science and Innovation*, a recent academic review of U.S. pharmaceutical research in the 1980s, "The generation of new drugs depends in large measure on activities that occur at the outset of the research-and-development process. Early research stages play a more meaningful role than in other industries, and they are the most creative steps of the drug innovation cycle."[7]

Over the past two decades, the U.S.–funded research establishment in government, universities, and medical schools has developed an extremely efficient conveyor belt for moving the patented products and processes of these "most creative steps" into the private sector. Virtually the entire biotechnology industry is made up of firms begun when an individual investigator or group of investigators decided to try to get rich using the patents they took out on their government-funded inventions. There's nothing wrong with that. Indeed, it's the American way. The technology commercialization conveyor belt is the product of a deliberate government policy adopted in 1980 to foster innovation in medicine as it has in other high-technology fields.

But when the senior citizen medical insurance system is headed for bankruptcy; when the cost of health care, largely driven by the high and rising price of drugs, is taking up a greater and greater share of the overall economy; and when a growing number of Americans cannot afford the fruits of the pharmaceutical innovation system they funded—then the public has the right to ask how rich the commercial side of the partnership needs to be to ensure their continued participation in the system. The drug industry consistently reports profit margins approaching 30 percent of revenue. And while the industry also spends slightly more than 20 percent of its revenue on research and development, this book shows that nearly half of that research is more properly categorized as either a marketing expense or of minor medical significance aimed only at coming up with drugs that replicate the action of those already on the market. Indeed, the financial press is filled with dire accounts about a looming industry crisis precisely because the industry's vaunted research and development pipelines have not generated the medical break-throughs promised to investors and consumers alike.

In the immediate aftermath of World War II, George W. Merck, the patrician head of the most research-oriented firm in the industry, laid out a credo for his scientists. "We try never to forget that medicine is for the people. It is not for the profits. The profits follow, and if we have remembered that, they have never failed to appear. The better we have remembered that, the larger they have been."[8] The company still puts his words in its annual report, and makes them the centerpiece of its displays at medical conventions and scientific meetings.

But a half-century later, the former head of global research and development at Hoffmann–La Roche, Inc., after surveying the pharmaceutical industry's research landscape, reported just how far the industry had drifted from Merck's ideal. Jürgen Drews raised the specter of large pharmaceutical companies disappearing from the face of the earth, like the dinosaurs. "There can be no doubt that drugs could be discovered and developed outside the pharmaceutical industry," Drews concluded in his 1999 book *In Quest of Tomorrow's Medicines*. He suggested that public institutions such as NIH, the Medical Research Council (England's NIH equivalent), or the German state-funded institutes could pick up the mantle of drug commercialization, relying on the same contract organizations that industry now uses for many of its research tasks. "An industry that becomes disconnected from its true purpose will gradually become replaceable," he said.[9]

Amgen's brief history is a good place to start in understanding how the drug industry got into this fix. But to understand its early successes and more recent disappointments, one must first travel to Chicago, where a bull-headed scientist working at the dawn of the biotechnology era made a discovery that would provide hope, energy, and extended life for millions of people, and from which he would never earn a dime in royalties.

PART ONE

BIOHYPE

1

The Longest Search

Eugene Goldwasser retired in 2002 after a forty-seven-year career as a biochemistry professor at the University of Chicago. Like most academicians, he spent most of his working years laboring in obscurity. The primary focus of his research, his obsession really, resulted in just one major discovery. His colleagues admired his dedication. But some whispered about what he didn't receive over his long career—the fame, the glory, and the money that rightfully should have been his from being one of the leading medical pioneers of the second half of the twentieth century. His discovery has prevented tens of thousands of deaths from tainted blood transfusions and enabled millions of cancer and dialysis patients to live longer and more productive lives. Yet he never won any prestigious awards. And very few people—certainly not the general public, nor the patients he helped—even know his name.

Goldwasser, a soft-spoken academician whose unassuming manner hides a ruthless intolerance for scientific error, spent more than two decades pursuing a single hormone. It is a tiny molecule that swims briefly in the bloodstream, stimulates red blood cell production, and then disappears. He knew from the outset of his search that the protein would help anemia patients if he could find it and produce it in sufficient quantities. Yet the pharmaceutical industry, through all his lonely years of halting progress and heartbreaking setbacks, scorned and ignored him.

After he finally succeeded in isolating the protein, Goldwasser shared the fruits of his research with Applied Molecular Genetics Inc., which later became known as Amgen. He was instrumental in transforming the firm from a struggling start-up into the largest and most profitable biotechnology company in the world.

The interplay of Goldwasser's search for erythropoietin, or Epo, as it is affectionately known by physicians who work in the field, and Amgen's success in turning it into a hugely profitable drug is a paradigm for the modern drug industry. Goldwasser's career spanned the half-century after World War II, which witnessed an extraordinary explosion in the basic knowledge about the biochemical processes that make up life on earth. Hundreds of drug and biotechnology companies are seeking to mine that knowledge in their search for new therapies. The commercialization of Goldwasser's work on Epo is only one piece of that vast mosaic. But it was one of the first therapies of the biotechnology era, and it turned Amgen into the biotechnology company that every struggling start-up would like to become.

The Epo story is instructive for everyone concerned about the rising cost of medicine. After the artificial version of Epo entered the marketplace, its story turned into a sordid tale of endless patent litigation, adroit marketing, and political fixing designed to discourage rivals, promote the overuse of the drug, and maintain its high price, which is largely paid by the federal government's Medicare program. Like all drug companies, Amgen claims that the high price of Epo is necessary to fund its search for innovative new drugs. Yet a close look at Amgen's research performance during the fifteen years after Epo's arrival reveals a company whose labs were unproductive by every measure. Its biggest success was coming up with a slightly modified version of the original Epo molecule, which enabled it to go after other companies' markets. This is the classic "me-too" behavior of large pharmaceutical companies, which innovative start-ups like Amgen were supposed to supplant.

It took decades for Goldwasser to find and purify the first small vial of human erythropoietin. Private companies rarely support that kind of research. It takes too long, and the odds of success are even longer. Every step of Goldwasser's journey was funded by the federal government. His journey was typical in that regard, too. Virtually all the basic science that enables modern medicine to move forward takes place in the nonprofit sector—at universities, research institutes, and government labs. And governments, in particular the U.S. government, are by far its largest financiers.

The pharmaceutical industry and its biotechnology stepchild occasionally contribute to the basic scientific understanding of disease. But the private sector's main role is to develop and commercialize therapies based on that knowledge. It is called applied research. But as we shall see in subsequent chapters, even in this arena the public sector plays a large and sometimes dominant role. The Goldwasser-Amgen story provides an excellent opening snapshot of the complicated relationship between basic and applied research in the public and private sectors and shows how private firms rely on public research to come up with important new drugs. And this particular story, in the time-honored tradition of scientific serendipity, also reveals how one man's solitary quest helped jump-start an industry.

Eugene Goldwasser was born in 1922 in Brooklyn, where his father ran a small clothing manufacturing business. In the middle of the Depression, the shop failed, and his father, desperate for work, moved the family to Kansas City, where an uncle owned another small clothing factory. The move forced Goldwasser's older brother, a science major at New York University, to drop out of school to work in the family business. His loss became the younger brother's gain. While still in high school, Eugene read his brother's copy of Sinclair Lewis's *Arrowsmith* (1925), a novel about an idealistic doctor, and Paul de Kruif's *Microbe Hunters* (1926), a popular account of pioneering microbiologists such as Louis Pasteur. He decided to pursue a career in science. He excelled at the local community college, which he attended for free, and won a scholarship to the University of Chicago, where he majored in biological sciences.[1]

After Japan's attack on Pearl Harbor, Goldwasser took a full-time job in the university's toxicity lab, which had been deemed an essential industry because of its top-secret investigation into antidotes for chemical warfare agents. After graduation in 1944, he was drafted and sent to Fort Detrick, Maryland, where he worked on anthrax. When the war ended, he returned to Chicago to complete a doctorate in biochemistry, and in 1952, married with a young son, he took a job as a research associate at the Argonne Cancer Research Hospital (later part of the University of Chicago hospital system).

At Argonne Hospital, Goldwasser was reunited with Leon Jacobson, the noted hematologist who had run the toxicity lab during the war. Jacobson had been deeply involved in a top-secret program to study mustard gas, which the army's Chemical Warfare Service feared would be deployed by Germany and Japan. Soldiers in World War I who had been exposed to nitrogen mustard died horrible deaths, ravaged within days by a multitude of infections after the gas suppressed the bone marrow's ability to produce infection-fighting white blood cells. The fear that the Axis nations would use the banned gas never materialized. But like so many government programs from the war years, the mustard gas research project had a major spin-off. Jacobson, among others, speculated that nitrogen mustard in minute doses might prove useful in fighting leukemia and lymphoma, which are characterized by a proliferation of the mutant white blood cells. Alfred Gilman and Louis Goodman, who would later write a famous textbook on clinical pharmacology, conducted similar experiments at Yale University.[2] Researchers at both schools found that tests on a handful of subjects generated brief remissions. These results were the first stirrings of cancer chemotherapy and generated tremendous excitement throughout the medical community.[3]

By the time Goldwasser joined Jacobson's lab as a full-time researcher, the senior scientist's priorities had shifted to the new threat—nuclear war. The Atomic Energy Commission wanted to find ways to counter radiation sickness, which, like mustard gas, severely compromised the body's ability to produce blood cells. As early as 1906 scientists had speculated there must be something in the blood that signaled bone marrow to replace red blood cells, which wore out while ferrying oxygen around the body. Scientists had already given the molecular trigger a name—erythropoietin, after erythropoiesis, the medical term for red blood cell formation. But no one had ever found Epo, much less isolated it for study.

In 1955, Jacobson challenged Goldwasser, new to academic life, to find the elusive protein. If the molecule could be purified in large quantities—perhaps from animals, as had been done with insulin—it might prove useful in treating people suffering from radiation sickness. "You'll be rich and famous," Jacobson told his young protégé. "This was a time when everyone was scared to death and children in the schools were taught to crouch under their desks," Goldwasser recalled. "It was a time of foolish panic, but it gave me every young investigator's dream. I had all the money and space I needed. And I didn't have to write any reports. I thought it would take about three months."

The search would last more than twenty years. The average person produces two to three million red blood cells a second—more than a thousand pounds of blood over the course of a lifetime. But researchers could dry the amount of Epo needed to produce that lifetime supply and form it into a tablet no larger than an aspirin. Moreover, the blood contains more than two hundred proteins, and Epo puts in only a brief appearance. Looking for Epo in the blood was like looking for dimes on a long stretch of sandy beach.

Goldwasser spent the first several years of his search trying to figure out what part of the body produced Epo. His research team carefully removed different organs from laboratory rats until they determined that the absence of kidneys triggered anemia. They next made animals anemic, under the assumption that their kidneys would overproduce Epo in an attempt to end the red blood cell deficiency. This overexpression, they speculated, would leave recoverable traces of Epo in the blood.

In the late 1950s, Goldwasser and members of his small team began taking regular trips to a slaughterhouse in Bradley, Illinois, an hour's drive from Chicago. They injected soon-to-be-slaughtered sheep with a chemical that destroyed their red blood cells and made them anemic. They waited a day before capturing their blood serum, assuming the sheep kidneys would overexpress Epo into the blood to correct the imbalance. Back in the lab, they distilled the blood serum into fractions they hoped were relatively pure, and then injected each one into anemic rats to see if any improved their red blood cell count. From time to time, there were tantalizing hints of activity from the trace amounts of Epo in one of the fractions. But he could never isolate it, much less get enough to test in humans.

The sheep experiments dragged on for fifteen years. Goldwasser received tenure and raised a family. He and his young son used to spend holidays and weekends in his University of Chicago labs injecting laboratory rats and testing their blood, but his son, frustrated by the glacial pace of scientific progress, eventually left for college to study German literature. He wasn't the only one frustrated by the endless sheep experiments. Rival investigators in Chile and at the California Institute of Technology published papers showing that excess Epo showed up in urine, not blood. The sheep had led Goldwasser down a blind alley.

Depressed, thinking his life's work amounted to nothing, Goldwasser unexpectedly received a letter in early 1973 from a Japanese scholar named Takaji Miyake. The Kumamoto University researcher had read the handful of papers that Goldwasser had generated during his long, fruitless hunt for Epo. Miyake explained that a number of patients near his university on the southern island of Kyushu suffered from aplastic anemia. The bone marrow of aplastic anemia patients does not work properly. Miyake didn't know what caused the defect in these patients, but he suspected they would be ideal candidates for Goldwasser's research. He offered to collect urine specimens and bring them to the United States so they could be tested in Goldwasser's lab, which, Miyake knew, had the most experience in the world in breaking down bodily fluids and searching for the rare molecule.

Over the next two years, Miyake and his colleagues collected urine samples from the island's aplastic anemia patients while Goldwasser sought a grant from the National Institutes of Health (NIH) to bring Miyake to the United States. The industrious Japanese scholar eventually collected 2,550 liters from his patients. The grant came through in the fall of 1975. When the two men met in the lobby of the Palmer House, the elegant neoclassical hotel in the heart of Chicago's Loop, the Japanese scholar bowed low and held out a foot-square package that had been carefully wrapped in a brightly colored piece of fine Japanese silk. Goldwasser later learned this was a *furoshiki*, the ritual covering for gifts given to special friends and colleagues. Inside was the dried urine.

Goldwasser, along with his chief assistant, Charles Kung, and Miyake, immediately set about the painstaking process of chemically searching for Epo. They subjected the urine to a seven-step purification procedure that had been perfected over years of sheep experiments. A framed X-ray photograph still hangs over Goldwasser's desk, capturing the final results of the eighteen-month experiment. "We got the fraction off that last column and put it to a test for homogeneity that we had used for the sheep material. There was only a single dark-stained band. All the previous fractions had many bands. The thought was bingo!" Years later he slapped his hand on his desk as he gleefully recalled the moment. "We did everything we could to disprove it was a single component. Then we put it in [the anemic] rats, and it worked like a charm with the highest potency we had ever seen."

The 2,550 liters of urine were eventually reduced to eight milligrams of pure human Epo, barely enough to fill a small vial. The results of that experiment were published in the August 1977 *Journal of Biological Chemistry*.[4] "I was walking on air," Goldwasser remembered. "We finally had something we could work with."

Finding someone to work with, however, proved almost as difficult as the final experiment. In the mid-1970s Goldwasser had tried to attract the interest of scientists at Parke-Davis, a medium-sized drug company based in Michigan. He wanted to show that kidney cells could be tricked into producing Epo when cultured outside the body, a process similar to the one that had been used to coax insulin from pancreas cells. Some initial efforts had shown promise. But the experiment could not be repeated, and Parke-Davis lost interest in the program. Goldwasser then traveled to Chicago's north suburbs where he tried to cajole Abbott Laboratories, one of the Midwest's largest pharmaceutical companies, into supporting his work. They rejected his repeated entreaties.

Desperate to interest someone in becoming his partner, Goldwasser launched a human clinical trial. He applied to the Food and Drug Administration (FDA) for permission to administer a portion of his tiny stash of Epo to three dialysis patients at the University of Chicago hospital. People with malfunctioning kidneys require constant blood transfusions because they don't produce enough Epo, thus making them ideal candidates for Epo therapy. "If we could demonstrate an effect in a patient with anemia of chronic renal disease, funding for our future research would be assured," he wrote.[5]

He also put the university on notice that he was sitting on top of a patentable invention. The disclosure was required by the Department of Energy and NIH, which had funded his research over the years. In the late 1970s, the government was increasingly concerned about the stagnant U.S. economy and the competitive threat posed by Japanese and German rivals. One cure for that disease was to get government-funded innovations out of America's basic science labs and into the marketplace. Patent disclosure was supposed to facilitate the process.

Those policy debates never crossed Goldwasser's mind as he filled out the paperwork. When he didn't hear back from the university or the government, he forgot about patenting his discovery and its use in dialysis therapy. Years later, as he prepared to answer a subpoena in the endless patent litigation between Amgen and other firms that wanted to manufacture artificial Epo, he uncovered the oversight. "I was going through all my boxes of files. There were dozens of them. I found this letter that had been sent to the agency funding us, asking them to file a patent. They never responded, and I didn't follow up. I forgot all about it. I was too busy doing science," he said.

The clinical trial's results were tantalizing but inconclusive. One patient showed a small increase in red blood cell count and a major increase in the formation of red blood cell precursors. But the dose was too small, and continuing the experiment would have dissipated his entire Epo supply. He dropped the trial and began searching for someone to work with. Luckily, by 1980 there were a host of new players ready to listen to his story.

The success of Eugene Goldwasser's protracted search for Epo coincided with a turning point in medical history. In the late 1970s and early 1980s, an entrepreneurial revolution swept through the once staid world of academic medical research. Dreams of Nobel glory were gradually replaced by dreams of high-tech riches, and a number of new biotechnology firms were eager to jump on his discovery. A quick side tour reveals the origin of this new industry: The core technologies of biotechnology were themselves products of university-based scientists who used public funding in the United States and in England to foment a revolution.

Biotechnology can trace its roots to 1953, when James Watson and Francis Crick, building on years of discoveries and the unheralded work of X-ray diffraction expert Rosalind Franklin, unraveled the double-helix structure of deoxyribonucleic acid (DNA), which makes up the genetic code for all forms of life. They showed how the broad diversity and complexity of life could be transmitted from generation to generation through a biochemical code contained inside an organism's cells. The code's mechanism was simple. It used just two complimentary pairs of molecules called base nucleotides. The order of these base pairs along strands of DNA expressed all the genetic information that makes up life on this planet. The code also provided a language for generating new combinations, thus explaining evolution. Many observers compared Watson and Crick's discovery to the emerging field of computer programming. If life was a computer program, why not use the information to recreate the building blocks of life, or even reprogram them?

The same year, Frederick Sanger of Cambridge University in England determined that all proteins, the workhorses of life, were made up of strings of the twenty-two different amino acids that were expressed by the genetic codes contained on DNA. He also figured out a chemical process for mapping the sequence of amino acids, and then did it for insulin.

The Nobel Prize–winning work of Watson, Crick, and Sanger began a worldwide quest to develop the tools needed to understand, manipulate, and eventually reproduce life's genetic code and the proteins it expressed. Scientists identified chemical scalpels, known as restriction enzymes, to snip DNA and proteins into small pieces. They developed chemicals for reconstructing proteins one amino acid at a time to determine their sequence.

In 1973, Stanley Cohen of Stanford University and Herbert Boyer of the University of California at San Francisco stitched together nearly twenty years of discoveries into a fitting climax: the invention of recombinant DNA engineering. Their breakthrough—actually the last step in a long string of academic science advances—led directly to the creation of the biotechnology industry. Recombinant DNA engineering enabled scientists to use biological and chemical processes to manufacture large quantities of proteins by splicing the genetic fragments that expressed those proteins onto the DNA of fast-growing bacteria or mammalian ovary cells. Unlike previous attempts at gene splicing that required complicated chemistry and the laborious manipulation of viruses, the Cohen-Boyer method "was so simple that high school pupils could easily learn it."[6]

A few venture capitalists in the San Francisco Bay Area immediately saw commercial possibilities in the new technology. So did Niels Reimers, head of Stanford's office of technology licensing. He begged the two scientists to apply for a patent on their invention, which they did after a short but heated debate. Cohen initially opposed patenting. In those days his attitude was common among academic scientists, whose incentives had not yet been influenced by the stock market fever of the 1980s and 1990s. Most scientists were still more interested in winning intellectual competitions and disseminating knowledge broadly than in commercializing their work. Cohen was especially leery of patenting a scientific tool like recombinant engineering since it might inhibit further research. He relented after Reimers argued that licensing recombinant DNA technology to all comers would be the fastest way to deploy it broadly.[7]

Boyer, on the other hand, was not reticent about chasing riches, especially after meeting Robert Swanson, a twenty-seven-year-old operative at Kleiner-Perkins, the venture capital fund responsible for many of the start-ups that would soon turn the southern half of the San Francisco Bay Area into Silicon Valley. Swanson, who earned chemistry and business degrees at the Massachusetts Institute of Technology, was eager to plunge into the new world of biotechnology after reading about the recombinant engineering breakthrough in the newspapers. He immediately called Boyer and asked if he was interested in starting a company. They met in a San Francisco bar and by January 1976 had created the business plan for a firm called Genetic Engineering Technology, or Genentech, which became the technological leader of the new field. Within a few years, there were a handful of other firms, mostly around

San Francisco and Boston, that were seeking to put the new technology to commercial use.

Two other events in 1980 transformed the environment for the nascent biotechnology industry. In Washington, Congress passed the Bayh-Dole Act, named after Senator Birch Bayh, a leading Democrat from Indiana, and Senator Robert Dole, a leading Republican from Kansas. The new law reflected the bipartisan concern that the U.S. economy was rapidly losing ground to its overseas rivals. The bill encouraged federally funded researchers and their university sponsors to license their patented discoveries to industry by giving them clear title to the patents. The debate behind the new law was focused on speeding innovation from the lab to the computer, auto, and steel industries. But the major beneficiaries of the bill turned out to be researchers on the frontiers of medical science.

The second major event of that year took place on Wall Street. In March, Cetus Corporation, one of the nation's first biotech start-ups, raised $108 million through an initial public stock offering (IPO). It was the largest IPO in the history of the American stock market to that time. In the fall, Genentech issued its IPO, raising $36 million. The Boyer-Swanson venture was hot on the trail of interferon, the "miracle" cancer cure that had generated intense media coverage. The stock, which opened at $35 a share, closed that first day of trading at $71.25.[8]

Biotech fever soon gripped most of the nation's leading molecular biology labs. William Bowes, an investment banker who sat on the Cetus board of directors, called Winston Salser, a highly regarded biologist and cancer researcher at the University of California at Los Angeles. Salser didn't need much prodding. In the mid-1970s, his entrepreneurial energies had gone into real estate ventures, most of which had failed. But biotech was something he knew about. At Bowes's urging, Salser formed Applied Molecular Genetics, later shortened to Amgen, and recruited an all-star cast from Southern California to join his scientific advisory board. The group included Leroy Hood of CalTech, whose government-funded lab had just invented the first gene sequencing machine. (The machine would later be featured in Michael Crichton's *Jurassic Park*. The government's decision to develop an advanced version to speed the completion of the Human Genome Project is the subject of chapter 3.) Hood's machine speeded up the laborious process of identifying the chemical structure of proteins and the genes that expressed them.

Amgen began with nothing more than a letterhead and a list of possible research projects. The company was typical of the dozens of start-up companies launched in that era. Its list of commercial targets covered the biotech waterfront. Interferon was hot, so it made the list. The company also wanted to create oil-eating bacteria and genetically modified organisms that could transform oil shale into oil. One particularly alluring target was chicken growth hormone for the poultry industry. Salser, a social liberal, also listed tropical diseases such as malaria and sleeping sickness as potential targets. Artificial erythropoietin made Salser's wish list, but only because one of his postdoctoral researchers had worked with Goldwasser and wanted it there.

Salser knew science. But he knew little about raising the money needed to hire scientists to work on his projects. His backers suggested he hire a chief executive officer who understood venture capital markets and marketing as well as science. That fall, George Rathmann, vice president of research at Abbott Labs in North Chicago, traveled to the West Coast to scout out biotech investment opportunities for his employer. Though able to understand the arcane chattering of senior scientists—he had earned his Ph.D. in physical chemistry from Princeton University—Rathmann had long since left the labs for the executive suite. After spending twenty-one years at 3M Corporation and several years with the medical systems division of Litton Industries, he had joined Abbott as vice president in charge of its research and development program.

The emerging biotech world intrigued Rathmann. But dragging the stodgy maker of pharmaceuticals and medical diagnostic kits into the modern age was proving a daunting task. Abbott manufactured a hepatitis test kit using blood factors, and contaminated blood sometimes infected the tests and its users. If the company could produce the blood factor for the diagnostic kits through genetic engineering, that danger would be eliminated and give the firm a marketing advantage over its rivals. But Abbott's efforts to develop its biotech capabilities were going nowhere fast, largely because of fears about safety. During the first years of the gene-splicing revolution, there were widespread fears that genetically engineered microbes might escape from a lab and devastate humanity. Even Cambridge, Massachusetts, had banned gene splicing for a short while. "People were so frightened to carry out recombinant DNA engineering in Lake County, outside Chicago," Rathmann said. "Abbott just viewed it as a potential scandal if somebody in the local community found out that we were doing something potentially dangerous." The company built an air-lock system for handling biotech materials. Inside the lab, workers wore moon suits.[9]

Rathmann decided to take a sabbatical to learn more about the technology behind recombinant genetic engineering. Phil Whitcome, Abbott's cardiovascular product manager, had trained at UCLA under Salser and mentioned his lab as a possible site. For six months, Rathmann parked himself at a desk in UCLA's Molecular Biology Institute. And in October 1980, he joined Salser's new company as its first chief executive. Whitcome soon followed.

Abbott's officials, including Kirk Raab, who later became chief executive officer of Genentech, begged him to stay. They offered to spin off their biotech lab into a separate company that could sell stock. But there was a caveat. Abbott would remain the majority shareholder. "After thinking about it for three days, I realized that it didn't have the upside," Rathmann recalled. "The guys at Genentech were talking about becoming millionaires. People [out west] were thinking in terms of infinite upsides."

To hedge their bets, Abbott officials offered to invest in Rathmann's new venture. But first they wanted to know the company's potential products. Rathmann ticked off the six or seven projects then under consideration. Last on his list was Epo. "Oh no, not Epo," said the head of Abbott's research division. "Gene Goldwasser has been beating us on the head about that for five years." Abbott invested $5 million in Amgen anyway, a stake they would sell a decade later for fifty times that amount. But its value to Rathmann at the time was incalculable. It signaled to West Coast venture capitalists that this start-up should be taken seriously. Several firms offered another $12 million, and Amgen was up and running.

The firm started hiring scientists. In early 1981, Fu-Kuen Lin, a journeyman bench scientist who had wended his way through a half-dozen academic labs on two continents, answered an ad in *Science* magazine and became the seventh scientist to join the firm. Lin was the fifth of seven children of a Chinese herb doctor. He came to the United States in the 1960s to study plant pathology at the University of Illinois, and did his postdoctoral work at Purdue University and the University of Nebraska before returning to his native Taiwan in 1975. Two years later, he was back in the United States. He worked for a while in the nucleic acid biochemistry lab at Louisiana State University before moving on to conduct genetic engineering experiments at the Medical University of South Carolina. To the peripatetic Lin, moving to an isolated industrial park on the far outskirts of the Los Angeles metropolitan area, where Amgen had located its offices, was a welcome change from the insular South. On his first day on the job he was given Amgen's target list and asked which project he wanted to work on. He chose Epo. The choice was easy. "We had the protein. A lot of other projects didn't have the protein," he said.[10]

Goldwasser, who held the world's sole supply of Epo, had decided to work exclusively with Amgen. At least two other biotech start-ups had already entered the race to develop an artificial version of Epo and were desperate to get their hands on his supply. Biogen, the Swiss-American firm that was briefly run by Nobel laureate Walter Gilbert, was the first to approach Goldwasser. Gilbert, a former Harvard professor, wanted access to Epo so the firm could begin searching for its gene. Finding the gene was key to producing a genetically engineered version of the molecule, and the obvious next step if the protein was going to be produced in the bulk quantities needed for clinical trials and sale. The two men met at a scientific meeting and went to dinner to discuss a possible partnership.

The dinner got off to a rocky start. Goldwasser was not impressed by Gilbert's invitation to join his all-star team. Biogen had loaded its scientific advisory board with virtually every scientist in the country with any connection to Epo. "He picked out just about every blockhead in the field. I said there was no way I was going to work with those people," Goldwasser recalled. After dinner, Gilbert didn't offer to pick up Goldwasser's half of the check. When he got home, the threadbare academic crossed Biogen off his list.

Genetics Institute, a Cambridge-based firm that had spun out of Harvard in 1980, also wanted to get into the Epo game. But Genetics Institute thought it didn't need the Chicago scientist. Before Goldwasser signed on to work with Amgen, he sent some of his Epo stash to Hood's CalTech lab for sequencing to determine its amino acid structure. The work was done by Rodney Hewick, one of the co-inventors of the machine. Once he had the results, Hewick quit, and on September 1, 1981, he arrived in Cambridge to become Genetic Institute's senior protein chemist. It was a logical strategy from a commercial standpoint, if questionable ethically. Natural Epo and its potential medical use remained unpatented since neither the government nor Goldwasser had thought to file an application in the wake of his initial discovery. Therefore, the first firm to patent its recombinant manufacture would get the gold, and for that, all one needed was the Epo sequence. Hewick had it.

There was one flaw in the strategy, though. Hewick and the CalTech team had made mistakes in transcribing the sequence, getting at least three of the protein's 166 amino acids wrong. Moreover, Genetics Institute didn't have any more Epo to double check the work. The errors would befuddle Genetics Institute's gene hunters for more than two years.[11]

Goldwasser, meanwhile, looked west. Salser invited him to join Hood on Amgen's scientific advisory board. He declined, choosing instead to work for Amgen as a consultant. Lin arrived on the scene just about the time Goldwasser decided to make his small Epo supply available to the firm on an exclusive basis.

In the fall of 1981, Lin and one assistant began the workmanlike task of sequencing the protein. Hood's machine had vastly simplified the process from the 1950s and 1960s, when Fred Sanger, in his second Nobel Prize–winning effort, had chemically sequenced the fifty-one amino acids of insulin. And unlike Hewick, Lin had a supply of Epo, which allowed him to recheck his work. But having the correct code for the 166 amino acids that made up Epo did not solve Lin's problem. How would he find the gene that expressed those amino acids along the vast expanse of human DNA? It was the equivalent of finding a single sentence in the *Encyclopaedia Britannica*.

It took Lin two years to figure out a process. During those two years, Goldwasser attended numerous Amgen meetings where every adviser and the other members of the scientific staff voted to kill the Epo program, even though there were only two scientists and an assistant working on it. Lin later testified he felt like a "lonesome soldier because the company felt so frustrated with the Epo project and felt it was dead; no one at the company wanted to touch it."[12] Goldwasser couldn't understand how a private company could be so impatient. He'd spent two decades looking for the molecule. They were ready to quit in less than two years.

Daniel Vapnek, who quit his job as University of Georgia professor of molecular genetics to become Amgen's director of research in 1981, was one of those who questioned continuing with the program. "Epo was a very difficult area to work in. It had a long history of people who worked on it and made up data." The single-minded Chicago scientist hedged his bets with the small team Vapnek put on the Epo project. "The biggest issue we had was getting enough material from him," Vapnek said. "He had a limited amount and he wanted to be certain we were in fact going to be able to do the microsequencing."[13] Rathmann listened carefully to the wrangling between his key outside consultant and his in-house research chief. At each meeting, he cast the deciding vote in favor of continuing the program.

Lin finally came up with an ingenious probe process for isolating the gene. The Pharmaceutical Research and Manufacturers Association (Pharma), which granted Lin its top science award in 1995, described Lin's frustrating two years. "He did not know if he would be successful in isolating the Epo gene. . . . Lin was on a fishing expedition in the human genome, searching, as it were, for a single specific fish in a sea of hundreds of thousands." Following Pharma's lead, Vice President Al Gore awarded Amgen and Lin the National Medal of Technology, calling him "a true national hero."[14] Lin's probe involved creating 128 radioactive fragments of Epo and matching them against a library of human DNA fragments. Once he had his probe, it took him only a few weeks to find the gene. It took another year to sequence and clone it using fast-growing Chinese hamster ovary cells, a technology that had recently been invented and patented by Richard Axel and two colleagues at Columbia University.[15] He filed his first patent on December 13, 1983. A year later, the company filed for the key patent on the process for producing recombinant Epo, which effectively limited other firms from doing the same.

Lin may have been first, but his approach was hardly unique. Genetics Institute and Biogen scientists were also using sophisticated probes to hunt for the gene. The other companies had also picked up on this quantum leap in how to search for genes from academics who were experimenting with the technique. Their problem was they didn't have Epo or its proper amino acid sequence. "The limiting factor in Biogen's effort to clone the gene was not having an adequate amount of protein sequence from which to derive good probes," said Richard Flavell, who was president of Biogen's Cambridge facility from 1982 to 1988. "Erythropoietin was a rather rare commodity and the major person who had that material was Dr. Goldwasser." Biogen finally succeeded in sequencing and cloning Epo in mid-1985, but it was too late. The vast riches that would flow from the molecule would go to another firm. But at least the gamble hadn't cost that much. According to Flavell, the three-year search for the Epo gene had cost the company just $4 to $6 million.[16]

Once Genetics Institute scientists recognized Hewick's mistake, they began scrambling for alternative sources of Epo. The company contacted several scientists who had received small samples of Goldwasser's stash, but soon realized they didn't have enough for sequencing. It next contacted Miyake, who had returned to Japan. He initially demanded a large fee for replicating his earlier work, but they turned him down. In

1983, he changed his mind and a year later Genetics Institute scientists got their first sample of purified Epo. Within a few months, they had sequenced and cloned it. On December 17, 1984, Genetics Institute scooped Amgen when their team submitted an article to *Nature* describing the isolation and characterization of the clones of human Epo.[17] But Lin had filed for a patent on his work a year earlier. Litigation over the matter would drag out until the mid-1990s when the Supreme Court finally determined that Amgen's Lin had won the race to the Patent and Trademark Office. In the emerging world of biotech, that was all that mattered.[18]

Once Amgen could make artificial Epo, the road was clear to prove it worked in curing anemia. Clinical trials, the second phase of drug research, are more costly than developing new molecules. Since 1962, when Congress reformed the nation's drug laws in the wake of the thalidomide scare (pregnant women who took the drug gave birth to horribly deformed babies), companies have had to prove that a new drug is effective as well as safe before offering it for sale. Companies usually go through three sets of clinical trials to clear the FDA hurdle. The first-phase trials are conducted on a small number of volunteers who receive an escalating dose of the experimental drug. They are designed to ensure the drug is safe, and to find the maximum tolerable dose that leaves enough of the drug in the bloodstream to carry out its task. The second-phase clinical trials, also done on a small number of patients, are designed to show that the drug is having an impact on the disease. The third and final phase of a drug's trials, usually conducted on hundreds or even thousands of patients, is designed to prove to regulators that the drug works on a significant number of the patients who take it. Third-phase trials are often double-blind and placebo-controlled trials, meaning neither doctor nor patients know who is getting the real deal or a fake. A drug is deemed efficacious when trial results of the drug group are significantly better than those of the placebo group.

As Epogen—the trade name for the artificial protein—neared its clinical-trial phase, Rathmann needed to raise more cash. He began selling off Epo's potential markets. In mid-1984, the company received $24 million from Kirin Brewery Company of Japan in exchange for the rights to market the drug in Japan. A year later it signed a similar deal with Johnson and Johnson's Ortho-Biotech division, which took European rights and all U.S. uses except dialysis. In exchange, Amgen received an immediate $6 million and the promise of future payments as the company passed milestones on the drug's road to approval. In November 1985, Amgen filed an application with the FDA to begin testing its experimental drug in people whose kidneys had failed. To cut its development time, the company opted to do a combined first- and second-phase trial.

The first results came in a little more than a year later. They were nothing short of spectacular. Writing later in the *New England Journal of Medicine,* kidney specialist Joseph Eschbach and hematologist John Adamson from the University of Washington reported that all of the eighteen patients who received the drug in the trial showed a sharp increase in red blood cell counts. Two-thirds of them no longer needed blood transfusions. The energy levels and sense of well-being among the dialysis patients had increased markedly. "These results demonstrate that recombinant human erythropoietin is effective, can eliminate the need for transfusions . . . and can restore the hematocrit (red blood cell count) to normal in many patients with the anemia of end-stage renal disease."[19]

The report sent the company's stock price soaring. Amgen immediately launched a larger trial with three hundred patients, which showed similar results. In November 1987, the company applied to the FDA for final approval to market what it now called Epogen. On June 1, 1989, the agency gave its go-ahead, just three and a half years after the initial new drug application. The relatively rapid turnaround was testimony to the extraordinary efficacy of the new drug.

Many observers have called Epogen and a handful of similar drugs the low-hanging fruit of the biotechnology era. The issue is worth exploring because it helps explain why, despite the hype of the past two decades, the biotechnology revolution has produced so few significant therapies like Epo. Epo is a single hormone whose absence results in a well-defined illness, in its case, anemia. Insulin, Factor VIII (the blood-clotting factor missing in some hemophiliacs), and granulocyte colony-stimulating factor (which triggers white blood cell formation and, after its gene was licensed from Memorial Sloan-Kettering Hospital in New York, became the basis for Amgen's second best-selling drug) are similar. If these proteins are missing, a person gets sick. If they are replaced, a patient gets better. Once researchers identified the functions of these proteins and found the genes needed to manufacture them, it became a relatively simple matter to make them in bulk to treat people who suffered from their absence. It didn't matter whether that absence was caused by illness (kidney failure, for instance) or genetic inheritance.

Unfortunately, not many diseases have this direct cause-and-effect relationship with a missing protein. People who inherit malfunctioning genes that cause protein-deficiency diseases are in fact quite rare. Inherited disorders such as Gaucher, Tay-Sachs, and Fabry disease occur in just one in every fifty thousand to one hundred thousand births (that's three to six thousand potential patients in a population of 300 million). Just one in ten thousand get Huntington's disease; just one in twenty-three hundred have cystic fibrosis. Scientists in the early 1990s identified two mutant genes associated with some forms of breast cancer, but they are present in only 4 to 10 percent of cases. Discovery of the genetic code for those exceptions has proven valuable for diagnostic purposes, but it has provided nothing in the way of a cure.

And even when a genetic flaw causes disease, it doesn't automatically mean that it can be treated by replacing the defective or missing protein with its biotechnologically created equivalent. Cystic fibrosis is the classic example. *Science* magazine put the face of a four-year-old patient on its September 1, 1989, cover when scientists at three institutions—one of them was University of Michigan's Francis Collins, who later ran the government's Human Genome Project—breathlessly announced the discovery of the malfunctioning gene that caused the disabling lung disease. Collins predicted there would be a cure within five to ten years. However, efforts to produce the missing protein and inject it into patients by university researchers and biotech companies repeatedly failed. The patients' immune systems rejected proteins perceived as foreign. Next came years of gene therapy experiments, where physicians attempt to insert cells with a properly working version of the gene into a patient. These, too, have not borne fruit. "We're still many years away from having a really promising result," Collins said a dozen years after his initial discovery, and "we won't get there without a lot of scientific creativity and ingenuity."[20]

The diseases that account for most early deaths and suffering in the advanced industrial world—heart disease, cancer, stroke, Alzheimer's, arthritis—are rarely genetically determined. Their cause has been variously attributed to everything from genetic predisposition to environmental pollution, from viruses to immune system malfunction, from diet to the process of aging itself. Scientists can be found on each side of every question. In recent years billions of dollars of basic research has focused on learning the biochemical processes of each disease and identifying the complex interplay of dozens of genes and proteins that, over time, leads to disease through either genetic mutation or malfunctioning.

But even after scientists have identified the biochemical cascade of a disease, intervention remains extremely difficult. Most proteins play multiple roles in the body; enhancing or limiting their action may have no net effect and will almost always have unintended side effects. "It is testament to the power of the idea of genetic engineering that the limits to its therapeutic potential were not appreciated earlier, but the reason is quite obvious," James Le Fanu, a British physician, wrote in 1999 in his critical study *The Rise and Fall of Modern Medicine*.

> Biotechnology may be a technically dazzling way of making drugs, but it is severely constrained by the fact that the only things that genes can make are proteins, so the only therapeutic use for biotechnology products are [sic] conditions where either a protein is deficient and needs replacing (such as the use of insulin in diabetes) or where it is hoped that giving a protein in large enough doses might in some way or other influence a disease, such as cancer.[21]

But when artificial Epo, one of the first miracle treatments of the biotechnology revolution, was approved, hopes soared among the scientists who had formed hundreds of biotech start-ups. Amgen's windfall, it was believed, would rapidly lead to many more such successes. The only thing that stood in the way was the private capital needed to finance the search for the cures. Amgen set the price for its new product with that thought in mind. It had nothing to do with the cost of developing the drug.

When Epogen was approved by the FDA, there were just under one hundred thousand Americans on dialysis for kidney failure, and a third of them were getting regular blood transfusions. Most patients received their treatment courtesy of the federal government, whose Medicare program paid for dialysis and related drugs. After initially setting its price low, Amgen negotiated a new price with Medicare that would generate anywhere from four to eight thousand dollars per year per patient. When the results of the first clinical trials had come out in 1987, Wall Street analysts had pegged the company's potential sales at $150 million a year.[22] After it got its hefty price hike from the George H. W. Bush administration, the analysts' estimates quickly soared toward $1 billion.

Medicare's rapidly escalating expenditures on Epogen eventually caught the attention of watchdogs on Capitol Hill. At a House Ways and Means Committee meeting in October 1991, Rep. Pete Stark of California grilled Health and Human Services (HHS) secretary Louis Sullivan about Epogen's price, since his department had negotiated the figure with Amgen. The liberal Democrat had gotten his hands on an internal HHS study that showed the drug had cost Amgen at most $170 million to develop. Yet the government had already paid Amgen $460 million during its first two years on the market, and manufacturing the drug exhausted just 5 percent of revenue. The number of patients on dialysis was rising rapidly: By the mid-1990s, it would double to two hundred thousand, and by the end of the century it had risen to nearly three hundred thousand, largely because of poorly treated diabetes and hypertension among overweight and out-of-shape Americans. Epogen was heading toward becoming the most expensive drug in the government's medicine chest.

Stark, who would wage a fruitless ten-year battle to lower the cost of Epogen, read to Sullivan from his own introduction to the report. "Medicare's coverage and payment decision for Epo could have had a serious impact on the financial markets of other companies involved in raising capital to finance research on other genetically engineered products. Because investment in drugs, especially those related to biotechnology, is a new, highly speculative business, venture capitalists expect a higher than average return on such investment." Stark was outraged. "Is it in fact the policy of this administration to use Medicare as a form of industrial policy to help ensure the profitability of the biotech industry?" Sullivan agreed that Amgen's return on investment was high. "I can assure you that [it] was not the intent of the administration to have an excessive return," he said, "but we have a policy of trying to have an adequate return to encourage companies to develop such drugs."[23]

A decade later, the results of that policy are in. Epogen and its successor drug accounted for more than half of Amgen's $5 billion in revenue in 2002, and most of that came from the taxpayers. Most of the rest of the company's sales came from Neupogen, the white blood cell factor licensed from Sloan-Kettering and approved in 1991. On paper, Sullivan's goal of spurring Amgen to conduct research had been achieved. The company spent more than $1 billion on research in 2002. That was well short of the company's profits, but it was a hefty sum by any measure.

What were the results of that private research drawn largely from federal payments? In the decade after Neupogen was approved in 1991, Amgen received FDA approval for four new drugs. Two were less effective versions of drugs produced by other firms, while the other two drugs approved in 2001 were new versions of the company's first two blockbusters. They had been slightly modified to stay in the body for a longer period of time.

Amgen's biggest laboratory success was Aranesp, which the company touted as its most significant medical advance since its first two drugs. Aranesp, like Epogen, was for anemia. But it was not a dramatic new treatment for the debilitating condition. Aranesp did exactly the same thing that Epogen had been doing since it was approved in 1989: it raised red blood cell counts by stimulating the bone marrow. What made Aranesp unique? By fiddling with some of the side chemicals on the original Epogen molecule, Amgen chemists discovered how to keep Aranesp in the blood stream three times longer than Epogen. Even if it worked as advertised, Aranesp would provide no medical benefits to the hundreds of thousands of people on dialysis. Those patients were hooked up to dialysis machines three times a week and received their erythropoietin during the sessions. Aranesp would provide no lifestyle benefits for them.

The real purpose of Amgen's new drug was to have something to sell to cancer and AIDS patients, who needed erythropoietin because their bone marrow's ability to produce red blood cells was suppressed by the drugs flowing through their bloodstreams to fight those diseases. Extra erythropoietin can lessen the fatigue that accompanies chemotherapy and has become a key component of cancer and AIDS therapy. But chemotherapy and AIDS patients did not take Amgen's Epogen. They receive injections of Procrit, which was the recombinant form of erythropoietin sold by Johnson and Johnson's Ortho-Biotech division.

Why were two companies selling identical versions of a patented product under different labels? When Amgen was a struggling start-up, it had to sign away half its market to Johnson and Johnson to raise cash. It received just a few tens of millions of dollars. Amgen has regretted that decision ever since. In 2002, Johnson and Johnson generated more than $2 billion a year from Procrit, making it a more lucrative market than the dialysis market. With FDA approval for once-a-week Aranesp under its belt, Amgen's sales force finally had ammunition to attack Johnson and Johnson's market.

However, Johnson and Johnson's detailers— the drug industry's name for its sales personnel—fought back. They spread the word among cancer physicians what some have long known. You can give Procrit once a week simply by increasing the dose. Johnson and Johnson asked Howard Grossman, an HIV/AIDS specialist on the faculty of Columbia University's College of Physicians and Surgeons, to give the higher doses of Procrit once per week to his AIDS patients over a sixteen-week period, and compare their red blood cells counts to patients who still received the lower dose three times a week. "There was no significant difference," Grossman said.[24]

The paucity of significant new therapies coming out of Amgen's investment in research and development came as no surprise to former Amgen research director Daniel Vapnek, who left the company in 1997. He said the culture inside Amgen changed dramatically after sales of Epogen began to skyrocket. In 1990, Rathmann stepped aside and was replaced as chairman and chief executive officer by Gordon Binder, who came up through the financing side of the operation. "The company generated a tremendous amount of money, and a lot of that was spent on buying back their own stock rather than finding out how they could invest in new technology," Vapnek said. "The management of earnings-per-share growth became very important rather than being really innovative. It never really developed a culture of taking risks, and became more interested in managing the existing products."[25]

The company used its research budget to pursue an odd assortment of possible therapies during the 1990s. The company gained a measure of notoriety when it licensed the so-called fat gene. Rockefeller University scientists in New York had discovered the gene that produced leptin, a signaling protein that is involved in the body's metabolism of fat. In early 1995, Amgen licensed the rights to the gene for $20 million and went hunting for every drug manufacturer's dream—a pill that would get people to stop eating. Preliminary tests on mice—genetically engineered to be grossly obese—showed dramatic results. Within weeks of receiving regular doses of artificial leptin, the mice were refusing to eat and running in circles around their cages. The company's press release triggered a flood of media coverage. Hundreds of overweight people besieged the company with requests for the experimental drug. The company's market value soared by nearly a billion dollars.[26]

Almost immediately, independent researchers began throwing cold water on the idea that obesity could be affected by manipulating the level of a single protein. Doctors at Thomas Jefferson University in Philadelphia tested eight overweight people and eight lean people for their leptin levels, and found to their amazement that heavier people had significantly more. It is possible that "a small, but as yet unstudied fraction of obese humans will display a functionally significant mutation in the obesity gene," the researchers concluded, but it was clear that obesity was a complex disorder in humans. It was "unlikely that any single gene mutation will describe the entire genetic contribution to this disease."[27]

Amgen ignored the warnings. Over the next few years the company poured tens of millions of dollars into the project. By 1999, the company had come to the same conclusion. Putting artificial leptin in mice that had been genetically engineered to produce none was one thing. Putting additional leptin into overweight humans who already produced it had no effect. Moreover, many of the dozens of patients in Amgen's test balked at getting daily injections of the bulky protein. "The great hope for leptin has not held up," said Jules Hirsch, the obesity researcher at Rockefeller University who codiscovered the gene.[28]

Amgen also spent a lot of its newfound riches acquiring promising drug candidates from other biotechnology companies. In December 1994, it purchased Synergen, a Boulder, Colorado, firm that was experimenting with artificial proteins believed to play a role in Parkinson's disease and Lou Gehrig's disease. Neither drug panned out.

Amgen next turned to developing another Synergen molecule, which would eventually be approved as a secondary treatment for rheumatoid arthritis. But Amgen's drug was only for patients who didn't respond to standard therapy, and turned out to be much less effective than comparable therapies that arrived on the market around the same time. Rheumatoid arthritis, where the immune system goes awry and attacks a person's own joints, affects more than two million middle-aged adults in the United States, with women twice as likely to get it as men. For decades, doctors have been prescribing methotrexate, a nine-hundred-dollars-a-year generic drug derived from naturally occurring cortisone. It has some success in limiting the painful swelling, especially if sufferers begin using it shortly after they get the disease. But doctors had no idea why it worked.

Throughout the 1970s and 1980s, basic science researchers worked to identify the signaling proteins in the immune system that caused inflammation after an injury. By the early 1990s, a number of biotech companies were racing to develop artificial versions of other signaling proteins that called off their action and could thus reduce swelling. Though many clinicians questioned the wisdom of tinkering with the body's immune system, Amgen became one of three firms that won approval in 2001 for a protein drug to fight rheumatoid arthritis. It was called Kineret. But at the same time, Immunex introduced Embrel and Centocor introduced Remicade. The new drugs each cost twelve thousand dollars a year.

Amgen's molecule was the least effective of the three. So, flush with cash from its Epogen sales, the company made a $16-billion offer to purchase Immunex, the biggest merger in biotech's brief history.[29] While the deal was highly touted on Wall Street, many physicians were openly skeptical of using these drugs as the first-line therapy for fighting the painful disease. They feared what else might happen when they inhibited the action of a naturally occurring immune-system agent. Embrel inhibits a protein called tumor necrosis factor (TNF). A number of "serious, life-threatening infections" occurred among patients in the clinical trials for Embrel (its generic name is etanercept), even though the exclusion of patients with active infections had "markedly diminished the risk," an article warned in the *New England Journal of Medicine*.[30] "We have to realize that TNF is not put into our biological system to cause rheumatoid arthritis," said Doyt Conn, a professor of rheumatology at Emory University and vice president of medical affairs at the Arthritis Foundation. "What will be the problems down the road by inhibiting it completely? There will be infections, and there may be other problems. The strategy should be short-term use, not long-term use. But that's not what the drug companies want of course."[31]

Meanwhile, Amgen in-house research had begun to drift away from genetically engineered products, which was supposedly its area of expertise. It hired medicinal chemists to come up with organic compounds that might treat a disease, the province of traditional pharmaceutical firms. It even began licensing some promising drugs. In 1999 it signed a deal with Praexis Pharmaceutical Inc. to market a prostate cancer drug still under development. But two years later that deal got cancelled when the drug proved ineffective. "We thought we could uncover other drug targets that no one had done before. We had a medicinal chemistry group all of a sudden," Vapnek said. "Amgen started to look like a pharmaceutical company. There was just a limited number of proteins that turned out to be therapeutics, like Epo . . . and that was what our technology was based on."

Amgen's research is not limited to looking for new drugs. It also spends millions of dollars sponsoring medical investigators who are willing to promote increased use of its biggest seller, Epogen. When the FDA first approved the drug, it suggested physicians give their patients enough Epo to raise their red blood cell counts to about 80 percent of normal. That had been the standard in the blood transfusion era. It also was the standard used in Amgen's clinical trials. But once the drug was out in the marketplace, Amgen salesmen quickly realized that they could sell a lot more Epogen if the dialysis centers aimed for higher red blood cell counts. In fact, raising red blood cell counts to normal could double or even triple the amount sold. Amgen began funding academic researchers around the country to test patients at the higher levels for mental alertness, energy levels, and similar hard-to-quantify standards. The company simultaneously funded the National Kidney Foundation, the main patient advocacy group, to conduct a major review of all treatment standards for dialysis. It was released in 1997. The physicians on the review board, several of whom were paid consultants for Amgen or on its scientific advisory board, recommended raising the standard to about 90 percent of normal.

Amgen sales agents fanned out across the country to spread the new gospel. Medicare's payments for Epogen soared. In 1997 the agency that oversees the program, the Health Care Finance Administration (HCFA), tried to set a maximum limit on reimbursements for the drug. Amgen hired a phalanx of top Washington lobbyists, including former Republican National Committee chairman Haley Barbour and former Senate majority leader Robert Dole, to beat back the effort. During hearings on HCFA's budget, Senator Arlen Specter, a Republican from Pennsylvania whose state contains the operations of a number of major pharmaceutical firms, ordered the agency to rescind the limit or face a sharp cut in its budget. The Clinton administration officials who ran the agency relented, and Medicare's Epogen payments continued their upward march.[32]

The company continued to pour its research dollars into scientific experiments aimed at justifying the increase in red blood cell counts for dialysis patients to normal rates, even though at least one clinical trial showed that in some cases it caused excess deaths from heart attacks and strokes. Allen Nissenson of UCLA, a past president of the Renal Physicians Association who sits on Amgen's medical advisory board and receives substantial research funding from the firm, is a chief proponent of this point of view. "Why shouldn't dialysis patients have the same hematocrit as everyone else?" he said. "That's the way the body is designed. There's a tiny bit of evidence that higher hematocrits might be beneficial."[33]

When I spoke with Eugene Goldwasser in his University of Chicago office in late 2000, he was recovering from a three-day deposition in Amgen's latest patent litigation fight, this one a suit by the biotech behemoth against a company called Transkaryotic Therapies Inc. (TKT) of Cambridge, Massachusetts, which wanted to make and sell its own version of Epo. TKT's founders have developed a method of making proteins using human cells, not the Chinese hamster cells used by Amgen. If TKT had succeeded in court, it would have subjected all biotechnology products to technological competition. But in January 2001, the same federal judge in Boston who ruled in the Genetics Institute case declared that TKT had infringed on Amgen's patents. One Wall Street analyst quipped that the company was "a brilliant legal department that happened to develop drugs."[34]

Goldwasser didn't want to talk about the constant courtroom squabbling that drained so much of his time. He wanted to tell me about the problems he had funding his own research. His work during the 1990s had focused on the kidney cells that produced Epo. He thought that if he could decipher the kidneys' internal mechanisms for producing the enzyme, it might be possible to repair damaged kidneys. But like most basic research, it would take time, more time than Goldwasser probably had. Moreover, with a wildly successful therapy on the market, NIH had lost interest in his work. Amgen had donated thirty thousand dollars a year to support his lab over the years, but it was far short of the three hundred thousand dollars he needed if he was going to continue his sixth decade of work on Epo.

As he gave me a tour of his lab, he pointed to the outdated electrophoresis machines, beakers, centrifuges, and incubators that had been the tools of his great discovery. Unless he came up with a major grant, he would soon dismantle and sell them, probably to some high school, or perhaps to a developing country that could only afford technologies that are several generations old. I asked him if he had any regrets about not patenting his discovery. It would have generated millions of dollars a year in royalties. He looked at the machines wistfully. "If I had 1 percent of a billion dollars," he said, "I could buy a new pair of shoes."

2

Rare Profits

In the waning days of World War II, President Franklin D. Roosevelt asked Vannevar Bush, the former dean of the Massachusetts Institute of Technology and his science adviser, to draw up a blueprint for how government should fund science in the postwar world. In *Science, the Endless Frontier*, which came out after Roosevelt's death, Bush argued that government should limit its support to basic research, leaving use-oriented applied research to the private sector.[1] This would give university-based scientists freedom to pursue their intellectual curiosity. The report assured the president that if scientists came up with something novel and useful, the private sector would be perfectly capable of turning it to commercial use.

There has always been a countervailing view to the Bush paradigm, especially in the health sciences. From the vantage point of elected leaders funneling billions of dollars into medical research and patient populations suffering from incurable ailments, a government that simply funded a pure and detached scientific establishment without taking into account the health needs of the public would be shirking its duty. In their view, the government needed to spend its research dollars on finding cures to specific medical problems. It needed to engage in targeted or directed research.

Over the years, the federal government has done both. If Goldwasser represents the pure science ideal, Roscoe Brady reflects the many targeted research programs inside the National Institutes of Health (NIH). For nearly half a century, Brady has studied rare diseases at NIH's sprawling campus in Bethesda, outside Washington. An estimated twenty-four million Americans suffer from five to six thousand rare illnesses, many of them like the genetic disorder made famous by the movie *Lorenzo's Oil*. Patients with a rare disease—legally defined as affecting fewer than two hundred thousand patients—represent a limited market, and at best can count on spotty attention from the pharmaceutical industry. The search for treatments or cures usually falls to the doctors and researchers who have dedicated their careers to studying that particular disease.

Brady's work on a subset of rare diseases is highlighted in a museum display on the ground floor of Building 10 of the NIH complex. Building 10 houses NIH's crown jewel, the renowned Clinical Center, which sits in the middle of a maze of buildings and parking lots on the agency's 306-acre main campus. NIH is the federal government's fastest growing nondefense agency. Congress doubled the NIH budget during the 1980s and doubled it again in the 1990s. Misshapen Building 10 stands as an architectural monument to the bipartisan support on Capitol Hill for pouring money into biomedical research. It looks like an amoeba in the center of a petri dish filled with nutrients, sprouting additional hospital wings on every side.

The display in the lobby celebrates Brady's discovery of the cause and treatment for Gaucher disease, a rare metabolic disorder that affects about ten thousand people around the world. Gaucher sufferers have a defective gene that fails to produce the enzyme needed to break down the fatty remnants of exhausted blood cells. The fats accumulate in the spleen and liver, leaving sufferers in excruciating pain. Most are Ashkenazi Jews. About one-third reside in the United States. The display's timeline traces Brady's work at NIH from its fumbling beginnings in 1956 to the FDA approving his enzyme replacement therapy in 1991. The display also mentions how Brady discovered the causes of about a half-dozen similar disorders, including Niemann-Pick, Pompe, Tay-Sachs, and Fabry diseases, which, like Gaucher, are inherited. Though the natural course of each disease differs, they all result in organ destruction, lifelong disabilities, and, in most cases, early and painful deaths.

A handful of drug companies are on the verge of winning FDA approval for treatments for some of these disorders. Notably absent from the display, though, is any mention of those companies. In particular, there's no mention of Genzyme Corporation, the Cambridge-based biotechnology firm that commercialized Brady's first breakthrough. The omission is understandable. Brady and his colleagues helped Genzyme—one of the most successful biotechnology firms in the nation with sales well over one billion dollars a year—overcome every obstacle it encountered in the development of enzyme replacement therapy for Gaucher disease.

Yet in the mid-1990s, when confronted with protests over the price on the drug that made it the most expensive in the world, Genzyme took sole credit for its development. Years later, when Genzyme finally got around to developing a very similar drug for Fabry disease, it went around Brady because he didn't have a key patent. Though in his mid-70s, Brady went around Genzyme and worked with another firm that had a different technology for manufacturing the missing enzyme. The result was that the FDA got to consider the rarest of rarities—two competing therapies for combating a rare disease.

There has been a lot of grousing over the years by Congress, patient groups, and some scientists that NIH spends too much money on basic science and not enough on curing disease. From the polar opposite side of the spectrum, some critics have argued that NIH's twenty-seven separate institutes and centers should get out of the business of developing treatments altogether.[2] The agency's defenders counter that it must do both. In fact, most of the 80 percent of NIH money spent on outside research at universities and nonprofit institutes—the so-called extramural program—goes toward developing a basic understanding of the biochemistry of the human body. A substantial portion of in-house research—known as intramural research—does as well. But ever mindful of the political pressure emanating from Capitol Hill, NIH officials have always justified their in-house priorities in both basic and applied research—and lobbied for higher budgets—by claiming the government's medical scientists were working tirelessly to promote the health of the American people. Even science critics have to admit that over the years "fighting disease was clearly a dominant personal motivation in the community of NIH scientists."[3]

Brady helped shape that mold. His pioneering work over five decades into the causes of lysosomal storage disorders never lost sight of the goal that his work should one day be used to develop treatments. (The lysosome, sometimes called the police force of the cell, stores powerful enzymes for breaking down old cells, food, and bacteria.) Many of the dozens of researchers who now populate the field passed through his labs, and many of the physicians who treat the patients spent time in the

NIH clinics under his tutelage. As he approached his eightieth birthday, he continued to report to his lab nearly every day and consulted with most of the companies pursuing therapies based on his research. "Brady is an amazing character, yet I would never describe him as a driven person," said John Barranger, a professor of molecular genetics at the University of Pittsburgh and one of Brady's protégés. "He was always pretty laid back."[4]

Brady was born in 1923 to a suburban Philadelphia druggist and spent his after-school hours during the Depression tending the soda fountain in his father's corner drugstore. Though his father hoped that he would enroll in the local pharmacy college to follow in his footsteps, Brady opted for Pennsylvania State University to study medicine. When war broke out, he rushed through his studies to attend Harvard Medical School on a military scholarship.

Brady encountered the exasperating world of medical research for the first time in Cambridge. His first-year biochemistry professor asked him to replicate a recently published experiment that had claimed that alcoholic mice could be cured with vitamin injections. He thought the experiment would take three months. Four years later, Brady proved that vitamins provided only temporary relief from alcohol dependency. His reward for years of working with tipsy mice was Harvard's top award for student research. "Ha! I learned something from that experiment," Brady recalled. A tall, slender man, Brady often precedes his comments with a short, barking laugh. "It taught me how long research takes."[5]

After graduating from medical school, he accepted an internship and then a two-year fellowship at the University of Pennsylvania, where he studied under Samuel Gurin, a biochemist researching the body's lipid system and its relationship to heart disease. Gurin would later consult closely with scientists at Merck and Company as they developed lovastatin, the first cholesterol-lowering drug. After the Korean War started, Brady was called up and given a choice. They wanted the draftee to run a clinic at the Navy Medical Research Institute in Bethesda. But if he wasn't interested in research, he could report to a base hospital on an island in the South Pacific. He chose Bethesda. NIH, which had just thirteen hundred employees at the end of World War II, was expanding rapidly in the postwar years. Congress created a new institute almost every year. Brady began spending his nights and weekends working on experiments at the National Institute of Neurological Disorders and Blindness. When that war ended and he received his discharge, he joined its staff, where has remained ever since (*Blindness* having been replaced with *Stroke* at the institute).

Noting his prior experience at Penn, the director put him to work studying lipids (the insoluble fatty parts of cells) in the brain and nerves. But within a few years Brady gravitated to the disorders caused by excess lipid buildup in the body's major organs. Many of the lysosomal storage disorders had been discovered in the late nineteenth and early twentieth centuries by scientists who gave them their eponymous names, but little was known about their causes. Did the body create too much of a particular lipid? Was it failing to break it down properly when cells died and were replaced? Was there a genetic defect—these diseases were all known to pass through families—causing them to make the wrong lipid-dissolving enzyme entirely? Whatever the cause, the effects were disheartening to see in the clinic. People with Gaucher disease, for instance, often had distended bellies from their enlarged spleens and livers, where an excess of a lipid called glucocerebroside wound up. It also wormed its way into bone marrow, and symptoms included anemia, bone pain, and a propensity to bleed uncontrollably and suffer bone fractures. Fabry patients built up lipids in the walls of small blood vessels, which led to unbearable pain in the feet and hands, kidney and heart failure, and almost always early death. The average life expectancy for a Fabry disease sufferer was forty-one years.

Brady spent his first two decades at NIH unraveling the mysteries of these diseases. He eventually discovered that each disease was caused by a missing enzyme, which broke down the lipids in normal people. Some people were missing the enzymes due to either genetic inheritance or a mutation at conception. The first breakthrough came in 1964 when Brady and his team of scientists identified the missing enzyme for Gaucher disease. "It was a biochemical Rosetta stone," he said. "Once we knew this was the basis of Gaucher disease, we had the key to all the single lipid storage disorders." By the early 1970s, Brady's team had done similar work on Niemann-Pick, Fabry, and Tay-Sachs diseases and other lysosomal storage disorders. They also worked on mucopolysaccharide diseases, where build-ups of jellylike sugars inhibit normal growth and mental development. "There are about thirteen of them and it was the same principle," Brady said. "They don't have enzymes to start the breakdown."

With much of the basic science under his belt, Brady turned to treatment. "I started with a very simple concept. If this enzyme is not as active as it should be, can you purify it from some source and put it into a patient to make him better? I wanted to try and purify glucocerebrosidase [the missing enzyme in Gaucher disease] from some human source, to reduce the possibility of humans rejecting it when it came in." One night, while out to dinner with the father of two children with Gaucher disease, it came to him in a flash. Why not human placentas? They were fresh tissues and would likely have higher than normal concentrations of the rare proteins. It took another half-decade to work out the procedure for purifying the enzyme from the placentas. Brady and a team of scientists spent nights and weekends liquefying placentas with a hand-cranked grinder in the cold room next door to their lab. NIH would get a patent for the process in 1975.[6]

Two years before the patent was granted, Brady and his team had enough enzyme to attempt their first clinical trial. But tests on several patients had spotty results, largely because they didn't have enough enzyme to maintain large enough doses over a long enough period of time. They also learned that something occurred to the enzyme during purification that made it difficult to absorb. It wasn't getting into the cells that had built up excess levels of lipids.[7]

Brady and his colleagues solved the first dilemma by seeking outside help in purifying the enzyme. They contracted with Henry Blair, who had worked at NIH with Brady but left to form the New England Enzyme Center at Tufts University Medical School in Boston. Supported solely by contracts from Brady's lab, Blair set up a lab for large-scale purification and began collecting fresh placentas. In 1981, with NIH getting ready to move into larger clinical trials and biotechnology fever exploding all around him, Blair privatized his venture. He launched Genzyme, with the NIH contract as its major source of revenue.

But just as the company was getting off the ground, the new venture stumbled. Animal experiments showed the enzyme wasn't getting to the cells where the excess lipids were stored. Brady assigned several researchers to the problem, including Barranger and Scott Furbish, who later went to work for Genzyme. They discovered that the purification process stripped away the end of the enzyme that stuck to the lipid-storing cells. So they developed a process for restoring the sticky end of the purified enzyme and gave it to Genzyme. The company was back in business. Over the next decade, Genzyme received nearly $10 million in contracts to produce the enzyme for NIH, giving the start-up company a major lift in its formative years. Blair eventually hired a young economist named Henri Termeer to run the firm. A 1992 study by the Office of Technology Assessment (OTA) estimated that at least a fifth of all the direct research costs in developing enzyme replacement therapy for Gaucher disease was represented by that one government contract.[8]

After solving the purification problem, Brady's team moved on to the next logical step: discovering the gene. Harvesting placentas would always be a time-consuming and expensive proposition. Manufacturing the enzyme through the brand new recombinant methods of biotechnology would be preferable. "Once we had this pure protein that worked, it was an impetus to have the gene in hand in order to make protein," Barranger said. "If you had pure protein, and we were sure ours was pretty pure, you could fish out from expression libraries the [gene] sequences that corresponded to the protein." It didn't take them very long. Barranger and his colleague Edward Ginns identified the gene that produced glucocerebrosidase in 1984. (Ernest Beutler, now at the Scripps Research Institute in La Jolla, California, deserves credit for similar work, also NIH-funded, which he performed at the City of Hope in the early 1980s.)[9] They neglected to patent it. "In those days, you didn't patent genes," Barranger said.[10]

While that work was going on, Brady focused on the clinic. With a properly targeted placenta-derived enzyme in hand, he asked the FDA for permission to use it on a patient. He didn't have to go far to find one. Robin Ely Berman, an Orthodox Jewish physician from nearby Potomac, Maryland, had quit her practice to volunteer in Brady's lab a few years earlier. Three of her six children had Gaucher disease, and four-year-old Brian was faring the worst. His overloaded organs had swollen his abdomen to several times its normal size. His desperate parents were about to have his spleen taken out. On a late December morning in 1983, the boy received the first of seven weekly treatments. "It was absolutely amazing. It was movie amazing," she recalled. "Every week his stomach got smaller and smaller and smaller. He put on some weight. Then we ran out of enzyme. For another seven weeks, he got nothing. He went all the way back down to the bottom, which was absolutely agonizing and wonderful. Agonizing because you watched your kid get ill again. And wonderful because we realized the drug was having some effect."[11]

To do a full-blown first-stage clinical trial—which is designed to determine safety and proper dosing—Brady needed a lot more enzyme. NIH began pouring money into Genzyme to produce it. It took until 1986 before they had stockpiled enough to begin enrolling patients. The clinicians in Brady's lab eventually infused single doses of the drug into nearly two dozen patients at the NIH Clinical Center. Fearful of harming their already ill clientele, the government scientists at first provided extremely low doses of the enzyme. It had no measurable effect. Finally, they infused eight patients—seven adults and one child—with a much higher dose. None of the adults showed any improvement, but the child, like the young Berman, showed a marked reduction in his lipid levels.

Genzyme's scientific advisory board, focusing on the effects in adults, wanted to cancel the program. But Brady convinced chief executive officer Termeer that the only problem was the dose. Termeer, with Robin Ely Berman in tow, began making the rounds of venture capitalists to raise money for a larger purification facility. She would show slides of her son's miraculous (albeit short-term) recovery, and Termeer would make the pitch for cash. He raised $10 million to construct a plant that could produce enough placenta-derived enzyme to supply a long-running clinical trial and support eventual commercial production.[12]

Though Genzyme's name was now on the paperwork at FDA, the company continued to rely on Brady's team for the final clinical trial. A dozen patients were given biweekly treatments over a year's time at NIH. The results at high doses showed adults clearing some of the excess lipids from their livers and spleens, just like the children had done in the earlier tests. The FDA approved Ceredase—Genzyme's trade name for placenta-derived glucocerebrosidase—in April 1991. The approval gave the company the exclusive rights to market the drug because it had been designated as an orphan drug, under a law signed by President Ronald Reagan in January 1983, which grants seven years of market exclusivity to newly approved drugs for diseases that affect fewer than two hundred thousand people.

Getting drug companies to develop treatments for rare diseases has always bedeviled patient advocacy groups, which are often run by people like Robin Berman. When just several thousand or even a few tens of thousands of people suffer from a disease, most drug companies are unwilling to invest the time and money needed to come up with potential therapies. Even when most of the work on a rare disease—like Brady's treatment for Gaucher disease—is done in an NIH-funded lab, drug companies often don't want to get involved. There's just not that much money in it.

Conditions were worse before passage of the Orphan Drug Act. A survey of NIH in the early 1980s found there were more than one hundred potential therapies for rare diseases languishing in its labs. But the scientists who had come up with them were usually more concerned with publishing their results in medical and academic journals than in rushing off to get a patent. That put the intellectual property in the public domain, available to anyone, so no drug company wanted to get involved. Why commercialize these so-called orphan drugs when another company could make it once it had been shown to work in patients?

Several government panels highlighted the problem in the late 1970s, but legislation to create special incentives for drug companies went nowhere until a 1981 *Los Angeles Times* article sparked the interest of Jack Klugman, the star of television's *Quincy*. He dedicated one of his shows to the woes of a Los Angeles youngster with Tourette's syndrome. The problem of orphan drugs "was catapulted from an insider's dialogue conducted mainly in medical journals and federal offices to a nationally recognized tragedy."[13] Rep. Henry Waxman, a liberal California Democrat, introduced legislation in the next session of Congress to give industry special tax breaks for research in rare diseases and a seven-year exclusive market for orphan drugs. Heavy lobbying by the newly created patient advocacy group, the National Organization for Rare Disorders (NORD), and another episode of *Quincy* showing hundreds of angry patients marching on the Capitol—a case of art substituting for reality—pushed the bill through the House and Senate and onto the president's desk.

The bill gave the orphan drug field a major boost. The number of companies, especially biotechnology start-ups, willing to get involved in investigating drugs for rare diseases shot up dramatically. The agency made grants to companies to work on orphan drugs and provided technical advice to small firms wending their way through the drug approval maze for the first time. It is tempting to say that the pump priming worked. By the end of 2001 there were 229 FDA-approved drugs and devices aimed at rare diseases, up from just ten when the law was passed. Hundreds more were in the drug development process.[14]

But those incentives don't really explain why so many companies became willing to pursue orphan drugs and stick with them through the long development process. The seven years of exclusivity under the new law was far less time than the twenty years of exclusivity granted by a patent, and, as it turned out, most of the new therapies were protected by patents. The extra tax breaks for companies working on orphan drugs didn't mean much to start-ups that weren't earning money. And the law hadn't changed the size of the potential patient population for most of these drugs, which was still quite small.

The real answer was much simpler: price. After Genzyme won FDA approval for Ceredase, it set a price on its new drug that set tongues to wagging across the industry. The initial cost of Ceredase therapy, which didn't include the office visits for the twice-monthly infusions, was $350,000 a year for an average-sized male (the dose was weight-dependent). After a few years, when the build-up of lipids was under control, the dose could be reduced. But even the maintenance dose cost nearly $200,000 a year.

The lives of Gaucher patients on enzyme replacement therapy—which they would need for the rest of their lives—became a constant scramble for insurance coverage. The company did provide the drug free of charge when people exhausted their benefits, but that left them without medical coverage for any other health problem. "Genzyme's pricing is similar in its consequences to a policy in which patients are offered a lifetime supply of aglucerase [the generic name for Ceredase] in exchange for the value of their remaining insurance coverage," the federal OTA study concluded.[15] "There was no rationale for Genzyme's high price. It was beyond belief," said Abbey Meyers, the mother of three children with Tourette's syndrome who has run NORD since its inception. "Ceredase was discovered and developed by the NIH."[16] Even Brady was shocked. "I was appalled it was that expensive," he said.

The outrage over the high price of Ceredase reached Capitol Hill shortly after the drug was approved. Rep. Pete Stark, the California Democrat, introduced legislation in the House to tax windfall profits generated through the Orphan Drug Act. Senators Nancy Kassebaum, a Republican from Kansas, and Howard Metzenbaum, a Democrat from Ohio, introduced similar legislation. Comparing Genzyme's annual profits, which in 1992 had already soared over $200 million, to the cost of developing the drug, which the federal study had estimated to be less than $30 million, Stark asked, "To stimulate research that we all desire, is it required that we pay any price? Is this sustainable if we are to attack more than one disease afflicting our population? Is this return necessary to stimulate subsequent research?"[17] Writing in the *Washington Post*, the two senators said the Orphan Drug Act was designed "to provide incentives for the development of drugs with small markets, drugs that would otherwise not be produced. Orphan drugs that are, in fact, of tremendous commercial value don't deserve—and were never intended to receive—seven years' worth of protection from the price competition that would make them more affordable for victims of rare disease."[18]

Genzyme's Termeer fired back in the pages of the *Wall Street Journal*. The marketplace will provide an answer, he declared.

> Since Genzyme developed Ceredase, other companies have jumped into Gaucher's disease research. We are now competing with a company working on a variation of our drug, and two others are competing with us to

develop gene-therapy approaches. There could be as many as four or five treatments for Gaucher's disease on the market within the next four years. If we hadn't taken the first step, there would be no market and no additional research on the disease.[19]

The published statement was not only disingenuous about who invented the drug, but the company had already taken steps to ensure the promised competition never came to pass—at least, not for a long, long time. Using the unpatented gene uncovered by Barranger and others in Brady's lab, Genzyme scientists in August 1991 applied for a patent on the recombinant manufacturing of glucocerebrosidase and its use in treating Gaucher disease, and three months later won orphan designation from the FDA for that form of treatment.[20] They immediately put this new drug into clinical trials. The FDA approved it a little more than a year after Termeer predicted that intense competition was just around the corner. The new drug effectively precluded other firms from using biotechnology to develop alternatives until well into the twenty-first century. And even though recombinant manufacturing meant the new drug, dubbed Cerezyme, cost far less to manufacture than placenta-derived Ceredase, the price to patients and their insurers didn't change.

Brady didn't dwell on the exorbitant price tag placed on his therapy. Once Ceredase was approved, Brady turned his attention to the other lysosomal storage disorders. A quarter-century earlier, his discovery of the Gaucher enzyme defect had been the template for deciphering similar diseases. In 1991, with sales of Ceredase taking off, the senior NIH scientist traveled to Genzyme's Cambridge headquarters to encourage the firm to use its cash flow from Ceredase to pursue enzyme replacement therapies for the other diseases.

Fabry disease, though it probably struck half as many patients as Gaucher disease, had the harshest impact on patients' lives. Youngsters often discovered they had it when they experienced shooting pain in their hands and feet while running or jumping. They didn't sweat and couldn't stand heat. By the time they were in their twenties, many Fabry sufferers found themselves in dialysis clinics and on kidney-transplant waiting lists. The downhill spiral ended in coronary heart disease, strokes, and heart attacks, usually by the time they were in their early forties. Many victims never knew the cause of their suffering.

Brady's visit to Genzyme didn't go well. "I had a list of diseases they should address next, and Fabry was at the top," Brady said as he reached for one of the file cabinets in his cubbyhole office at NIH. "Ha! I can show you the slide [from his presentation]. If they didn't know it before, they certainly knew it after I told them. Why they didn't do something about it is their business."[21] In fact, Genzyme was quite aware of Fabry disease. As early as January 1988, the company had applied to the FDA for orphan drug status for an experimental drug called trihexosidase-alpha, which was its name for the placenta-derived enzyme missing in Fabry patients.[22]

Brady's touchy relationship with Genzyme regarding Fabry disease was understandable. He had tried enzyme replacement therapy for a few Fabry patients in the early 1970s, but the Fabry enzyme was much harder to purify than the Gaucher enzyme so he had to put the project on hold. In any case, by the early 1990s the era of enzyme purification from natural sources was nearing its end. Genzyme was already in the process of switching to the recombinant form of the Gaucher enzyme. Any company that wanted to get involved in Fabry disease research was either going to make the missing enzyme through recombinant technology or try gene therapy, which was the hot new item in biotechnology circles. But recombinant manufacturing required a patent on the process of making the enzyme from its gene, and Brady didn't have it.

The process for manufacturing the missing enzyme in Fabry disease belonged to Robert J. Desnick, the chairman of the human genetics department at Mt. Sinai School of Medicine on Manhattan's Upper East Side. If Brady was the king of the lysosomal storage disease world, Desnick was its crown prince, towering over the rest of the small field's roster of academic researchers. A 1971 graduate of the University of Minnesota Medical School, Desnick devoted his career to studying rare genetic disorders. By the early 1980s he had built a large department devoted to the disorders at Mt. Sinai in New York, where he moved because of its proximity to a large number of patients. Desnick, whose broad forehead and dark-knitted eyebrows command immediate respect, depended heavily on the government for support. For more than a decade, he received more than a million dollars a year from NIH to study Fabry disease, grants that lasted well into the 1990s, according to agency records.

Like Brady, he helped train many of the leading clinicians in the field. Unlike Brady, he seems to have made numerous enemies along the way. Desnick turned down many requests for an interview, at first citing the ongoing clinical trials for his patented treatment for Fabry disease, and after they were concluded, his own desire to write a book on the subject.

But based on a half-dozen interviews with former colleagues, there can be no doubt that he engenders as much fear as respect from others in the field. "You can't quote me; I have to make a living," pleaded one former associate, "but he's the emperor over there." Meyers, the blunt-talking head of NORD, was more direct. "He's not a good-hearted researcher," she declared. "A lot of people discover genes and don't patent them. They think scientific discovery belongs to science."[23]

The scientific name for the missing enzyme in Fabry disease is alpha-galactosidase. Like Brady, Desnick had purified a small amount of the enzyme in the 1970s. He had even injected it into two patients, although his test trailed Brady's by a couple of years. But he ran into the same problem as the senior NIH scientist. It was impossible to come up with enough enzyme to pursue effective therapy. By the early 1980s, recombinant technology was making headlines, and Desnick immediately saw the possibilities. In August 1981, David Calhoun, a biochemist at Mt. Sinai, was taking a week off at his home in Leonia, New Jersey, when Desnick called. "Desnick asked me to talk to him about Fabry disease," Calhoun said. "I knew how to sequence genes. His laboratory had no experience in that area. They were medical geneticists. They worked with lipids, grew cells in culture, and did enzyme assays. Nobody in that department had experience cloning and sequencing genes. It seemed like an interesting project to me. If we cloned, sequenced, and produced it in the laboratory, the gene product could be used therapeutically."[24]

Relying on graduate students in his and Desnick's lab, Calhoun began searching for the gene that produced alpha-galactosidase. They experimented with the probe technology then being used by commercial scientists at Amgen and Genetics Institute to hunt for the erythropoietin gene, but eventually fell back on the traditional chemical means developed in the 1950s by the field's pioneer, Frederick Sanger. Mary Jean Quinn, a doctoral candidate in Calhoun's lab, logged long hours testing the results in thousands of test tubes as they mapped the enzyme's genetic sequence. "I was standing there at the computer as she read me the final sequence," Calhoun recalled. "We knew we had it." They uncorked a bottle of champagne kept in the lab's refrigerator for the occasion to celebrate the culmination of three years' work.

Unlike Barranger, the NIH scientist who had uncovered the Gaucher gene, Calhoun was very aware of the economic potential of his discovery. The tectonic shifts in the world of biomedical research had reached Mt. Sinai. Calhoun, who'd received his academic training at the University of Alabama, wanted to jump on the plate moving toward commercialization and private gain. But in the mid-1980s, Mt. Sinai as an institution wasn't ready. The medical school hadn't yet established an office dedicated to carrying out the 1980 Bayh-Dole Act, which encouraged universities to patent technologies developed in their labs so they could be licensed to commercial partners. "Even though I wanted to do it, there was nobody at Mt. Sinai to work with me," Calhoun said. Instead, Desnick's lab, with Calhoun as the lead author, described the gene in a paper published in the proceedings of the National Academy of Science in November 1985.[25] Publication, according to U.S. patent law, starts the clock ticking on the year when authors can file for a patent. It passed without event.

NIH continued pouring money into Desnick's lab for Fabry studies. The senior scientist assigned Calhoun and a slew of other researchers the task of using the gene to develop a recombinant form of the enzyme. Yiannis Ioannou, a native of Cyprus who had come to New York to attend college, began his graduate studies in Desnick's lab in 1986. He immediately went to work on the project, which would dominate the next eight years of his life. So would Desnick. "He had a very tight leash on everything," Ioannou said. "He always bothered me. He likes to be on top of everything to the point where he could try and manage every small aspect of day-to-day activity that doesn't necessarily need supervision."[26] Ioannou, perhaps because he was familiar with the rigid hierarchies of European universities, was able to deal with it. Others couldn't. Calhoun left in 1987 to join nearby City College, where he began tinkering with producing the Fabry enzyme from insect cell lines.

Desnick's lab, meanwhile, used the fast-replicating and long-lived cells from Chinese hamster ovaries (CHO cells), the technology developed at nearby Columbia, which by that time had become the standard methodology in the biotechnology field for recombinant manufacturing. Over the next few years, they refined their process, constantly comparing their manufactured enzyme to purified human enzyme and adjusting the process until their hamster-derived molecule came out almost the same. Even the slightest change in the sugars attached to the molecule could render it ineffective. In October 1990—right around the time Brady was concluding his Gaucher clinical trial—Desnick, Ioannou, and David Bishop, who was Desnick's chief lieutenant in the lab, filed for a patent on a process for producing large quantities of the Fabry enzyme. They also claimed its use in treating the disease.[27] Even before they filed for a patent, Desnick contacted the FDA and requested orphan drug status for an investigational new drug he called Fabrase.[28] It was granted on July 20, 1990.

Desnick was making all the right moves. He had closely followed Brady's work with Genzyme and Ceredase, which was nearing FDA approval. Mt. Sinai had one of the largest Gaucher patient populations in the world, and Desnick was their primary care physician (although he usually saw them only once and then turned their care over to clinicians on his staff).[29] Desnick's work on Fabry disease, which Brady had put to the side while pursuing Gaucher therapy, gave his lab a lock on the right to make the drug recombinantly. Indeed, all the pieces were in place for taking Desnick's Fabrase into clinical trials. All he needed was a company willing to do it.

Clinical trials on CHO cell-derived alpha-galactosidase wouldn't start for another seven years, even though Mt. Sinai received nearly a half-million dollars from the FDA's Orphan Drug Development office between 1990 and 1992. Desnick and officials at Genzyme, which eventually licensed his invention, were not willing to talk about the long delay. Frank Landsberger, who launched Mt. Sinai's technology transfer office in 1992, recalled that Desnick's demands complicated the negotiations with Genzyme, which dragged on for several years. "There were discussions about the licensee paying to have research done at Mt. Sinai. Desnick wanted to do some of the research at Mt. Sinai, certainly the clinical trials. . . . You have a conflict of interest—this is a generic problem in the industry—because Desnick would benefit financially from the outcome of the clinical trials," he said.[30] With those negotiations moving slowly, Desnick and Landsberger approached other firms. Desnick on his own initiative talked to Genetics Institute, which, despite the Gaucher example, turned him down.[31]

Landsberger approached Transkaryotic Therapies Inc. (TKT), a small biotechnology firm that was also in Cambridge. Harvard-trained Richard Selden had launched TKT in 1988 and shortly thereafter issued press releases stating it was experimenting with gene therapy cures for Fabry disease. TKT became a logical target for Landsberger's efforts. But the struggling start-up wasn't willing to meet Desnick's demands, and talks broke off after two years of negotiations.[32]

Desnick and Genzyme finally cut a deal, but Fabry treatment was hardly a high priority at the firm. In 1994, for instance, the company spent $55 million or nearly a quarter of its revenue (which was mostly from Ceredase sales) on research. But in the rare disease arena, its target was cystic fibrosis, a genetic disease of the lungs that had ten times as many potential patients as Fabry disease. It also sought a toehold in the mainstream of medical markets by developing nonscarring products for postsurgical tissue repair. At the time, financial analysts lauded the move as a much-needed effort at diversification. Instead of making Fabry disease a priority, the company gave grants to Desnick and Mt. Sinai, expecting them to carry the ball.

With Genzyme now their main revenue source instead of NIH, Desnick and his team launched a full-scale effort to cure mice. They spent two years developing a strain of mice with Fabry disease, and then treated them with the enzyme. The work was largely done by graduate students. "I had three or four people working full time on the mouse studies, generating data, trying to figure out what would go into the IND [investigational new drug application]," Ioannou said. "There was no question who we were working for. We got to publish our results, and they [Genzyme] got to use them to go to the FDA."[33] The leisurely pace seemed to suit everyone involved, except, of course, Desnick's Fabry patients, who had no idea what was going on inside their physician's lab.

Brady, without a patent and cut off by the firm that had brought his Gaucher treatment to market, was hardly ready to throw in the towel. NIH had its own Fabry patient population, and the number of researchers and clinicians abandoning Desnick's ship was growing rapidly. He first linked up with City College's Calhoun, who in 1991 earned a patent for producing alpha-galactosidase from insect cells. Calhoun was already working with a small company called Orphan Medical of Minnetonka, Minnesota. They would produce the enzyme, while Brady would conduct the clinical trials. But the start-up company stumbled as it clambered up the learning curve of recombinant manufacturing.

Desperate for a capable partner, Brady called Calhoun and told him he wanted out. He had been approached by Selden of TKT, who wanted to start Fabry disease clinical trials. The offer came totally out of the blue. Brady knew TKT was interested in Fabry disease. But the company had been pursuing treatments that relied on gene therapy, not enzyme replacement. But in the early 1990s, Selden's firm had stumbled onto an exciting discovery. TKT had learned how to produce proteins by turning on inactive human genes in cell cultures outside the body, a process he called gene activation. If allowed by the patent courts, the humanized process posed a threat to every biotechnology product on the market since the existing products were all made from animal cell lines.

Selden didn't look the part of a man who wanted to overturn the entire biotechnology field. Sitting at a small table in one of Cambridge's old brick industrial buildings between Harvard and MIT that have been turned into biotechnology laboratories, he struggled to explain the complicated process of gene activation to a visitor. Though still in his early forties, his curly red hair was already half gray and receding rapidly. He wore topsiders and casual slacks. His knit tie dangled at half-mast.

Since every cell contains every gene, every cell has the potential to make any protein, Selden explained. But in any particular cell, only some genes are turned on. The insulin gene, for instance, is only turned on in the pancreas, not in the brain. Each gene has sequences that keep the gene either turned on or off, depending on where it is in the body. TKT researchers had come up with a way of taking the sequences that turned on a particular gene from active cells and splicing them into other, fast-growing human cells, which could then be cultured en masse outside the body to produce whatever protein the turned-on gene expressed. Biotechnologists would no longer be dependent on hamsters or insects to produce proteins. They could now use human cells.

"There are several advantages," Selden said. "It's much more efficient in terms of a production system than working with conventional technology. You're ending up using the gene in its natural location with all of the synthesis machinery that is supposed to be involved in the first place," he continued. "The second thing is that many genes are really too big to manipulate in the conventional approach. You can use this method to make enormous proteins that are difficult to manufacture. But probably the most important thing is that the proteins that come out have the potential to be more effective."[34]

By 1995, TKT had used gene activation to produce alpha-galactosidase. Selden immediately called Brady to see if he would run the young company's clinical trials. "I felt and feel to this day that Dr. Brady is the leader in this field," Selden said. "He has done a phenomenal amount of work since the 1950s to understand Fabry's disease and other diseases as well. It was an honor when Brady said yes. When I was in college, he was somebody I looked up to."[35] In 1996, TKT and NIH signed a cooperative research and development agreement (CRADA) to develop human-derived alpha-galactosidase, a drug that TKT would soon call Replagal. In late summer, TKT raised $37.5 million in an initial public stock offering. The Securities and Exchange Commission (SEC) document revealed to the world that the upstart company was not only chasing gene therapy cures for Fabry disease—which was well known in Cambridge biotechnology circles—but enzyme replacement therapy as well. It also announced plans to start the first phase of clinical trials before the end of the year.[36]

The news sent shock waves through Genzyme and Desnick's Mt. Sinai lab. In the spring of 1997, Genzyme for the first time mentioned in its annual filings with the SEC that it was in " preclinical" research on Fabry disease. "To date, it has successfully produced the recombinant α-Gal enzyme in mammalian cells and has shown it can reduce lipid levels in the plasma and tissues of a Fabry mouse model. The development program is currently focused on producing sufficient quantities of enzyme for pilot clinical studies, which are expected to begin in late 1997 or early 1998," the company said.[37] A year later they revealed they were testing a new drug for Fabry disease dubbed Fabrazyme.

The race was on. Two companies were chasing a therapy for a patient population that was no more than ten thousand persons worldwide. They both quickly leaped over the early safety and dosing hurdles. But then they faced a critical juncture. How should they design the final efficacy trial that would be submitted to the FDA? Measuring improvements from enzyme replacement therapy for Fabry disease was much more difficult than detecting them in patients with Gaucher disease. The lipid buildup in Fabry disease took place in the kidneys, heart, and brain, organs that were difficult to scrutinize without invasive and potentially dangerous biopsies. The reduction in spleen size in Gaucher patients, on the other hand, had been easily measured with magnetic resonance imaging machines. Moreover, reduction in the intermittent pain that afflicted Fabry sufferers, a major potential benefit of treatment, could only be shown through a survey, which the FDA might interpret as a highly subjective measure.

TKT's clinicians, led by Raphael Schiffmann at NIH, opted to measure pain reduction as the primary test of Replagal after lengthy negotiations with the FDA. In 1999, the government lab enrolled twenty-six patients for the final study. The NIH clinicians also measured lipid levels in the blood as a secondary test of the new drug. Genzyme's clinicians, meanwhile, led by Christine M. Eng, who worked in Desnick's division throughout the 1990s before moving to Baylor University Medical School, chose lipid reduction in the kidneys as the primary measure. It was a more limited approach, but one that would more easily pass FDA muster if the agency was willing to accept a surrogate marker. Genzyme tested Fabrazyme on fifty-eight patients recruited from eight clinics in Europe and the United States, including Mt. Sinai. They also surveyed their patients to measure pain reduction. Both studies were double-blind and placebo controlled—neither the patients nor the doctors knew which group was getting the real drug and which the placebo. Both lasted twenty weeks.

The results, according to the academic literature, were extremely positive for both sides. Patients in the TKT test showed reduced pain and lower lipids in the blood compared to those in the placebo group. The Genzyme test cleared lipid deposits from the kidneys, heart, and skin, "the chief clinical manifestations of this disease." There were major differences between the drugs, however. The TKT/NIH team infused their patients for only forty minutes compared to four to six hours for patients in the Genzyme/Desnick trial. Moreover, TKT's human-derived protein generated far fewer reactions and didn't require premedication to curb them.[38]

Did that make Replagal better? "TKT, by activating a gene in human cells, [has] raised the technology to the next level, the next step," said Gregory Pastores, a physician who worked with Desnick for a decade before leaving Mt. Sinai in 1997 to join New York University, where he treats hundreds of patients for rare genetic disorders. He participated in neither company's trial, although he has done work for both companies in the past. "It's like cow's milk and mother's milk. We all feel instinctively that there are advantages to mother's milk."[39]

TKT beat Genzyme to the FDA, filing its license application on June 16, 2000. Genzyme's application followed a week later.[40] The larger company also tried to win the war in patent court. A month after filing with the FDA, Genzyme accused TKT of violating Desnick's patent. Over their three decades of competition, Desnick had never beaten Brady on an issue of scientific or medical significance except in winning his Fabry patent. Here was his chance to play the trump card. But on December 17, 2001, the U.S. District Court in Delaware dismissed the case.

Less than six months after the two applications arrived at the FDA, Mike Russo discovered he had Fabry disease. A freelance journalist turned manuscript editor, Russo was always aware there was something wrong with him while growing up near Greece, New York. He didn't sweat as a child. When he joined his high school golf team, he would have to beg off competing on hot days. "What's the matter now," his father, the coach, would ask. "It's too hot," Russo complained, even though it was barely past eighty degrees. He took up swimming instead. By his early twenties, doctors diagnosed high protein levels in his urine, a sign his kidneys weren't functioning properly. His doctors took a wait-and-see approach. He suffered periodic bouts of joint swelling and itchy skin. His doctors treated the pain with steroids.

In late 2000, just past his thirty-fifth birthday, Russo received a Friday afternoon call from his nephrologist. The creatinine levels in his urine and blood were soaring, a sign his kidneys were beginning to fail. They had done some extra blood work. Could he come in Monday to discuss the results? "This is my life," he said, and rushed over with his wife. They told him he had Fabry disease, "which we're just finding out about." Russo spent the weekend scouring the Internet to learn more about the rare disorder that was ruining his life. He learned that it was an X-chromosome genetic disorder. His mother had given it to him. His two daughters were carriers. He also learned that researchers had been working on the disease for a long time, and that clinical trials on a possible treatment were underway in Desnick's lab in New York. He called. He wanted to get involved.[41]

In 1991, the FDA had approved Ceredase for Gaucher patients just six months after the end of a clinical trial on twelve patients that lasted a year. Nearly a decade later—a decade that has seen several waves of drug-industry-driven liberalization wash over the agency—things had changed, but apparently not in favor of patients when they had two companies competing to treat their rare disease. Six months after TKT and Genzyme submitted applications, the regulators sent letters to both companies indicating their data was inadequate. Desnick assigned Russo to his follow-up trial.

By late 2002, Mike Russo was an angry, frustrated young man. He had been fired from his job for poor performance about a year after he began taking time off every two weeks to go to New York City for his infusions. He was convinced he was on placebo, since none of his symptoms had improved. His kidneys were continuing their downhill slide toward a date with dialysis. While he waited, both drugs had been approved by the European Union (EU) and a half-dozen other countries. With two firms competing to sell in their market, the EU priced enzyme replacement therapy at $160,000 a year to start—substantially below the price Genzyme had placed on its Gaucher treatments. "They can get it in the Czech Republic but not here," Russo said. "There are people out there who need it more than I do. Some of these people have died since. I don't understand how other countries can get it approved so quickly, and the United States, where are you would think. . . ." His voice trailed off.[42]

A few months later, in January 2003, an FDA advisory committee, whose recommendations are invariably followed by the agency, met over two days to consider the two drug applications. A parade of patients testified to the vast improvements in their lives—especially the reduction in pain—since taking the regular infusions of replacement enzyme. But the FDA examiners are rarely swayed by such emotional outpourings. They need numbers. The academics on the advisory committee questioned Genzyme's assertions that lowering lipid levels would eventually improve patients' health status. But in the end the committee gave an overwhelming endorsement to the surrogate marker.

The next day the same group came down hard on TKT's data presentation. The pain studies were not adequately controlled, and the company had not submitted enough data to show that Replagal had the same lipid lowering effect as Fabrazyme. The panel narrowly voted to send TKT back to do more studies, or to retest its slides to show the same thing that Genzyme had showed. "We shot for the moon," Schiffmann, the NIH scientist in charge of the trial, moaned. "They were just smarter in their approach with the FDA."[43] Desnick had defeated Brady at last.

The competition between Genzyme and TKT presented a startling new paradigm for orphan drug development, indeed, for all drug development in the postgenome era. The U.S. Orphan Drug Law was premised on the idea that no one was interested in developing drugs for tiny markets. Commercial firms, it was believed, wouldn't touch therapies developed in government labs or in universities that were either unpatented or protected by weak process patents. The law granted seven years exclusivity to overcome that barrier. Of course, it never precluded another company from coming along and getting its drug approved for the same orphan disease if the manufacturer proved its drug was better. In fact, the FDA had twice withdrawn orphan status for interferon treatments for multiple sclerosis when superior versions came along.[44]

The race to develop a Fabry treatment blew the old paradigm apart. Largely because of the high prices set on orphan drugs, two companies found it worth their while to pursue different versions of the same therapy. In the years ahead, feisty start-up biotechnology firms like TKT will inevitably come up with even better and more innovative ways of building proteins and molecules. Will they be prevented from entering the market? As Senator Dole wrote in the early 1990s, the Orphan Drug Act was never meant to prevent competition.

However, there are forces at work to frustrate the application of new technologies like Selden's for decades. TKT would have never had a chance to pursue enzyme replacement therapy if Desnick and his team had patented the Fabry gene in the late 1980s. But as the new millennium dawned, the days when scientists thought more about publication than patenting were long over. Across the country, companies and academic researchers ran gene sequencing machines overtime as they sought to stake their claims to the human genome. It was a great gene grab, the fencing of the human commons. And it was all made possible by machines whose invention—the subject of the next chapter—had come at taxpayer expense.

3

The Source of the New Machine

onday, June 26, 2000—Human Genome Day in the nation's capital. The rhetoric inside the White House East Room rivaled the steamy weather outside as an ebullient President Clinton welcomed the three scientists who symbolized the race to complete the Human Genome Project: James Watson, the cantankerous geneticist who had codiscovered the double helix structure of DNA a half-century earlier; Francis S. Collins, a gene hunter whose discovery of the cystic fibrosis gene a decade earlier had catapulted him into the front ranks of the nation's genetic scientists and atop the massive federal program; and J. Craig Venter, the erstwhile government researcher who had launched Celera Genomics, a private firm, with the expressed intent of beating the government at its own game.

The president first turned to Watson, who had kick-started the effort to map the genome in the late 1980s and more than any single individual was responsible for the government pouring $3 billion into the project. "Without a doubt, this is the most important, most wondrous map ever produced by humankind. . . . Thank you, sir," the president said. Gazing toward the heavens, the president noted that Galileo had described the planets circling the sun as the language of God's creation. "Today we are learning the language in which God created life. We are gaining ever more awe for the complexity, the beauty, the wonder of God's most divine and sacred gift."[1]

Clinton then shifted gears. He downplayed the controversy surrounding the race to complete the genome. The personalities of the two men who epitomized the race reflected their funding sources. Collins, with a droopy mustache and quiet and avuncular speaking style, was a role model for self-effacing bureaucrats. He rarely spoke about his involvement in the high-profile hunts for therapeutically significant genes. A physician by training, he preferred talking about the potential medical breakthroughs that might come from finding them. Collins rode to work on a motorcycle and played guitar in a pickup rock band.

The flamboyant Venter had been a mediocre student and California surfing fanatic before his life was transformed by his experience as a medic in Vietnam. He returned to the United States as a serious science student, focusing on the technical side of scientific questions. He eventually turned to genomics, and by all accounts professed little interest in the eventual uses of the genomic information he had dedicated his life to generating. His meteoric research career was marked by his willingness to upset authority and challenge established wisdom. And he had the knack, which so many of his peers lacked, of generating media attention. He carefully cultivated an image of a bold scientist turned brash entrepreneur. By the late 1990s, his face had graced the cover of numerous business magazines. His rivals in the government-funded program resented his ability to seize center stage. On the eve of his great triumph, one used the cloak of anonymity to brand him an "asshole," an "idiot," and an "egomaniac" in an unflattering *New Yorker* magazine profile.[2]

But on this, the human genome's unveiling day, Clinton proved he could gloss over bitter conflicts in science almost as well as in politics. He welcomed the grand compromise that had enabled the joint announcement and praised both sides' pledge to publish their results simultaneously and cooperate in the completion of the still-unfinished project.

In a final comment, the president sought to reassure Wall Street, whose 1990s bubble was starting to burst. Three months earlier, the president and British prime minister Tony Blair had sent biotechnology stocks tumbling when they seemed to suggest that they opposed patenting the genes that were being uncovered by the Human Genome Project. This time, Clinton wanted to make sure that the volatile stock market didn't get mixed signals as he outlined the tasks still ahead. It would take years of research to identify the genes in the three-billion-plus letters of the genetic code, the proteins they encode, and their cellular functions—

and then turn that knowledge into medical treatments. "I want to emphasize that biotechnology companies are absolutely essential in this endeavor," the president said. "For it is they who will bring to the market the life-enhancing applications of the information from the human genome. And for that reason this administration is committed to helping them to make the kind of long-term investments that will change the face of medicine forever."[3]

The president had neatly finessed the many controversies surrounding gene patents, which had swirled for more than a decade and were still being hotly contested at the Patent and Trademark Office (PTO). But the questions couldn't be dodged a few hours later when the public and private sector protagonists gathered at the nearby Capitol Hilton Hotel's Congressional Room for a joint press conference. Unlike the semiprivate White House event, hundreds of reporters, researchers, and interested hangers-on filled the cavernous ballroom. Dozens of television cameras cast their glare over the crowd. The lineup on stage reflected the tensions in the room. Venter and his team from Celera Genomics sat on one side of the podium. Collins and the leaders of the government's team, including Watson, sat on the other. In a fitting gesture, Aristides Patrinos of the Department of Energy (DOE) presided. The energy agency, renowned for championing big science projects, had originated the idea of mapping the human genome. To avoid a public spat in its final hours, Patrinos had gotten Collins and Venter together in his Rockville townhouse where, over pizza and beer, they finally agreed to the joint announcement.[4]

Collins, speaking first, sought to dismiss the notion there had been a competition between the two teams. "The only race we're interested in discussing today is the human race," he said, "and we want them to be the winners." But Venter exuded the same feistiness that had put him at odds with the genome's establishment for most of the previous decade. He spent much of his opening presentation heaping praise on Mike Hunkapillar, the president of the company that had put Celera in business. In 1998, Applied Biosystems, a small machinery maker headquartered in an industrial suburb south of San Francisco, introduced the advanced gene sequencing machine that made rapid completion of the human genome possible. Hunkapillar then recruited Venter to run a new subsidiary—Celera, named after the Latin word for speed—that used the machines to complete its own version of the genome. Venter claimed it was only Hunkapillar's willingness to sell the three-hundred-thousand-dollar machines—known as the ABI Prism 3700—to the half-dozen universities and institutes on the public-sector side that enabled the public sector to compete at all. "This is a triumph for new technology, assembling the genome with computers that did not exist two years ago," he said. "It enabled this small team of scientists to do in a few years what it was previously thought to take fifteen years and thousands of scientists." Proof of his company's goodwill came from the fact that Applied Biosystems had been "willing to make these same machines available to the public program." On this penultimate day, however, Hunkapillar was home with the chicken pox and could not be present to revel in a success story that was largely his. "I said if he came, he had to sit on the public side," Venter finished to loud guffaws.[5]

The laughter only came from one side of the room. The Applied Biosystems (later Applera) business plan was still sending shock waves through the scientific community. The company wanted to turn Celera into the Microsoft of the gene-hunting world, selling its version of the human genome to private or public gene hunters through a proprietary computer program.

But the first reporters to jump to the microphones weren't interested in the corporate source of Venter's new machines, nor his business plans (which had already made him a millionaire many times over). They wanted to know where both sides now stood on the issue of gene patents. The PTO planned to issue new guidelines by the end of the year, and officials at that obscure yet critical government agency were indicating they wanted to make it more difficult to patent genes. In the past, a simple definition of the amino acid sequence of a gene and the protein it expressed, coupled with some vague connection to a disease state, was sufficient to get a patent. Now, the PTO wanted "substantial, credible utility" to meet the statutory test that a patent be both innovative and useful. In layman's terms, the PTO seemed to be suggesting it wanted gene hunters to spell out exactly how the protein it expressed was involved in a disease before issuing a patent.

The National Institutes of Health (NIH), which ran the government gene hunting program, had vacillated on the issue of gene patenting over the previous decade. In 1980, the Supreme Court, in *Diamond v. Chakrabarty*, had opened the door to patenting life forms when it validated a patent on an oil-eating bacteria produced by a subsidiary of General Electric. Over the next decade, the PTO awarded a few gene patents to private companies or university researchers, but their therapeutic use, in the jargon of the patent office, their utility, was known. In 1991, though, the floodgates opened. The move to wider gene patenting was triggered, ironically enough, by then NIH director Bernadine Healy.

The agency's office of technology transfer pursued patents on the first genes—really just segments of genes called expressed sequence tags (ESTs)—that had been uncovered by the nascent Human Genome Project. The inventor was none other than Venter, who at that time was still at NIH. Speaking later about his first patent application for an EST, Venter admitted that he had "no idea what it does."[6] The application kicked off a firestorm of controversy that raged across the pages of science magazines and set off an arms race among profit-seeking researchers and companies like Human Genome Sciences and Incyte Genomics, which began seeking patents on genes whose functions were still unknown. "The NIH proposal for patents is only an extreme example of a widespread practice in biotechnology that seeks to control not discoveries but the means of making discoveries," Thomas D. Kiley, an attorney and director on several biotechnology ventures, wrote in *Science*. "Patents are being sought daily on insubstantial advances far removed from the marketplace. These patents cluster around the earliest imaginable observations on the long road toward practical benefit, while seeking to control what lies at the end of it."[7]

Under Harold Varmus, who was Clinton's appointee to run NIH, the government largely got out of the gene patenting business. In testimony on Capitol Hill throughout the 1990s, Varmus repeated the concerns of scientists who feared that vague gene patents would hamstring future research. The patents would discourage investigators driven by curiosity and not monetary gain, or they would burden them with either unreasonable fees or unnecessary paperwork when using those genes in future research. Varmus saw cloned fragments of DNA as research tools, whose patenting "changed the conduct of biomedical research in some ways that are not always consistent with the best interests of science," he testified.

> It has promoted the creation of sometimes aggressive and usually expensive offices at many academic institutions to protect intellectual property and to regulate the exchange of biological materials that would at one time have been freely shared among academic colleagues. It has encouraged some companies to make protected materials and methods available to the investigators under terms that seem unduly onerous. . . . It has fostered policies that have inhibited the use of new scientific findings, even in the not-for-profit sector, and has reduced open exchange of ideas and materials among academic scientists.[8]

Collins, codiscoverer of the cystic fibrosis gene in the late 1980s, knew firsthand how uncovering a gene was only the first step in the long process of understanding how a disease worked. He laid it out for reporters on Human Genome Day. "NIH has been concerned about an alternative approach where you attempt to apply patent protection to genes whose function is not determined," Collins said. "That's why the public project places all its information on the internet every twenty-four hours. It will take decades for everyone to figure out what this information . . . is, and [public disclosure] is the best way to ensure that happens."[9]

But those complaints from NIH and NIH-funded scientists had little influence on private firms, many of which were run by scientists who were once on public payrolls. Venter knew the scientific arguments against gene patenting, but he also knew that Celera was filing patent claims on hundreds of genes every month. The strategy suggested the company's long-term plans called for it getting into drug development, and its first priority was staking its claims during the gold rush as the mother lode of genetic information emerged. "New therapeutics like human insulin are only available to patients because Genentech and Eli Lilly and Company got a patent to the human insulin gene," Venter declared at the press conference. "Patents are a key part of the process of making sure that new therapeutics are made available to the American public."

Wall Street was paying close attention to the squabbling over gene patents. In March, Clinton and Blair's comments had sent Celera's stock tumbling from its bubble-inflated $234-per-share high down to around $70. Venter told reporters then that he wanted a strict test for gene patents. "If patents have the word 'like' in the title [as in this protein or gene is like others that are involved in treating a disease], [then the companies] got it from a quick computer search."[10] In June, he repeated those sentiments again. "You have to know what the use will be in therapeutics," he said. "We think that bar should be very high. The pharmaceutical industry does not want early patents."

Though the simmering controversy over gene patents dominated the press conference, it was largely forgotten by the time reporters sat down to write their stories for the evening news and the next day's papers. The coverage either repeated the president's laudatory rhetoric or emphasized the race ("Private firm and public project finish remarkable achievement in a dead heat," blazed the *Los Angeles Times*, covering both bases).[11] Collins and Venter donned white lab coats to pose for the cover of *Time*, and made the rounds of television talk shows to proselytize the public on the profound significance of publishing the equivalent of five hundred thousand pages of the letters A, C, G, and T, which are the symbols of the four nucleotide bases that make up the genome. Only insiders—the gene sequencers, the researchers, the patent lawyers, the drug and biotechnology companies, and the handful of reporters who closely followed their actions—knew that the real story of the Human Genome Project was about to begin. What did the genes identified in the Human Genome Project do and how did they interact? Who would get to lay claim to those genes and on what basis? How would those claims affect future research? And how would they affect the cost of any medicines based on their protein interactions?

Pondering those troubling questions, I got up to leave the Hilton ballroom. As I moved toward the exit, a lonely public relations man from DOE pressed a one-page press release into my hands. In the early 1980s, it had taken researchers—whether they were at NIH or biotech startups like Amgen and Genetics Institute—about two years to find a gene. Now, with Mike Hunkapillar's fabulous new machine, it took about two days. DOE wanted people to know who had developed the technologies inside the machine that made rapid sequencing, not to mention widespread gene patenting and Celera, possible. Contrary to Venter's statements at the press conference, it wasn't Applied Biosystems.

The moment in 1953 that Watson and Crick published their theoretical model of the double helix structure of DNA, scientists began a quest to unravel its content. The model showed each chromosome's long strand of DNA is shaped like a twisting ladder whose rungs are made up of two of four possible chemical bases—adenine, cytosine, guanine, and thymine or A, C, G, and T. They are arranged in matching pairs. A is always linked to T, and C is always linked to G. The DNA strand is also divided up into genes, which run anywhere from a few thousand to tens of thousands of base pairs in length. Before the genes express proteins, which actually do the work of the body, they go through a two-step process. First, the bonds of a gene's base pairs separate, and each half gathers up loose bases in the cell to makes a mirror-image of itself. This newly made reversed half (called messenger RNA) then penetrates a protein-making factory called the ribosome, where it gathers up matching amino acids. The end product of this molecular square dance is an independent protein capable of doing the cell's work.

During the 1950s, Frederick Sanger of Cambridge University in England, who was hunting for the chemical structure of insulin, developed a chemical process for identifying the order of bases in an expressed protein. That work won him the 1958 Nobel Prize. He repeated the trick in the 1970s when he came up with a chemical method of identifying the order of bases in DNA. His methods depended on the DNA replication process, which takes place one base at a time along the inside of the ladder. He found four chemicals that acted just like A, C, G, and T in that they bound to their opposite mate. But unlike the real bases, these "terminator" bases halted the replication process. By tagging his terminators with radioisotopes that could be read on X-rays, Sanger had his tool for mapping genetic sequences. In an autobiographical article published years later, Sanger praised the Medical Research Council—Britain's equivalent of NIH—for its farsighted support of his research over many decades. "I was not under the usual obligation of having to produce a regular output of publishable material, with the result that I could afford to attack problems that were more 'way out' and longer-term."[12] He wasn't alone. On the other side of the pond in the New World's Cambridge, Allan Maxam and Walter Gilbert of Harvard University discovered an alternative method. They found four chemicals that broke apart DNA at the four different bases, thus giving scientists another way of mapping its genetic code.

Using chemical methods to decipher DNA was slow, tedious work. Graduate students or technicians would mix reagents in tiny wells filled with droplets of fluid, and then spend hours pouring over X-rays. It was hardly a recipe for keeping the best and brightest in the field. The California Institute of Technology was one of the few schools interested in the problem. In the late 1960s, CalTech molecular biologist William J. Dreyer had worked with Beckman Instruments to develop an automatic protein sequencer using Sanger's original chemistry. The school quickly emerged as the academic leader of the small field dedicated to sequencing machinery. They built a machinery fabrication shop for developing prototype machines and developed a corps of sixty-five to one hundred (the higher number during summers) of young faculty, postdoctoral fellows, graduate students, and technicians who were interested in looking at the pressing problems of molecular biology through the prism of machinery.

By the end of the 1970s, the lab was focused on two major projects: automating gene sequencing; and improving the existing line of protein sequencing machines, which were manufactured by Beckman Instruments. Leroy Hood, who had been a quarterback on a state championship football team in his native Montana before earning his doctorate at CalTech under Dreyer, led the charge on DNA sequencing. Hood also held a medical degree from Johns Hopkins School of Medicine. His expertise was in immunology and fundraising. Well-established companies like Baxter-Travenol, Monsanto, and Upjohn, as well as the foundation run by Arnold Beckman, the chairman of Beckman Instruments, made major grants to CalTech's efforts.[13] Virtually all of the postdoctoral researchers in the lab worked on NIH grants. The National Science Foundation gave the university $1.8 million in 1985 specifically to develop a DNA sequencing machine. The foundation even joined CalTech for the 1986 press conference where the first machine was unveiled.[14]

But it was the team that wanted to improve protein sequencing machines that scored first. The team was led by Mike Hunkapillar, a graduate of a small Baptist college in Oklahoma who had gotten his doctorate at CalTech in 1974. When Hunkapillar threatened to return home in 1976, Hood convinced him to stay put by placing him in charge of the protein sequencing project. Over the next five years, Hunkapillar and his colleagues at CalTech developed a prototype protein sequencer that was faster and required less material than the previous generation of machines developed under Dreyer. When Hood tried to interest Beckman Instruments in licensing the new machine, the company's middle managers demurred. They didn't believe that piling on additional development expenses made sense when the company already dominated the market. Several other large equipment makers also rejected Hood's overtures.[15]

The exploding venture capital market for start-up biotechnology companies rode to their rescue. In 1981, a group of venture capitalists in the San Francisco Bay Area recruited several top managers from Hewlett-Packard to form a start-up company called Applied Biosystems to build new tools for the emerging biotechnology industry. It licensed the CalTech technology, and in the summer of 1983, just a year after starting development work and with still only sixty-five employees on its payroll, the company brought its first protein sequencing machines to market. Sales of the superior product immediately took off. Applied Biosystems' machines largely displaced Beckman in the market to the consternation of its namesake chairman, whose philanthropy had helped launch the competition. The start-up was also immediately profitable—not because of the machine's price tag, which was $42,500, but from the $3,600 every machine generated every month in chemical and reagent sales. Selling sequencers, it turned out, was like selling razors. The big money was in the blades. That summer, the new company raised $18 million in an initial public offering and Hunkapillar quit academia to join the firm.[16]

Before he left, Hunkapillar and two postdoctoral fellows studying at CalTech on NIH grants, Henry Huang and Lloyd M. Smith, began zeroing in on gene sequencing. Sanger's original scheme for reading the gene fragment sequences had relied on attaching radioactive trace elements to his chain terminators. Exposing the fragments to X-ray film allowed researchers to read the length of each fragment, but the labor-intensive, eye-straining process was prone to human error. The three men eventually hit on a solution. They attached colored dyes to the chain terminators that could be read by a laser. Huang, who left CalTech in 1982 to begin his teaching career at Washington University in St. Louis, later claimed he was the one who came up with the idea of attaching different colored chemical dyes to the DNA chain terminators, and then sending the negatively charged fragments down a capillary tube using electrophoresis. Since the speed of the fragments as they traveled down the tube would be determined by their weight and length, the order in which they came off the end of the line—which would be read by a color-sensitive laser attached to a computer—would provide an accurate readout of the fragment's genetic sequence.[17]

Shortly after Huang left the lab, Smith realized his colored dyes weren't bright enough for even the best lasers. He spent the next two years searching for better fluorescent dyes that could be attached to the chain terminators. The CalTech team also had trouble getting the DNA fragments to flow evenly through the tiny capillary tubes. They switched to a gel sandwiched between two glass plates, and eventually put sixteen lanes on a one-by-two-foot slab. Each run took twelve or more hours, so a single machine could only measure sixteen fragments of DNA, each about five hundred bases in length, in a day. The technology was licensed by Applied Biosystems in 1986, and a year later the first sixteen-lane slab-gel gene sequencer hit the market. Over the next decade, the company made gradual improvements to the technology, eventually putting a forty-eight-lane machine on the market with small improvements in the run times. They cost one hundred thousand dollars.

In the late 1990s, the federal government launched an investigation into the funding behind the technologies inside the original gene sequencing machines. The government believed NIH- and Medicare-funded clinics that had purchased the machines should have been charged less because of federal sponsorship of their development. Top officials at CalTech, which received royalties from sale of the machines, denied that government grants were instrumental in their work. But Smith recalled that the lab would not have been able to complete its work without government help. "The whole environment of the lab was permeated with federal funds," he said.[18]

CalTech's first gene sequencing machine helped provide the impetus to the academic biologists and the scientists inside the federal bureaucracy who were pushing the idea of mapping the three-billion-plus bases of the human genome. Robert Sinsheimer, a biologist and chancellor of the University of California at Santa Cruz, had planted the seed in 1985 while scrambling to come up with a government- or foundation-funded big science project to put his university on the map. He organized a meeting on the West Coast that attracted many of the leading lights of the field, including Watson, Hood, and Gilbert. At the start of the decade, Gilbert, who had already won the Nobel Prize for his work on sequencing, had shocked the academic world when he left Harvard to run Biogen. But he was ill-suited to the world of biotech start-ups, as his run-in with Eugene Goldwasser attested, and he returned to his teaching post two years later.

Gilbert and Watson gave the nascent genome project the media cachet it needed to gain traction in Washington, and Gilbert emerged as a main spokesman. Gilbert claimed that mapping the human genome was the holy grail of human genetics, and "an incomparable tool for the investigation of every aspect of human function." Virtually every major researcher in the field signed on to the quest. Gilbert, in a fit of back-of-the-envelope prescience, also gave the project its estimated cost: about $3 billion, or $1 for every letter of the genetic code. "The Grail myth conjured up an apt image," said Robert Cook-Deegan, the historian of those early years of the project. "Each of the Knights of the Round Table set off in quest of an object whose shape was indeterminate, whose history was obscure, and whose function was controversial—except that it related somehow to restoring health and virility to the Fisher King, and hence to his kingdom."[19]

There were a number of scientists in key government agencies who were ready to listen. Indeed, the roots of the government's involvement in the Human Genome Project can be traced to the original government big science project: the building of the atomic bomb. In the immediate postwar years, the Atomic Energy Commission emerged as a major supporter of genetics research in its efforts to develop ways to counter radiation sickness. It was, for instance, the original supporter of Goldwasser's search for erythropoietin. By the mid-1980s, the agency, now part of DOE, was still involved in the long-term study of Japanese atomic bomb survivors. Other agencies of the federal government were grappling with the public policy implications of inherited genetic mutations caused by exposure to carcinogens like Agent Orange, environmental toxins, and low-level radiation.

Charles DeLisi, a former genetics researcher at the National Cancer Institute, pulled together these various strands of genetic research. Shortly after becoming head of DOE's Office of Health and Environmental Research, DeLisi read a 1986 Office of Technology Assessment report entitled "Technologies for Detecting Heritable Mutations in Human Beings," which included a long section on the new sequencing machines. He immediately saw that the new machines would make a large-scale project dedicated to DNA sequencing feasible. He set the bureaucratic wheels in motion to get it funded.

By mid-1986, DeLisi had a memo on the desks of all the top officials of DOE, outlining the biological equivalent of a ten-year moon shot. The first half-decade would be devoted to three simultaneous projects: mapping all the human chromosomes that contained the genes that would be eventually sequenced; developing better machinery for sequencing them; and developing better computers and computer programs for analyzing the data. Phase II of the project—the actual high-speed sequencing—could then be implemented. DeLisi was well aware of the technical limitations of the existing sequencers developed in Hood's lab. He knew it would take better machines to complete the project in a reasonable time frame and at a reasonable cost. Given the time it would take to develop better machines, his original memo estimated the overall project would take at least a decade or more.

By the end of 1989, Congress had signed off on the Human Genome Project and created a new agency inside NIH run by James Watson. (He would leave in a huff two years later after opposing NIH's endorsement of gene patenting.) Though DOE would eventually be shunted off to the side in the bureaucratic maneuvering, the two agencies published a joint five-year plan in April 1990. It was remarkably similar to DeLisi's original memo. The projected completion date was initially set at 2005. The need to move beyond the existing machines dictated the snail-like pace.

DOE took responsibility for the technology initiative aimed at revolutionizing automated sequencing. "We needed better dyes, better enzymes, better constituents for everything going into sequencing," recalled Marvin Stodolsky, a molecular biologist who moved to DOE from Argonne National Laboratory in 1985 to become part of the nascent program. The agency advertised in scientific publications and attracted thousands of proposals. Over the next decade, DOE granted nearly $1 billion to hundreds of scientists working on improving instrumentation technologies, about one dollar for every two spent by NIH on sequencing.[20]

Smith, who left CalTech for the University of Wisconsin in 1987, remained a central figure as the technology evolved. In 1990, he published papers outlining what would become the core concept behind the next generation of machines. He resuscitated the original idea of using ultra-thin capillaries for transporting the DNA fragments. This concept would eventually allow scientists to run ninety-six samples at a time (up from forty-eight on the slab-gel machines) and cut the cycle time (the amount of time it took the DNA fragments to run down the tubes) to two to three hours from the previous twelve hours. It was a tenfold improvement in the number of bases that a single machine could read in a day. The capillaries would also eliminate a major source of errors in the slab-gel system. In the old machines, the DNA fragments had a tendency to wander outside their lanes as they scampered down the glass plates, thus corrupting the readouts at the end of the line.

Several problems needed solving before the capillary technology could be made practical. "The capillary work we did was not cost effective the way we did it," Smith said. "We used a gel in the capillaries that was difficult to pour and left bubbles in the capillaries. What were you going to do? Throw them away every time? That was too expensive. So a lot of money from DOE and NIH went into creating polymer liquids to pump into the capillaries." Barry Karger, a chemist at Northeastern University, eventually solved the problem. He came up with a liquid that could carry the microscopic genetic material through the tiny capillaries without ruining them.[21]

Reading the fluorescent tags in this miniaturized environment was another major hurdle. That problem was solved by several scientists, including Richard Mathies of the University of California at Berkeley. He developed a new set of fluorescent dyes that when attached to the end of the molecules could be read by a laser that focused its beam on the inside of the capillaries. Norman Dovichi, a Canadian chemist at the University of Alberta, developed an alternative laser optics system that read the fluorescent tags the moment the molecules emerged from the capillaries. Publicly funded scientists weren't the only ones working on the problem. Hitachi, the Japanese electronics giant that also had a biology instrumentation division, developed a laser-reading system that was identical to Dovichi's. Applied Biosystems eventually licensed both.

By early 1996, DOE officials realized they had solved most of the technical puzzles. They asked Joseph Jaklevic at Lawrence Berkeley National Laboratory to use them to build a prototype machine. The national lab complex, which lines a winding roadway in the foothills behind the Berkeley campus, is best known as home for the nation's first cyclotron. But by the mid-1990s, the demise of the Superconducting Supercollider Project had left many of its best scientists looking for alternative projects. Some focused on biology and earth sciences. "One of our funding managers at DOE said, 'You're engineers. Can you take these various ideas and get us moving toward a prototype? We want to get these into the hands of sequencers,'" Jaklevic said.[22]

During a visit to his lab five years after making the first prototype, Jaklevic took me to a building on the far side of the complex. Once inside, I found myself inside a warehouse filled with what looked like old high school science experiments. The room's tabletops and shelves held dozens of machines whose protruding wires, glass tubing, and metal housings gave no hint to their intended function. We eventually halted at a waist-high table no larger than a bedroom end table with a small machine on it. Its interior contained an array of ninety-six copper-colored tubes, their combined width no greater than two fists butted together. A small laser sat above the array on a glide path. I immediately recognized the configuration. I had seen it two months earlier when visiting a nonprofit gene sequencing research institute outside Washington that contained dozens of Applied Biosystems' Prism 3700 machines, the ninety-six-capillary gene sequencing machine that came out two years after Jaklevic built his prototype. "There's a lot of engineering that goes into making a machine that is reliable, that you can put in the box with an instructional manual and ship across the country," he told me during my Berkeley visit. "But once you know someone has done it, it makes it a lot easier."[23]

By the time Jaklevic and his team finished building the prototype, Applied Biosystems—renamed PE Biosystems after being purchased by the Connecticut-based semiconductor equipment manufacturer, Perkins Elmer—wasn't the only company pursuing advanced sequencing technology. Scientists from Mathies's lab, working just down the hill from Jaklevic on the Berkeley campus, had linked up with Molecular Dynamics of Sunnyvale. Its scientists also wanted to leapfrog Hunkapillar's slab-gel machine. "We made a presentation at a local biotech meeting in San Francisco and made contact with Molecular Dynamics," the Berkeley chemist recalled. "I saw one of their corporate people. We made a visit and everything started clicking."[24]

Molecular Dynamics teamed up with a relatively new company called Incyte Pharmaceuticals (later Incyte Genomics) to develop their new machine, which they eventually called the Megabase. Jingyue Ju, who had joined Mathies's lab as a postdoc on a DOE fellowship, developed and patented a number of reagents used in the process. He licensed them to Molecular Dynamics, and by early 1997 they had their first machines up and running. In September, Ju, now an Incyte employee, stunned the gene sequencing world at a meeting held in Hilton Head, South Carolina. The annual meeting brought together the Human Genome Project's leading players and was sponsored by the nonprofit research institute run by Venter, the Institute for Genomic Research, or TIGR. Ju presented the first data from the new Megabase machine. His presentation showed that, compared to the older machines, the new machines were capable of very large runs in very short periods of time with very few errors.[25] "It was a stunning presentation, and it was clear to everybody in the field that gel-based sequencing had no future," said Roy Whitfield, chairman of Incyte. "That was the day that [Applied Biosystems] realized it had to start playing in this new field or its whole franchise would be lost."[26]

Several participants recalled that Hunkapillar made a hurried presentation later in the week. His sketchy briefing suggested to the audience that his firm was clearly behind in the race to develop a ninety-six-lane capillary sequencing machine. Years later, Hunkapillar claimed his firm was already far along in the process. He cited the fact that the company had already come out with a single-capillary machine aimed at nongovernment markets. The focus on a single-capillary machine was understandable. His company had always sold far more slab-gel sequencing machines to diagnostic labs that screened patients for inherited disorders and to criminal labs that processed DNA evidence than it did to government-funded labs involved in the Human Genome Project. Under PE Biosystems' leadership, Applied Biosystems' in-house research staff focused on developing a single-capillary machine because that was what most of its customers wanted. "The impetus wasn't the Human Genome Project but our other customers," Hunkapillar said. "We were selling to clinical diagnostic labs and forensic labs. It was low throughput."[27]

Once kicked into motion by the Molecular Dynamics presentation, though, the company moved quickly. Hunkapillar licensed the technologies needed to build a ninety-six-lane capillary system and within a year had a prototype. As soon as the computers were finished reading out the first sequences that came through the capillaries, he realized that several hundred of the new machines, which were ten times faster than his old models, would be able to sequence the entire human DNA chain in a time frame that would make a shambles out of the government's 2005 schedule. A rough cut could be fashioned in a few weeks, and a final version that had very few gaps in just a few years.

Hunkapillar took his calculations to Tony White, the new chairman of the renamed PE Corporation. They decided to launch their own genomics company to sell the data from the human genome. If nothing else came of it, the new company—dubbed Celera—would at least buy hundreds of the machines. The plan called for making Celera a separately traded company so it could sell its story on Wall Street and raise capital for the machine purchases. All they needed was a good front man for the new venture. In late 1997, Hunkapillar called Venter, whose nonprofit institute had been one of the biggest purchasers of his earlier generation of machines. He asked him if he wanted to run the new venture. Venter at first said no, but a few months later accepted the offer.

The world quickly learned about Celera's plans. Nicholas Wade, a *New York Times* science reporter, had closely followed Venter's career since his early squabbles with the Human Genome Project's managers over gene patenting. He had also covered Venter's decision to leave the government and form TIGR using money supplied by Wallace Steinberg, the inventor of the Reach toothbrush and chairman of the venture fund HealthCare Investment Corporation. Steinberg put up $70 million over ten years (later raised to $85 million) in exchange for the first rights to any inventions that came out of its work.

In early May 1998, Wade scored another Venter-generated scoop when he splashed Celera's plan to sell the data from its own human genome sequence across the front pages of the Sunday paper. In the article, the Hunkapillar-Venter team bragged their version would be completed years ahead of the government project, and would only cost $300 million to complete. "If successful, the venture would outstrip and to some extent make redundant the government's $3-billion program to sequence the human genome by 2005," Wade concluded in the second paragraph of his story.[28]

Venter did not mention that a good portion of the government's billions—deemed a waste in print—had been spent on developing the machinery that made Celera possible. The article provoked howls of outrage from the scientists in the government-funded project. They thought Venter was trying to steal both the data and the scientific credit. A week later Venter added insult to injury when he told the government's gene sequencing establishment, who had gathered at Watson's federal lab in Cold Spring Harbor on Long Island for its annual meeting, that they should shift their efforts to sequencing the mouse genome. "He's Hitler," Watson said to anyone who would listen. "This should not be Munich."[29] It wasn't. The government's six sequencing centers quickly purchased hundreds of Prism 3700 and Megabase machines and the race to a final product was on. Two years later, on June 26, 2000, the president of the United States declared it a tie.

The race wasn't the only by-product of the technology created for the Human Genome Project. It set off a genetic gold rush. Though the patent office cannot provide an exact estimate, it is likely that no more than a few hundred applications for gene patents had been filed by the time the Prism 3700 and Megabase machines hit the market. The number of gene patents actually granted was probably a small fraction of that. Over the next few years, though, private companies and university-based researchers, after sifting through the data pouring off the new machines, filed tens of thousands of gene patent applications. The less commercially oriented scientists working in universities around the world cried foul. John Sulston, who ran England's Sanger Center, spoke for many of them when he called genome sequencing for commercial gain "totally immoral and disgusting. I find it a terrible shame that this important moment in human history is being sullied by this act." Genes should not be patented because they are "intrinsically a part of every human being, a common heritage in which we should all share equally . . . Craig [Venter] has gone morally wrong," he concluded.[30]

That was not the attitude at the U.S. patent office, however. As of mid-2002, more than thirteen hundred patents had been granted. It was as if the manufacturer of the lunar lander had staked a claim on the surface of the moon. The vast majority of gene patent applications were filed by Celera and Incyte, the genomics information companies tied to sequencing machinery makers. And despite the patent office's pledge to reject patent applications lacking a clear medical use, officials admitted a great many were slipping through that were based largely on literature searches on genes' potential utility. "There's plenty of paper patents out there that are not based on hard bench science," said John Doll, chief of the biotechnology section of the PTO.[31]

As the glamour of the race faded, Celera quietly shifted business strategies. A number of companies and universities had signed up to use its proprietary programs for sifting through its genomic information—its original business plan. But the government's GenBank provided much the same data at no cost. The telling blow came in the spring of 2001 when the completed genomes were simultaneously published in *Science* and *Nature*, the world's preeminent science journals. At a joint press conference announcing publication, again in the cavernous ballroom of the Capitol Hilton Hotel, the humbled authors from the Celera and government teams admitted that the finished genome contained just thirty thousand genes, about a third of the anticipated number. More significantly, those genes produced as many as three hundred thousand proteins, and the evidence suggested that different genes may produce different proteins at different stages in life. The one-gene/one-protein paradigm that had ruled biology for decades—and underpinned hopes that mapping the genome would quickly lead to medical progress against the major diseases—was no longer operative. "We now know the notion that one gene leads to one protein, and perhaps one disease, is false," Venter said. "One gene leads to many different protein products that can change dramatically once they are produced. We know that some of the regions that are not genes may be some of the keys to the complexity that we see in ourselves. We now know that the environment acting on our biological steps may be as important in making us what we are as our genetic code."[32]

More cautious scientists had long issued warnings that the number of diseases whose courses might be directly affected by the new tools of biotechnology were few and far between. Biotech's biggest sellers, like Epogen or Cerezyme, were the exceptions, not the rule. When failing kidneys did not produce enough erythropoietin, recombinant technology could make it and introduce it artificially into the bloodstream. But what happens if the dozens of genes involved in the complex interactions of brain chemistry begin malfunctioning? Some might be producing at less than their appropriate rate. Some might be producing at more than their appropriate rate. And that over- or underexpression might be a cause, or it might only be an effect. It will take decades of biological investigation and experimentation to sort out the complex factors behind diseases like Alzheimer's or the more than one hundred forms of cancer, and it is highly unlikely that a drug that affects a single protein will halt their progression. Even when a disease is caused by a single disorder in a single gene, it is usually not treatable by simple addition or subtraction. Lysosomal storage disorders like Fabry disease are the rare exception that can be treated with a recombinantly made enzyme. But as Francis Collins and other scientists who discovered the genetic defect responsible for cystic fibrosis eventually learned, the effects of a single mutation were often complex. It would take decades of basic scientific research to develop therapies based on that piece of knowledge.

As soon as the hope faded that gene mapping would lead to rapid medical progress, the genomics companies moved on to the next frontier—mapping and patenting the three hundred thousand proteins. Myriad Genetics Inc. of Salt Lake City announced a joint venture with Hitachi, a machinery maker, and Oracle Corporation, the software developer, to create the human proteome. Like Celera before them, they planned to market the database to pharmaceutical companies for use in drug development. Celera and several other companies announced similar plans.[33] Many of the companies were filing patent claims on the proteins and their chemical structures, even though their function was poorly known.

Once again there was a conflict between the private expropriators and public-spirited scientists. Rutgers University's Protein Data Bank sought to compile a comprehensive, publicly accessible database of all three-dimensional structures in the human proteome. Those structures were derived using standard laboratory X-ray crystallography or spectroscopy procedures. But many companies, citing their patent claims, refused to put their information in the database unless they could put restrictions on access to that data.[34]

Other companies filed patent claims on single nucleotide polymorphisms (SNPs), the slight variations in genetic code that account for human differences. SNPs not only determine a person's eye, hair, or skin color but may also determine a person's susceptibility to drugs. These so-called pharmacogenomic markers may one day be useful in screening people for drugs that are the most effective for their genotype.

In the SNP case, the opposition to the privatization of basic science information came from large pharmaceutical firms. From their perspective, the small biotechnology companies and universities that filed patents on SNPs were simply laying claims on future revenue without discovering new drugs. To combat this incursion, the big pharmaceutical companies launched their own nonprofit database—the SNP Consortium—and encouraged their members to publicly disclose to prevent others from filing patents on them. "Although it may seem extraordinary for firms that usually sing the praises of the patent system to collaborate in a concerted effort to put new discoveries in the public domain, it makes perfect sense from the perspective of the pharmaceutical industry," wrote Rebecca S. Eisenberg, a law professor at the University of Michigan and an expert on pharmaceutical intellectual property issues. "The patents that matter to pharmaceutical firms are the drug patents that secure the revenues that fill the pharmaceutical feeding trough. Patents on the many prior discoveries that facilitate drug development look like siphons, diverting those revenues to the troughs of other firms."[35]

The bottom line was that basic biomedical research that was once open to all in the public domain has been quietly converted into the intellectual property of private-sector actors who may or may not be doing something useful with the information. Indeed, as the PTO widened the intellectual property possibilities, academic researchers and their institutions, most of which once operated exclusively on government grants but have increasingly turned to small companies for research support, have licensed their "inventions" to small biotechnology firms in hopes of one day collecting a toll from anyone who uses that knowledge while looking for a therapy. "From the perspective of the pharmaceutical industry, biotech firms and universities that hold patents on these research inputs are like so many tax collectors, diluting their anticipated profits on potential new products," Eisenberg said.[36]

The new paradigm was dramatically illustrated in June 2002 when the PTO issued a patent on a crucial signaling protein to a dozen researchers at the Massachusetts Institute of Technology, the Whitehead Institute for Biomedical Research, and Harvard University. More than five thousand academic papers had been written over the years about the protein NF-KB, which sits on the surface of cells and triggers a response to specific external stimuli. Yet the academic institutions that first identified it immediately licensed their patent to Cambridge-based Ariad Pharmaceuticals, which turned around and sued Eli Lilly for infringement. Two of the giant pharmaceutical's company biggest selling drugs—raloxifene (Evista) for osteoporosis and drotrecogin alfa (Xigris) for septic shock—made use of the signaling protein in carrying out their actions, Ariad's suit said. Patent attorneys who reviewed the patent expressed surprise at the overly broad claims allowed by the PTO. "Just about anything that blocks the activity of NF-KB would appear to come under this claim," Michael Farber, a Harvard-trained scientist and patent lawyer, said. "All you have to do is block the activity of this factor at the transcriptional level, the translational level, the protein level, or any combination of mechanisms, and this patent is implicated."[37]

Celera parted ways with Craig Venter less than a year after it switched business strategies. The company was sitting on nearly a billion dollars in stock market–raised cash, and its genetic information business had clearly peaked. "In the long run the genome sequence just wanted to be public," Francis Collins, director of the public project, said. "It would not for long be sustainable inside any kind of boundaries." The new strategy involved using the intellectual property the company had amassed from its gene patents to pursue drugs, or, perhaps, to collect tolls from those who might be infringing on its "inventions." But to get into drug development, the company needed leadership that knew something about it. "A realistic assessment of Craig's background is that neither he nor I have ever developed a drug," said Tony White, the chairman of Celera's parent company. He made the announcement while Venter was off sailing his yacht in the Caribbean.[38]

Will Celera be able to turn its cash horde into a successful therapy? A quick perusal of its patent portfolio suggested that the firm, like other gene patent holders, was still years away from knowing what to do with its basic scientific discoveries. For instance, on June 25, 2002, the PTO awarded Celera's parent company U.S. Patent no. 6,410,294 for "isolated human kinase proteins, nucleic acid molecules encoding human kinase proteins, and uses thereof." The company had filed for the patent in December 2000, just six months after completion of the Human Genome Project.

About 2 percent of the human genome expresses kinases, which are proteins on the surface of cells that send and receive signals from other proteins. More than 670 have been identified by molecular biologists. A few months before completing his map of the genome, Venter had assured critics of gene patenting that his company would never pursue an unspecific patent with the word "like" in it. But according to the description in Patent No. 6,410,294, Celera's newly patented class of kinase proteins "are related to the SNF-like kinase subfamily." Experimental data in the patent, entirely drawn from the academic literature, indicated the newly patented kinases are expressed "in lung, liver, kidney, thyroid, brain, infant brain, fetal brain, placenta, bone marrow, germ cell tissue, germ cell tumor tissue, and primary cancers." These kinases, the patent concluded, could "serve as targets for the development of human therapeutic agents."[39]

A month after its issuance, I took a copy of the patent to Susan Taylor, a professor of biochemistry at the University of California at San Diego. She is one of the nation's foremost experts in human kinases. In 1991, she codiscovered the kinase protein that became the target for Novartis's Gleevec, which was approved by the FDA in 2001 to combat chronic myeloid leukemia amid much media hoopla (see chapter 7).[40] A member of the National Academy of Sciences and a past president of the American Society of Biochemistry, she has testified before Congress for increased funding for NIH, which is the primary source of funds for her lab. Her lab is located in a modern building across the street from Torrey Pines State Park, which overlooks the Pacific Ocean. But its enviable location isn't apparent from the inside of her windowless, basement office, where the concrete walls are lined with the pictures of her children, now in their late twenties, and the scientific posters for the lectures announcing her most significant discoveries. She wore blue jeans and a turtle neck, with her closely cropped graying hair accented by a set of dangling silver earrings.

After looking over the patent, she said, "All this says is these kinases are likely to be targets for diseases." "What diseases?" I asked. "I don't know," she replied. "There's nothing specific in this other than this is a gene family that's likely to be important."[41]

She explained how researchers used genetic information to generate the knowledge needed to speed the search for new drugs. Scientists can breed mice that lack a specific gene in order to study the impact of that absence. Or they can quickly create recombinant versions of the molecule and feed it to experimental animals to see what an excess will cause. Researchers who had identified the first kinases in the early 1990s had initially thought that the convoluted folds of the long-chain proteins would make finding drugs to inhibit them almost impossible. But, in fact, it turned out that the folds provided numerous sites where a drug might block a kinase's function, and thus there might be many potential inhibitors (presuming, of course, that scientists discover that blocking a particular kinase's function is a desirable thing during the course of a disease). "People in the field are against patenting genes like this," she continued. "This is basic research. And if they're saying anyone who works on these kinases and figures out what to do with it gives them some rights to that, [then] I don't agree. . . . Genes are supposed to be public information."

PART TWO

DIRECTED RESEARCH

4

A Public-Private Partnership

The discovery of a drug combination capable of controlling the human immunodeficiency virus (HIV) was one of the great triumphs of biomedical research in the postwar era. Over the last quarter of the twentieth century, no disease spread greater havoc across the globe than HIV-caused AIDS (Acquired Immune Deficiency Syndrome). At century's end, more than forty million people were infected, with AIDS threatening to devastate large swaths of the developing world, especially in sub-Saharan Africa. It is a mark of progress that public health officials and activists—who fought to bring the drugs to control AIDS into existence—have turned their attention to making drugs affordable in those parts of the world that have been hardest hit by the epidemic.

Developing AIDS drugs was not an easy or inexpensive task. Every step of the process was dogged by controversy, and success often seemed an unreachable goal. But in the end, the successful campaign represented the triumph of a simple idea, one that in recent years has been overshadowed by the public's infatuation with private sector ingenuity. Significant medical advances are almost always the product of collaborations between the public and private sectors, and in areas of the greatest public health concern, the government invariably plays the leading role.

Yet well into the 1990s, the public sector's effort to develop treatments for AIDS seemed doomed to failure. To much of the public, not to mention an aroused and desperate patient population, the government's effort seemed hopelessly misguided. Many Americans wrongly believed the disease was somehow caused by the hedonistic lifestyle of its victims and would remain resistant to the best efforts of medical science. Like tuberculosis in the nineteenth century or cancer for much of the twentieth century, AIDS was perceived by many as divine retribution. The metaphor insinuated itself into the scientific debate. To this day, the National Institutes of Health (NIH) feels compelled to refute that myth on its Web site by carefully documenting that AIDS is caused by a viral infection and is spread by the usual suspects for blood-borne pathogens: unprotected sex, tainted blood supplies, infected needles, and, tragically, during childbirth or breastfeeding if the mother carries the virus.

The AIDS metaphor could flourish for a simple reason: The virus, discovered in 1983 and thoroughly described and categorized by 1987, proved remarkably resistant to the best efforts of modern medicine to control or eliminate it once inside its human host. But thanks to the willingness of government and industry to pour billions of dollars into researching cures and vaccines, there are now drugs available that are somewhat effective in controlling the disease. They are cumbersome to take, have debilitating side effects, and are extraordinarily expensive, at least in the advanced industrial world, where they were initially researched, patented, and produced. Research today is focused on developing vaccines to prevent the spread of the disease and on producing new medications that are less toxic, easier to take, and more effective at preventing the wily virus's ability to mutate, survive, and spread.

The story behind the discovery of the first generation of drugs for controlling HIV involved thousands of scientists on three continents and housed in hundreds of public and private institutions. Those drugs' relatively rapid emergence came about in no small part because of the public health movement that arose among AIDS carriers and their advocates demanding that something be done about the epidemic. The following chapters are not an attempt to tell that entire story, but only one part of it: the emergence of a class of drugs called protease inhibitors, which, when used in combination with previously discovered drugs, showed that effective therapy was possible. The first protease inhibitor was approved by the Food and Drug Administration (FDA) in December 1995, with two more in March of the following year. These powerful new drug combinations proved capable of controlling the virus in most patients who became infected. Though drug resistance was and continues to be a major problem, the U.S. death toll was cut by two-thirds within two years of their introduction.

This tremendous victory could not have been achieved without the private sector, but over the course of more than fifteen years of research and development, governments in the United States, Europe, and Japan spent three times more money than private firms on the basic science, drug development, and clinical trials that led to the drugs that tamed the disease. It comes as no surprise then that the public sector's fingerprints are all over the final products of that research. What is surprising is how private pharmaceutical firms sought to wipe them away.

It is bracing to recall how grim the prospects for such a breakthrough appeared before the emergence of protease inhibitors. Indeed, if the AIDS epidemic had a darkest hour, the summer of 1993 was surely it. The Centers for Disease Control had just announced that more than a half million Americans were infected with the virus. The death toll in the United States alone that year reached a staggering 37,267, a majority of them young homosexual men. The obituary pages of the nation's leading newspapers read like a dirge for the worlds of high fashion, literature, and the arts, where many gay men had made their careers.

And to the consternation of many Americans, AIDS was no longer a disease limited to homosexuals. Los Angeles Lakers star Magic Johnson's forced retirement from basketball in 1991 had brought home to the heterosexual population that it, too, was at risk, just as the death of Ryan White, the eleven-year-old Indiana hemophiliac who had died in 1990 after receiving a tainted blood transfusion, made AIDS as all-American as apple pie. A disease that had announced its presence in 1981 when a Los Angeles physician noticed an outbreak of a rare skin cancer among five of his homosexual patients had become by 1993 a society-wide pandemic with no effective treatment or cure.

More than fourteen thousand scientists, activists, and media people gathered in Berlin that summer for the ninth International AIDS Conference. Hoping for good news from the frontlines of medical research, they came away bitterly disappointed. The low point among the eight hundred lectures and forty-five hundred poster presentations occurred when European physicians issued the final statistics from the so-called Concorde trial, which had compared the life expectancy of untreated AIDS patients to those on Burroughs Wellcome's drug zidovudine (AZT). AZT had been approved by the FDA in 1987, and for many years was the only drug for HIV. But according to Concorde's Anglo-

French authors, people who took AZT when their immune systems began to deteriorate fared no better in the long run than people who took no drug at all.

Researchers from NIH immediately went into damage control mode. Daniel Hoth, the director of the AIDS Clinical Trials Group (ACTG), a nationwide network of government-funded academic researchers, issued a press release claiming the Concorde study results were merely preliminary and did not contradict earlier ACTG studies. AZT, a drug that government scientists had discovered, screened, and cajoled Burroughs Wellcome into taking through the FDA approval process, at least delayed the onset of serious disease, Hoth insisted. "At this time, we see no basis for changing the current recommendation to initiate antiretroviral therapy for HIV-infected persons."[1] Moreover, there was good news from some patients in new trials combining AZT with other drugs that government-funded scientists had discovered and licensed to private drug firms. The two-drug combination therapy had slightly increased the number of disease-fighting white blood cells in some of the patients in those trials.

The hundreds of AIDS activists in attendance—many of whom privately referred to AZT as rat poison because of its side effects—weren't impressed. AIDS activists had radically transformed the traditionally paternalistic relationship between doctors and patients. Angry, aware, and articulate, people with AIDS had forced two successive conservative administrations to take the plague seriously. Their noisy protests and sit-ins at NIH, the FDA, and in the corporate suites of major drug manufacturers were largely responsible for the fact that by 1993 taxpayers were spending more than a billion dollars a year on AIDS research, dwarfing the efforts of private industry. The activists had even forced their way into scientific meetings and onto government panels, intruding on a medical world that preferred to operate in secrecy.

In Berlin, when the results of the latest studies became known, many of the AIDS activists had the sophistication to read between the lines of the government-funded studies. "Our deepest impression from the conference is that the most important and productive approach possible to saving the lives of those already infected was simply not on the table there—not among the scientists, not among the physicians, and not among the activists," wrote John James in *AIDS Treatment News*, the widely read newsletter in the AIDS activist community. "The greatest need, everyone did seem to agree, is for better drugs. . . . Existing drugs are largely useless."[2]

For those paying close attention at the Berlin conference, though, the news wasn't entirely grim. At the last minute, conference organizers allowed a number of drug companies to make presentations on early-stage protease inhibitors, which they hoped would become the next generation of AIDS medications. The first AIDS drugs—three had already been approved by the FDA—were called nucleosides because they directly interfered with an enzyme called reverse transcriptase that HIV needs to copy itself during reproduction. HIV comes from a class of viruses known as retroviruses, whose genetic material is made up of ribonucleic acid, or messenger RNA, and who reproduce in backward fashion. After invading a host white blood cell, the virus produces a mirror-image strand of deoxyribonucleic acid, or DNA. That strand in turn takes over the host cell's DNA and spawns a new RNA-based retrovirus. The evil genius of HIV is that it infects the white blood cells needed to fight off invaders. It is the arsonist that targets firehouses, to paraphrase one memorable metaphor.[3] The clinical trial results shown in Berlin proved what many AIDS patients already knew: The effects of nucleoside reverse transcriptase inhibitors were short-lived at best. The virus was mutating around them.

But scientists had long known that the HIV genome had other potential targets. Researchers by the mid-1980s knew that the retrovirus produced an enzyme called a protease, which cut the new genetic material of a reproducing retrovirus into little pieces before reassembling them into a new offspring. If scientists could find a chemical to block the action of the protease scissors, the infected cell would be unable to reproduce and would soon die. Since the late 1980s private drug firms and government-funded researchers had been searching for a protease inhibitor, which they hoped would be the "magic bullet" to kill HIV. By the summer of 1993, their efforts were beginning to bear fruit. A number of firms pushed to get their initial attempts onto the Berlin agenda.

Keith Bragman, Hoffmann–La Roche's top European clinical virologist, coordinated one of the presentations at the sparsely attended meetings on protease inhibitors. Bragman, a thin, retiring Englishman in his early forties, whose soft voice masked a fierce determination to leave a mark on AIDS research, had recruited doctors from three of Europe's top academic research institutes to test Roche's new protease inhibitor, known then only as Ro31-8959. It would eventually be called saquinavir. To anyone who understood the dynamics of pharmaceutical research, the Roche compound presented huge problems. The immense molecule was hard to absorb through the gut, or, to use the industrial term of art, it lacked bioavailability. Test subjects had to take a fistful of capsules before it began showing up in their bloodstreams. Although it was potent in the test tube—at the concentrations at which they had succeeded in getting it into the blood—it had only a minor ability to kill HIV and raise white blood cell counts. But at least it showed activity, the clinicians reported to the meeting. It was concrete evidence that a protease inhibitor actually worked in humans. All Bragman needed now was a better version of the drug.

Illinois-based Abbott Laboratories also pressed to get on the Berlin agenda, which was something of a surprise. The buttoned-down midwestern firm usually maintained a high level of secrecy about its operations, not unusual in the hush-hush world of industrial drug development. But John Leonard, who had been brought in from a small drug testing firm to run Abbott's AIDS program a year earlier, also felt pressure to show that his protease inhibitor could work. Abbott, though a large health care firm, was a bit player in pharmaceutical research, especially when compared to industry giants like Pfizer, Merck, or Hoffmann–La Roche. It had even sought federal government help to fund its initial protease inhibitor research. But that grant had recently run out, and Leonard was under strict orders from chief executive officer Duane Burnham to avoid all further contact with government-funded clinicians. He went to Europe instead, where scientists doing initial safety tests on drugs didn't have to divulge their experiments to the government. Leonard asked Sven Danner at the University of Amsterdam to test the company's initial protease inhibitor.

Danner's findings, unveiled at Berlin, attracted almost no attention and for good reason. Abbott's protease inhibitor candidate was so unwieldy it had to be given intravenously, and even then the liver cleared it from the body almost as fast as the doctors could pump it in. It also caused blood clots. "I felt so sorry for the guy having to present that embarrassing story," Leonard recalled.[4] But like Roche's drug, it seemed to inhibit viral replication in a handful of patients. It was the "proof of concept" that the Abbott scientists needed to convince top management to continue supporting their bare-bones AIDS drug discovery effort.

Several other companies made presentations about their preclinical protease research. Vertex Pharmaceuticals, a biotech start-up from Cambridge, Massachusetts, announced it had just come up with a protease inhibitor candidate. Though the young firm had attracted some of Merck's top AIDS research scientists in the late 1980s, the company had initially ignored AIDS research in order to hunt for drugs that would impede transplant rejections. But with chief executive Joshua Boger desperate to show progress to his Wall Street backers, the firm had suddenly shifted back into AIDS research and fairly quickly came up with a drug they thought would inhibit viral replication.[5] And since their drug candidate was small, it should, theoretically at least, have good bioavailability. Merck's joint venture with DuPont Pharmaceuticals also unveiled a potential drug. But neither Vertex's nor Merck-DuPont's drugs had entered human trials.

Pessimistic press accounts from the conference completely overshadowed the scanty news about protease inhibitors. Robert Yarchoan, one of the National Cancer Institute doctors who had played a key role in bringing the first AIDS drugs to market, was one of the few scientists who came away from Berlin in an upbeat mood. "People are too down about things," he recalled thinking at the time. "For the first time, a new class of drugs was shown to have activity."[6]

Three years later, those initial rays of hope would blossom into a significant medical breakthrough. In December 1995, Roche's saquinavir would become the first protease inhibitor approved by FDA; an Abbott drug derived from the one shown at Berlin would be second a few months later, with Merck's entry a close third. Vertex, the nimble biotech whose entrepreneurial zest was supposed to run circles around the traditional drug firms, wouldn't get its drug to market until April 1999, three years behind the old-line pharmaceutical firms.

The studies submitted to the FDA showed that protease inhibitors were not the magic bullets that cured AIDS. But when used in combination with at least two other antiretroviral drugs, HIV could be suppressed to near undetectable levels in most patients, and therefore prolong life. The annual U.S. death toll, which had soared to more than forty thousand in the mid-1990s, fell below fourteen thousand within two years.

In the years since protease inhibitors came on the market, huge problems have arisen with drug combinations to control HIV. Resistance arises in anywhere from a third to half of patients, usually among those who do not closely adhere to the complicated pill-popping regimens or had previous exposure to the individual drugs used in combination therapy. The protease inhibitors also turned out to have a host of unwanted side effects. They induced nausea, diarrhea, and fatigue. Prolonged usage also caused lipodystrophy, an unsightly condition where fat cells from the face, arms, and legs redistribute themselves to the abdomen and the back of the neck, leaving many on combination therapy looking like concentration camp survivors.

But throughout 1996, as word of the miraculous breakthrough spread through the subcultures that had been hardest hit by the AIDS epidemic, the idea that their world had been given a biomedical reprieve acted like an intoxicant. *Newsweek* proclaimed, "The End of AIDS." *Time* hailed David Ho, head of the Aaron Diamond AIDS Research Center in New York and a lead investigator for Abbott's protease inhibitor, as "Man of the Year." The *New York Times Magazine* carried an eight-thousand-word article entitled "When Plagues End" by former *New Republic* editor Andrew Sullivan, himself HIV-positive. "The power of the newest drugs, called protease inhibitors, and the even greater power of those now in the pipeline, is such that a diagnosis of HIV infection is not just different in degree today than, say, five years ago. It is different in kind. It no longer signifies death. It merely signifies illness." Larry Kramer, the radical playwright and founder of ACT UP (AIDS Coalition to Unleash Power), the most militant of the AIDS activist groups, signaled the next phase of the anti-AIDS struggle when he penned a long article complaining about the high price of drugs and their lack of affordability in the developing world, where most AIDS sufferers lived.[7]

In these and subsequent accounts, the emergence of protease inhibitors and cocktail therapy was portrayed as a triumph of private enterprise. Whether the writers lamented or endorsed the high price of the drugs, their accounts provided tacit endorsement of the drug industry's insistent claim that the high prices of AIDS medications were necessary to fund the extraordinarily expensive research and development behind them. "As the new protease inhibitors remind us, however, large corporations are in many cases the only organizations with the resources capable of providing us with the innovations we need," Louis Galambos, a drug industry historian at Johns Hopkins University, wrote in an op-ed article for the *Washington Post*. "In the case of AIDS, companies like Merck, Hoffmann–La Roche and Abbott started their programs when much of the basic research on the virus and the disease still remained to be done. Only companies with significant scientific resources could afford to mount sustained research-and-development campaigns under these conditions."[8] It was a tidy story. But it was misleading about the science and flat-out wrong about the economics.

John Erickson wasn't a typical employee at Abbott's research labs in a far northern suburb of Chicago. In the mid-1980s, Erickson wore long hair, a shaggy beard, and sandals. Raised by a physician and a social worker in Buffalo, he was more liberal and more academically inclined than most of his industry peers. Hungry for "medical relevance," he had started his academic career studying human viruses but switched to the biochemistry of plant pests while finishing his doctoral work at the University of Western Ontario. At the urging of his adviser, he accepted a postdoctoral fellowship with Purdue University's Michael Rossmann, who in the early 1980s was pioneering the use of X-ray crystallography to view biochemical interactions at the molecular level. There, the young scientist found his professional calling. The Rossmann-Erickson team would eventually come in second in the race to publish an accurate portrait of the virus that causes the common cold—then considered the moon shot of the tiny X-ray crystallographic world.

With his fellowship nearing its end, he accepted a teaching post at the University of Wisconsin at Milwaukee. But in late 1985, shortly after starting his teaching assignment, Erickson heard from a former Purdue colleague that Abbott wanted to put the new technique to work in its drug discovery division. X-ray crystallography, which was developed in academic labs with federal research dollars, was quickly becoming one of the key technologies behind the newly emerging field of structure-based drug design, sometimes called (to the consternation of traditional medicinal chemists) rational drug design.

For nearly a century, medicinal chemists working in public health labs or pharmaceutical firms pursued new drugs using methods that were not much different from those pioneered by German scientist Paul Ehrlich, the father of modern drug therapy. Ehrlich had cut his teeth in the 1890s in the laboratories of Robert Koch, who was himself following in the footsteps of Louis Pasteur, the discoverer of the microbes responsible for infectious diseases such as cholera, diphtheria, and tuberculosis. Ehrlich eventually shared the 1908 Nobel Prize for discovering how the immune system develops antibodies—"magic bullets"—to combat invading organisms. By that time he was running his own lab in Frankfurt and began experimenting with the dyes used to stain cell specimens that might be used as artificial magic bullets. Ehrlich surmised that since different colored dyes bound to particular cells, there must be unique receptors on cells. If he could find chemicals that bound to the receptors that played a role in a disease and at the same time blocked their action, physicians could use those chemicals as therapeutic agents. He spent the rest of his career searching for chemicals that would attack cellular interaction at the molecular level. Ehrlich would eventually become a household name and one of the early superstars of drug discovery when he and a Japanese assistant developed the first medicine for combating syphilis, a derivative of arsenic called arsphenamine.

Ehrlich's pioneering research revolutionized the tiny, turn-of-the-century drug industry, forcing it to move away from the quackery of patent medicine into the modern world of scientific drug discovery. The move proved far from a magic bullet for the firms. Medicinal chemists who followed in Ehrlich's footsteps would invariably screen hundreds of chemicals in their search for agents active against a disease, and their search more often that not proved fruitless. Even when they found a compound that showed some activity in a test tube, they often had to synthesize version after version (called analogues) to come up with one worthy of testing in animals, and if that proved nontoxic, in humans.

The commercialization of advanced X-ray crystallography techniques in the early 1980s promised to overthrow the screening regime by hastening the search for new drugs. Crystallographers sent high-powered X-rays through the tiny protein molecules in cells, whose atoms would bend the beams before they hit the film. The crystallographers then used computers to create a three-dimensional image of the molecules. When viewed through special 3-D glasses, the long, convoluted chains that made up the proteins looked like Lego contraptions. The hope was that by peering intently at the revealed structure, biochemists could design drugs that fit precisely into the proteins' chemical folds and block its action.

Always on the lookout for ways to make their research and development departments more efficient, most major companies jumped on the X-ray crystallography bandwagon. In late 1985, Erickson joined a small department at Abbott formed to experiment with the technology. But what would their first target be? Besides X-ray crystallographic expertise, Erickson brought his background in viruses to the firm. AIDS was the hottest topic in virology and a social problem of growing proportions. Abbott was already involved, having licensed an AIDS diagnostic kit from NIH. But Abbott had tried its hand at researching drugs for other viral diseases without success. So despite the millions it was making off the AIDS diagnostic kit, Abbott wasn't spending a dime to combat the disease. Erickson was appalled. "There was no virology," he recalled in 2001. "It was all bacteria and fungi. I thought to myself, As a drug company, shouldn't we have antivirals?"[9]

He began researching the literature. Scientific papers about the AIDS virus were already pouring out of dozens of government and academic labs and a handful of industry labs. The virus had been codiscovered in 1983 by Robert Gallo of the National Cancer Institute and Luc Montagnier of the Pasteur Institute in Paris, although their joint claim to the discovery remains a subject of heated controversy to this day. In

1987, President Ronald Reagan and Prime Minister Jacques Chirac of France signed an agreement that gave equal credit to the two scientists; they split the royalties from the AIDS diagnostic kits based on that discovery between the two governments. But that hardly put the matter to rest. A *Chicago Tribune* special section written by Pulitzer Prize–winning investigative reporter John Crewdson in November 1989 concluded that Gallo either stole the virus or had allowed his laboratory samples to become contaminated with the French isolate. His fifty-thousand-word article—later expanded into a book—launched a round of congressional investigations that proved inconclusive.

But from the point of view of scientific inquiry into the causes and potential cures for AIDS, the controversy was irrelevant. The virus's discovery led to the sequencing of its genes, which in turn enabled scientists to begin tearing apart its inner workings. They quickly discovered it was made up of at least nine genes, six of which contained information necessary for the HIV to reproduce itself. Their work was hastened by the knowledge that HIV was a retrovirus, a class of viruses that had been thoroughly studied during the 1970s by Gallo's Tumor Cell Biology lab at NCI during its largely fruitless hunt for viruses that caused cancer. (Some rare forms of leukemia were the exception.)

Retroviruses require several enzymes to reproduce themselves, all of which would eventually become drug targets. There was, of course, reverse transcriptase, the key building block for HIV. The fact that all retroviruses needed reverse transcriptase for reproduction had been discovered by Howard Temin of the University of Wisconsin and David Baltimore of the Massachusetts Institute of Technology in 1970. These NIH-funded scientists would win the Nobel Prize for their work five years later. The virus also produced an integrase enzyme, which it used to insert itself into the host white blood cell. There were genes that made the proteins for its viral offspring and genes that controlled the rate of reproduction. There were receptors that allowed the virus to insert itself into the target cell. And it produced a protease enzyme, which the virus needed in order to dice and splice its genetic material as it reproduced. It has often been called chemical scissors.

From the start, the HIV protease was a tempting target, especially for industry scientists. Drug industry researchers had spent much of the 1970s and 1980s investigating potential inhibitors of a scissorslike protease enzyme called renin, which helps regulate blood pressure. They had even synthesized many renin inhibitors. But those were more costly to make and harder to get into the blood stream than dozens of other blood pressure drugs already on the market, so it made no sense to take them into clinical trials. However, that failed program left behind a corps of industry scientists with protease knowledge and experience that could be tapped when the search for an HIV protease inhibitor came along.

A few of those industry scientists even contributed to the basic scientific understanding of HIV's protease. But most of the basic research and key breakthroughs came from academic labs. In September 1987 Laurence Pearl and William Taylor of Cambridge University published an article in *Nature,* the leading British science magazine, which laid bare the inner workings of the HIV protease scissors.[10] They proved that its chemistry was very similar to renin. But the two British scientists took the research one step further. They used computer simulations to predict that the HIV protease had two matching halves, like a clam shell. The implication to anyone reading the paper was clear. If a chemical could be found that would stick inside the clamshell and jam up the mechanism, the virus would be unable to reproduce itself.

At Abbott, Erickson had already gravitated to the HIV protease as his target. He independently figured out its chemistry by consulting with Steve Oroszlan, a Hungarian-born senior scientist in Gallo's NCI lab. Oroszlan had discovered the chemistry and structure of the protease in a leukemia retrovirus. By the time the Pearl-Taylor paper came out and confirmed his suspicions about the HIV protease, Erickson was already constructing crystallographic models on his computer. The next step was to get a chemist who could synthesize chemicals—potential drug candidates—that might stick to the innards of the protease and gum up the works. Company officials asked biochemist Dale Kempf, a Nebraska farm boy who had done his postdoctoral work at Columbia University after earning a doctorate at the University of Illinois, to help out on Erickson's project. At thirty-one, Kempf had already logged three years in Abbott's renin program. Perhaps he could try some of his renin inhibitors against the HIV protease. "I can design better ones," Kempf recalled telling his superiors.

But he couldn't do it by himself. Kempf needed meticulous bench scientists who wouldn't bungle the multiple steps needed to synthesize the complicated compounds. Erickson needed help, too, to tweak his computer simulations. In academia, when a professor needs help in his experiments, he recruits postdoctoral researchers. But in industry, one hires help. And at tight-fisted Abbott, help was not immediately forthcoming.

Through his contacts at NCI, Erickson learned about a new government program to develop drugs to combat AIDS. The National Institute for Allergies and Infectious Diseases (NIAID), which under Anthony Fauci had become the lead agency in the fight against AIDS, had just launched the National Cooperative Drug Development Grant (NCDDG) program. Over five years in the late 1980s and early 1990s, the NCDDG would spend about $100 million at both nonprofit and private-sector labs to develop drugs to fight HIV. The model for the program was NCI, which had spent years forging ties with both nonprofit and industry scientists to come up with anticancer chemotherapy agents. The government's managers had a clear picture in their own minds about how to foster innovation. "You fund competing groups and don't worry about overlap," recalled John McGowan, who was directing outside grant-making for NIAID at the time. "You try to get competition among them to get things moving faster to the market."[11]

Overcoming some initial skepticism inside the firm ("They don't give grants to industry," one executive scoffed), Erickson applied for a million-dollar-a-year grant to fund Abbott's protease inhibitor program over the next five years. It came through. Abbott wasn't the only company ready to jump onto the government payroll. Hoffmann–La Roche received a grant to pursue inhibitors of one of HIV's regulatory proteins. William Haseltine, a star researcher at Boston's Dana-Farber Cancer Institute who would go on to form Human Genome Sciences, hooked up with SmithKline and Beecham Research Laboratories to pursue a range of anti-HIV drug targets. Former NCI scientists at the University of Miami got a grant to begin testing Upjohn's repository of chemicals against AIDS. A number of independent academic investigators like Garland Marshall at Washington University in St. Louis received grants to develop protease inhibitor drug candidates, some of which were eventually licensed to private firms like G. D. Searle. By 1990, nearly a dozen firms had drug development programs aimed at HIV, with about half getting some form of direct government support.

When I met Kempf at Abbott's sprawling research campus north of Chicago more than a decade later, he had risen to become head of Abbott's antiviral research efforts and was considered one of the nation's best medicinal chemists in the anti-AIDS fight. I asked him to recall the significance of that original grant. He pushed back his wire-rim glasses, which make him look every inch of his Swiss-German heritage. "It was through that NIH funding that head count opened up and I was able to hire a postdoc and associate chemist. The three of us started working full-time on HIV chemistry," he said. "Before that, I was making HIV inhibitors on the side."[12]

Parroting ideas drawn from Vannevar Bush's 1946 study, *Science, The Endless Frontier*, business leaders and government officials tell a tidy story about government's role in technological innovation. It is government's job to fund basic research, the pure science conducted by inquisitive investigators at the nation's universities that advances the nation's storehouse of knowledge. Applied research—taking that science and fashioning it into products and processes for the marketplace—is industry's job.

During the war, Bush ran the Office of Scientific Research and Development (OSRD). The executive-branch agency's wartime mission had succeeded in tearing down the walls that separated pure science, conducted mainly in universities, and applied science, conducted mainly within private industry. It oversaw the development of a cornucopia of what science historian Daniel J. Kevles has called "military miracles": microwave radar, proximity fuses, solid-fuel rockets, and, in the most spectacular government-funded science project of all time, the Manhattan Project, which built the world's first atomic bomb.[13]

Less well known were the achievements of the OSRD's Committee on Medical Research, which spent a mere $25 million during the war. Its federally financed breakthroughs included the mass production of penicillin and the development of blood plasma, steroids, and cortisone. The penicillin breakthrough has often been claimed by the private firms that supplied the "miracle drug" to the troops abroad, but their efforts would have been impossible without the fermentation techniques developed at a federal lab in Peoria, Illinois.[14] Similarly, the federal government spent a half million dollars to turn blood plasma, which had been developed by the Rockefeller Foundation in 1938, into an industrial commodity so that it could be purchased from government contractors.[15]

With the end of the war in sight, Franklin Delano Roosevelt asked Bush, a Massachusetts minister's son whose prewar career was spent on the electrical engineering faculty at MIT, to draw up a blueprint for government support of science in the postwar world. Roosevelt wanted to continue the "unique experiment of team work and cooperation" that had been developed between academia and industry during the war. His seminal report was delivered to President Harry S. Truman on July 19, 1945.

Bush turned his back on the wartime experience and came down squarely on the side of those who saw a limited role for government in controlling the direction of scientific research. The report drew immediate opposition, spearheaded by Senator Harley Kilgore, a crusty West Virginia Democrat who happily admitted his ignorance of the technical side of science and technology. During the war, Kilgore complained that the government was being too generous in its reimbursements to university and industry for war-related research and development. He also worried about the government giving industry the patents to federally funded inventions, which he feared would be used to monopolize the exciting new markets for technological products that were sure to open up after the war. The New Dealer was also concerned with the future direction of government-funded science. He was the first to propose a National Science Foundation, but his 1944 vision put the government—not scientists—in charge of the agency. He wanted it involved in both basic and applied research and in the training of scientific personnel. He also wanted it to promote social goals, including small business promotion, pollution control, and rural electrification. Kilgore also wanted to give financial support to the soft social sciences such as sociology, economics, and political science.[16]

Bush, who before the war had helped turn MIT into the preeminent basic science research institution in the country, rejected such thinking out of hand. Government should use its money to support basic research alone, he wrote. Wartime breakthroughs had drawn down the capital stock of basic scientific understanding, which had to be rebuilt by funding pure science in the nation's universities. Bush scoffed at social science as thinly disguised political propaganda. He supported the idea of a National Science Foundation, but he wanted the agency to give out peer-reviewed grants that would promote intellectual innovation in hard sciences like chemistry, physics, mathematics, geology, and biology. Applied research, the report said, should be left to private industry, which was perfectly capable of sifting through the intellectual breakthroughs generated at publicly supported universities and federal labs to pick out the nuggets that would lead to technological and commercial innovation. Years later, science policy historian Donald E. Stokes, who spent his career managing major research centers at the University of Michigan and Princeton University, decried this separation of research from its uses. But he understood the economic and professional motivations of the men who designed the system. "The task Bush and his advisers set for themselves was to find a way to continue federal support of basic science while drastically curtailing the government's control of the performance of research," he wrote. "It [the scientific community] wanted, in other words, to restore the autonomy of science."[17]

Legislatively, Bush won. But while the creation of NIH in 1948 (before that there had been just the Public Health Service's National Institute of Health and the National Cancer Institute) and the National Science Foundation in 1950 were premised on Bush's vision, the rapidly escalating cold war got in the way of its faithful execution. Military spending dominated the government's research-and-development budgets during the 1950s. The vast majority of resources went to applied research and prototype development of military hardware. Basic research received substantial funding from the Pentagon, too, but often along lines that had military application. Throughout the 1950s, the Defense Department and the Atomic Energy Commission were by far the largest bankers of pure and applied scientific research in the United States, and by 1956 more than half of industrial research was military related. Many of the technologies had duel uses and thus spun off huge civilian industries— computers, nuclear power, jet airplanes, for instance—but the initial thrust of the research, whether in pure or applied science, was to achieve some prespecified military mission.[18]

NIH rode the rising tide of federal science budgets. Immediately after the war, the tiny agency—it had just eleven hundred employees on its Bethesda campus in suburban Washington—successfully avoided takeover by the soon-to-be-created National Science Foundation. It then won control of the military's medical research grant program. Congress, recognizing there was broad public support for medical research invariably billed as a war on disease, added institute after institute to the NIH roster. Budgets rose twenty-five-fold in the first decade after the war and tenfold again by 1967 when they topped the $1 billion mark for the first time. Most of the money, especially under James Shannon, who took over the agency in 1955, was distributed through the so-called extramural grant program, which came to represent four-fifths of the NIH budget. These grants to university and nonprofit researchers were based on peer review of proposals, just as Bush had envisioned it. Yet the institute heads at NIH, who each year trekked up to Capitol Hill to justify their rising budgets, told Congress that their research was mission oriented, which much of it was. "What emerged was a comprehensive strategy, unique in America's experience, of research investments that ... clearly centered on use-inspired basic science, an institutional strategy that has led at times to a kind of schizophrenia among both NIH staff and principal investigators," Stokes wrote. In policy circles, they stressed how they were going to cure disease, while in academic circles, "where the ideal of pure inquiry still burns brightly," they billed their research as pure science.[19]

Virtually every medical discipline benefited. Star academic researchers in the laboratories of the nation's leading medical schools were able to build small empires on NIH grants. No research enterprise benefited more than the emerging field of molecular biology, which used biology, chemistry, and physics to understand life through its biochemical interactions. Decades of scientific discovery in those fields eventually gave birth to the biotechnology industry.

But long before the practical application of scientific research electrified the public (and the nation's stock market), politicians and patient lobbyists had completely lost interest in the pure-science ideal. In 1966, a war-beleaguered President Johnson, hoping to extend his domestic legacy into a new arena, called all the NIH division heads into his office. "I think the time has come to zero in on the target—by trying to get our knowledge fully applied," he said. "We must make sure that no lifesaving discovery is locked up in the laboratory."[20]

The president had been influenced by New York philanthropist Mary Lasker, whose husband, an advertising executive, died of cancer in 1952. Using his substantial estate, she lavished support on the American Cancer Society but soon realized only the federal government had the ability and resources to coordinate a full-fledged assault on the disease. She launched the Citizen's Committee for the Conquest of Cancer, which, though short-lived, can safely be called the most influential patient lobbying group in the nation's history. On December 9, 1969, Lasker funded a full-page ad in the *New York Times*. "We are so close to a cure for cancer. We lack only the will and the kind of money . . . that went into putting a man on the moon." Within a year, a new president, Richard Nixon, declared war on cancer, and both houses of Congress resolved to find a cure by the nation's bicentennial. Congress passed the National Cancer Act in December 1971. NCI, whose budget was $190 million in 1970, would see its budget quadruple over the next five years.

NCI used the new infusion of funds to build on its long history of applied research. The agency poured billions of dollars into a wide-ranging search for anticancer drugs. Its scientists developed assays for testing drugs and screened thousands of natural and synthetic chemicals for anticancer activity. Through its grant system, the agency set up a clinical trials network at fifteen academic research centers to test therapeutic agents in cancer patients and, when they showed promise, developed the capability of taking them all the way through the final trials on hundreds of patients that were needed to win FDA approval.

It is popular, and in some ways accurate, to brand the government-funded war on cancer a failure (for a full discussion of the government's war on cancer, see chapter 7).[21] But the system set up during the in-house NCI hunt for cancer drugs also had its unforeseen successes, most notably against AIDS.

Just as the failed hunt for cancer viruses provided the expertise for the rapid discovery and characterization of the AIDS retrovirus, the NCI system for drug discovery and applied clinical research became the model for NIH as it geared up to combat the AIDS epidemic. The Reagan administration at first did not want to respond to the outbreak. Reagan press spokesman Larry Speakes was still making jokes about gay cruising as late as mid-1983.[22] Government spending on the "gay plague" was just $66 million a year in 1985. But as activists made inroads in Congress and promising research began to emerge from science laboratories, the government began taking the disease seriously. By the end of Reagan's second term, funding for AIDS research had jumped to $500 million a year.

The person who deserves the most credit for that change of heart is Samuel Broder, who was head of NCI when the AIDS epidemic began. Conventional wisdom—derived from years of research into retroviruses—suggested they couldn't be stopped with conventional drug therapy. Broder set out to prove the conventional wisdom wrong.

Broder, the diligent son of Jewish holocaust survivors, had grown up in postwar Detroit where his parents ran a diner. He won a scholarship to attend the University of Michigan, where he developed a passion for medicine. He received his medical training at Stanford before joining NCI in 1972.

Not long after Gallo identified the retrovirus that caused AIDS, Broder joined a special task force to fight the disease, with Gallo as scientific director and himself as head clinician. Throughout 1984, he called on drug companies across the country, asking them to send potential anti-AIDS compounds to the NCI labs in Bethesda. He wanted to screen them for antiviral activity. An assay for testing drugs had already been developed in-house by Hiroaki "Mitch" Mitsuya, a Japanese postdoc who had trained at Kumamoto University on the southern Japanese island of Kyushu, where his mentor had been Takaji Miyake, Eugene Goldwasser's collaborator in purifying erythropoietin (see chapter 1).

One of Broder's first stops was at Burroughs Wellcome, which had its main U.S. research facilities in Research Triangle Park, North Carolina. Broder knew Burroughs Wellcome had been home to Gertrude Elion, who had retired a year earlier after a dazzling career. Elion, who would eventually win the Nobel Prize, never earned her doctorate and was a high school chemistry teacher before joining Burroughs Wellcome in 1944. Her pioneering investigations into the biochemistry of viruses had culminated in the development of acyclovir for genital herpes, one of the few successful antiviral drugs on the market. Yet in the 1980s the top managers at Burroughs Wellcome weren't interested in drugs to fight AIDS, the most significant new viral disease to come along in years. Where was the market, they wanted to know. Broder persisted, as did AIDS researcher Dani Bolognesi at nearby Duke University. In meetings at Burroughs Wellcome's offices, the two men argued the disease would eventually spread far beyond the few tens of thousands of cases that had appeared thus far. In early 1985, Burroughs Wellcome became one of fifty companies sending compounds to NCI for testing.

In February 1985, Mitsuya passed Burroughs Wellcome's AZT through his assay. The chemical had been synthesized by Jerome Horwitz of the Detroit Institute for Cancer Research on an NCI grant in 1964, but it didn't have anticancer properties and as a result was never patented. It would later become one of the many chemicals Elion licensed at Burroughs Wellcome in her search for an antiherpes drug. Mitsuya saw that it was active in the test tube against HIV. In June, the company filed for a patent on how to use the drug against AIDS and applied to the FDA to begin investigating the drug for safety on patients recruited by NCI and Duke. Traditionally, drug companies conduct all the blood tests on patients in their clinical trials, even when they are done by academic investigators. But AIDS was a different story. Fearing for the safety of its lab personnel, Burroughs Wellcome backed out of the project at the last moment, leaving it to NCI researchers to conduct the blood tests themselves.

After safety tests established the maximum dosing levels at which AZT could be tolerated by patients, Burroughs Wellcome jumped back in the game. It arranged for a dozen academic medical centers to test AZT for efficacy. When those results began looking good, they expanded the trials and submitted an application for new drug approval to the FDA. Though FDA reviewers had serious questions about the toxicity of the drug, it was approved for general use on March 19, 1987, a scant twenty-two months after submission of the new drug application. "For drug development, that is the speed of light," Broder said.[23]

AIDS activists raised angry questions about AZT almost immediately. They complained about its toxicities, about its effectiveness, and, most of all, about its price, which came to the then unheard of total of ten thousand dollars a year to treat a single patient. Challenged in court a few years later by two generic manufacturers, Burroughs Wellcome successfully defended its use patent in a case that went all the way to the Supreme Court (in January 1996 the high court refused to hear a final appeal). NIH supported the suit against Burroughs Wellcome. In the late 1980s the company had begun claiming that it had developed the drug on its own. Responding to a letter from Burroughs Wellcome chairman T. E. Haigler Jr. to the *New York Times* making such a claim, Broder and four other NCI-funded scientists excoriated the audacity of the firm.

> The company specifically did not develop or provide the first application of the technology for determining whether a drug like AZT can suppress live AIDS virus in human cells, nor did it develop the technology to determine at what concentration such an effect might be achieved in humans. Moreover, it was not first to administer AZT to a human being with AIDS, nor did it perform the first clinical pharmacology studies in patients. It also did not perform the immunological and virological studies necessary to infer that the drug might work, and was therefore worth pursuing in further studies. All of these were accomplished by the staff of the National Cancer Institute working with staff at Duke University. Indeed, one of the key obstacles to the development of AZT was that Burroughs Wellcome did not work with live AIDS virus nor wish to receive samples from AIDS patients.[24]

For government scientists, the lesson drawn from AZT was clear: They had the capacity to bring drugs to market. "The key issue in that era, really my obsession, was to find something practical that would be shown at a clinical level to work," Broder later said. "I felt the fate of all future antiretroviral drug development programs would be linked to the success or failure of AZT. If AZT succeeded, then many other programs would be possible. If AZT failed, it would set the field back many years."[25]

After AZT gained FDA approval in early 1987, NIAID, which had only recently been designated the lead agency in the AIDS fight, began laying plans for a broader pharmaceutical assault on HIV. Borrowing pages wholesale from the NCI playbook, the agency set up a nationwide network of academic physicians to test new drugs. It became known as the AIDS Clinical Trials Group, or ACTG. "The ACTG established the ground rules, funded the people who continued the field, and provided all the basic mechanisms for conducting AIDS clinical trials," said Lawrence Corey of the University of Washington's School of Medicine, who headed its executive committee for its first four years. "Once the basic concepts were established, the companies went it alone."[26]

The agency also launched the National Cooperative Drug Development Program (NCDDG), again drawing on NCI's experience in developing anticancer drugs. The NCDDG had a lot on its plate. They were under pressure to come up with drugs to fight the numerous infections and cancers that ravaged AIDS patients once their immune systems collapsed. They also launched a high-profile hunt for a vaccine, which remains a priority for government-funded research. But a key part of the program encouraged academic investigators and private drug firms to come up with drug candidates that might block the virus's reproduction after it had entered its human host. How? By blocking the actions of its proteins, which in the previous two years had been identified in academic labs around the world.

The HIV protease was one of those proteins. Dan Hoth, who had moved from being chief of NCI's investigation drug branch to the new division of AIDS within NIAID, recalled walking into director Margaret Johnson's office shortly after she was appointed head of the NCDDG program. She held up an X-ray crystallographic picture of the HIV protease. "This is where I want to focus," Hoth recalls her saying.

That's where Merck wanted to focus, too. Whether drug development is taking place in the public or private sectors, a new therapy—at least the ones that are truly novel and represent a significant medical advance—almost always depends on the dogged determination of a committed researcher, a true believer who is willing to stake his or her career on bringing a particular drug to market because he or she fervently believes in its promise. For a brief period of time, Merck had such a person for its protease inhibitor program.

Because of its willingness to nurture such careers, Merck has had its share of breakthroughs over the years. Indeed, if corporations have personalities, Merck would have to be considered the aristocrat of the U.S. drug industry. The company traces its roots to Friedrich Jacob Merck, a seventeenth-century German apothecary, and has long professed the noblesse oblige characteristic of old money. Until its merger with Sharp and Dohme in 1952, the firm didn't even sell drugs directly. It simply researched, developed, and manufactured them before turning them over to other firms for marketing. In the 1940s, the firm worked closely with

Selman Waksman of Rutgers University to develop the antibiotic strepto-mycin and then donated a million dollars worth of the drug to re-searchers for clinical tests. When Waksman and university officials asked Merck to cancel its exclusive rights to the patent so it could be licensed to other firms to promote competition, chairman George W. Merck returned the patents "without demur." In short order, several companies began rapidly reproducing large quantities of streptomycin, the first great breakthrough in the treatment of tuberculosis.[27] The company's commitment to scientific research encouraged Vannevar Bush to join Merck's board of directors after he left government service. A *Fortune* poll in 1986 showed Merck had derailed IBM as America's most admired company, and a glowing profile in *Business Week* magazine on the eve of the 1987 stock market crash, when Merck's 30-percent profit margins made its stock market value the seventh largest in America despite hav-ing only $5 billion in annual sales, called it "The Miracle Company."

That same year, Merck chairman P. Roy Vagelos made a major cor-porate commitment to combat AIDS. Vagelos had been recruited in 1975 from Washington University in St. Louis to run Merck's famed Research Laboratories, then headquartered in grimy Rahway, New Jersey, where Vagelos grew up. He rebuilt Merck's drug discovery capabilities, which had suffered a dry spell in the early 1970s, and helped launch blockbuster drugs to lower cholesterol and blood pressure. Vagelos rode their success to become the company's chief executive. In 1982, he recruited Edward M. Scolnick from NCI to run its labs. Scolnick, a Harvard-trained physi-cian, had spent the prior decade in the government's huge but unsuc-cessful effort to uncover the viral causes of cancer and from 1982 to 1985 edited the *Journal of Virology,* a rare honor for an industry-based scientist. It gave him a front-row seat for watching the AIDS discovery drama unfold in government and academic labs.

Even before the company had committed itself to fighting AIDS, Scolnick had begun building up Merck's capabilities in virology and molecular genetics, his own specialties. Scolnick recruited Irving Sigal, a brilliant young scientist whose father had once run Eli Lilly's research department, and Emilio Emini, a recent Cornell graduate with a doctor-ate in microbiology. By 1986, with NCI chief Broder pushing the AZT through highly publicized clinical trials and the academic literature ex-ploding with information about HIV's viral mechanics, the firm was ready to jump into the AIDS fight. Emini was asked to spearhead the firm's push for a vaccine, an area where the company had substantial ex-pertise. Sigal would lead the drug discovery team. Scolnick later recalled

Sigal coming into his lab to discuss a scientific paper showing how HIV had a protease very similar to renin and asking for resources to develop potential inhibitors. "Great, go do it," Scolnick had said.[28]

Though they were initiating their antiretroviral research about the same time NIAID was launching its drug development program, Merck did not pursue government aid. The company was a firm believer in the Vannevar Bush model. Merck scientists took pride in their independent research skills, which were nurtured by Merck's surging sales and profits. In the early days of its hunt for a protease inhibitor, Nancy Kohl, a Merck scientist recruited by Sigal from MIT's Center for Cancer Research, conducted a series of experiments that proved inhibiting protease would inhibit replication of the virus in a test tube. Her findings appeared in the proceedings of the National Academy of Science in July 1988.

While that purely scientific work was interesting, the real work of the drug company was taking place in its chemistry labs. Sigal initiated a dual-track strategy for finding a molecule that would inhibit the HIV protease. He asked thirteen of Merck's medicinal chemists to begin developing analogues of its renin inhibitors to see if they could come up with one that halted the protease's action in a test tube. In the summer of 1988 they found one. But like Abbott's drug, it was so large that it had to be administered intravenously. Needing a better molecule, Sigal, a hard-charger prone to yelling at colleagues who couldn't meet his demanding deadlines, doubled the number of chemists on the job.[29] At the same time, he pushed Merck's X-ray crystallography department, headed by Manuel Navia, to come up with the structure of the protease so the chemists could design a better molecule. In February 1989 Navia became the first scientist to publish the HIV protease structure in the scientific literature, earning Merck's protease inhibitor program a front-page profile in the *Wall Street Journal* and Navia an appearance on NBC's *Today Show*.[30] While the scientists carefully couched their presentations—a cure could be years away, they cautioned—the media hoopla left the impression that private industry was well along the trail of a cure for AIDS.

The media attention also provided a temporary respite from the troubles plaguing Merck's protease inhibitor program. A month and a half earlier, Sigal had flown to London to attend a scientific meeting. He booked a flight back for December 22, but at the last minute decided to take the prior evening's flight out of Heathrow so he could spend more time with his family. Pan Am 103 never made it. A terrorist's bomb destroyed the plane thirty-one thousand feet over Lockerbie, Scotland, killing the 259 passengers and crew and 11 persons on the ground. "His death was devastating to the organization, but it didn't affect our protease inhibitor work at all," Emini recalled. "We just went on. It is always possible to say what things might have been if he had been here. Would we have done it differently? Would we have done it better? It's impossible to answer."[31]

Navia, the crystallographer, thought the post-Sigal program could have been run a lot better. A few months after his brief brush with media fame, he asked Merck's chemistry department to send down some more of their analogues so he could model them on his computers for potential antiprotease activity. The head chemist refused to cooperate. An outraged Navia protested to Scolnick, who eventually backed his media-savvy crystallographer. But the headstrong Navia quit in protest and a few months later moved on to Vertex, a biotech start-up run by another Merck refugee. He ignored entreaties to stay from both Scolnick and Vagelos.[32] Navia's potential for contributing to the hunt for a protease inhibitor disappeared with him. At Vertex, it would be two years before he returned to HIV work.

Crystallographers at other firms and in government labs, meanwhile, began puzzling over the structure that Navia had published in *Science*. He hadn't released any of the data points, so no one else could use it to design drugs. A little more than a year later, Alex Wlodawer, an X-ray crystallographer at NCI, published a complete portrait of the protease molecule. It was more accurate than the Navia model and included data on how it bound to the other HIV proteins as it carried out its mission. Unlike Navia and Merck, the government was more than happy to share its information with everyone. "I spent lots of time flying in 1989 and 1990 to every pharmaceutical company in the universe talking about our structure," Wlodawer told me in 2001. "They were trying to think how their drug development programs could benefit. I briefed their scientists. I went to Abbott. I went to Merck. They were trying to energize their own scientists."[33]

However, Merck scientists turned their backs on X-ray crystallography-based rational drug design and returned to traditional screening. In the spring of 1989 its chemists finally came up with a protease inhibitor candidate. But when safety experts tested the drug in dogs, it cut off bile flow. Some company officials speculated all protease inhibitors would be toxic.[34] With Sigal and Navia gone, there was no longer anyone around to champion alternative approaches. Scolnick, sensing depression setting in among his medicinal chemists, sharply cut back on the number of chemists working on protease inhibitors. He authorized Emini to begin chasing down reverse transcriptase inhibitors that might be an alternative to AZT. The focus of Merck's AIDS research shifted.

About the same time that Merck was deemphasizing its work on protease inhibitors, Hoffmann–La Roche scientists were ready to move their candidate into clinical trials. The pharmaceutical giant, based in Basel, Switzerland, was clearly in the lead. The company traced its roots to the merger of Fritz Hoffmann and Adele La Roche, who followed a Swiss custom of combining their names when they married. Fritz Hoffmann–La Roche was born in 1868 to wealthy Basel merchants and worked for a Belgian drug company before launching his own manufacturing firm at age twenty-eight. Over the next decade, the company spread across Europe and in 1905 established U.S. operations. On the eve of the Great Depression, the company opened a huge research and manufacturing complex in Nutley, New Jersey, which to this day remains the company's largest worldwide research and manufacturing facility.

Though proud of its research capabilities on both sides of the Atlantic, Hoffmann–La Roche has never been shy about forging collaborations with the public sector to pursue medical breakthroughs. Near the end of World War II, Elmer H. Bobst, whose legendary skill at marketing drugs to physicians made him president of Roche's U.S. operations, was getting ready to step down. Basel-based Roche officials sought out Lawrence D. Barney, the head of the Wisconsin Alumni Research Foundation, to replace Bobst. The foundation had been established in 1925 to help the land-grant university commercialize the food and vitamin patents pouring out of its labs and became the prototype for academic-industry collaborations enabled by the 1980 Bayh-Dole Act. Barney passed muster with his corporate interviewers when he rattled off the names of twelve pharmaceutical company chief executives whom he knew personally through his work at the foundation.[35] Over the ensuing decades, the firm's European operations maintained close ties with universities, especially in Switzerland, and with the government-sponsored Medical Research Council in the United Kingdom.

The company's willingness to engage government researchers on their turf enmeshed it in the earliest days of the AIDS fight. In 1983, NIAID officials contacted the firm to see if its interferon, an overhyped biotech product, might prove useful as an immune system booster.[36] The substance eventually proved marginally useful to AIDS patients by slowing the progression of opportunistic infections and combating hepatitis C. Another one of the company's biotech products—interleukin 2—was tested against AIDS and shown to be useless. The company also sold an early diagnostic test for AIDS after licensing the assays from the government.

These early experiences made the company a willing partner when Broder and his colleagues at NCI finished pushing Burroughs Wellcome's AZT through the FDA approval process in 1987. A coterie of scientists at Roche not only understood the disease, but was anxious to compete for the next antiretroviral coming out of NCI's labs. Broder and his team had not stopped at AZT. They kept looking for more effective drugs and, when they found something that worked in test tubes and passed animal toxicity tests, sent them out to private firms for clinical trials. Roche conducted the initial clinical testing of government-owned didanosine (ddI), which was eventually licensed to Bristol-Myers Squibb. It did the same for zalcitabine (ddC), the next reverse transcriptase inhibitor to emerge from NCI labs.

Indeed by late 1987 there was no shortage of companies willing to jump into the AIDS market. The price tag Burroughs Wellcome set on AZT made AIDS drugs financially attractive. When ddC came along, there were fifty companies competing for the right to develop it. NCI staged a beauty contest among the four finalists, and Roche won. "NCI saw itself as the incubator to get these drugs to a certain level but didn't have the infrastructure to move these drugs through the late clinical trials stage or commercial manufacturing," recalled Whaijen Soo, vice president for clinical sciences at Hoffmann–La Roche.[37]

The Taiwanese-born scientist had earned a doctorate in retrovirology and biochemistry at Berkeley and received his medical training at the University of California at San Francisco. He had treated some of the nation's first AIDS patients (in those days the disease was known as GRID, or Gay-Related Immune Disease) while in medical school and during his postdoctoral years at Harvard. By the mid-1980s, several of his mentors had become frontline physicians in the government clinical trials network. After moving to Roche, Soo gladly ran the clinical trials for ddC through the ACTG. It gained FDA approval in June 1992, the third nucleoside reverse transcriptase inhibitor approved to combat AIDS.

But long before that program got under way, Roche scientists were looking for ways to cooperate with the government. In early 1988, Ming-Chu Hsu, who also worked at the Nutley complex, applied to NIAID for a drug development grant to pursue inhibitors of an HIV gene (known as tatIII) whose proteins regulated replication of the virus once it was inside white blood cells. "The whole idea of attacking the regulatory proteins was still up in the air," Soo recalled, "and [Hsu] wanted to be academically known. Scientists in drug companies also want to be considered solid scientists and a peer that's well respected by academic scientists." Hsu's team eventually developed a tat inhibitor, but it foundered in early testing. While it slowed viral reproduction in a test tube, it didn't increase the white blood cell count in patients. The project was terminated when the company's protease inhibitor program, based at its UK facilities, began showing positive results.[38]

The Roche complex in Welwyn, England, was roped into the anti-AIDS fight by company scientists in the United States, who were worried about the severe side effects of ddC and ddI. They asked the Welwyn chemists to develop analogues that might be less toxic to patients. The Welwyn group immediately immersed themselves in the literature, which pushed them in a very different direction. They learned that HIV had a protease that was very similar to renin, the blood pressure protease. Like many drug companies, Roche had a renin inhibitor program, which was in Welwyn. In November 1986, the nascent AIDS team launched a protease inhibitor program and asked Noel Roberts, who had spent a dozen years in the fruitless hunt for a renin inhibitor, to run it.

It took the small Welwyn team of basic scientists nearly three years to come up with a viable drug candidate. The Pearl-Taylor paper in 1987 confirmed their suspicions that the HIV protease had a clamshell-like structure. They spent much of the next year developing assays to test drug candidates for antiviral activity. As more information about the protease appeared in the academic literature, house crystallographer Anthony Krohn began constructing a theoretical model of the protein, which, like Erickson's theoretical model at Abbott, could be used by company chemists to design inhibitors. When Merck's Navia published his paper in *Nature* in February 1989, Roberts pulled together the team to discuss the implications.[39] Were they on the wrong track? Krohn kept them waiting for fifteen minutes before bursting into the room and slamming the paper on the conference table. "The bloody bugger's got it wrong. It doesn't agree with my model," he exclaimed. Roberts told his team members to follow their own instincts. "It turned out [Krohn] was absolutely right. Merck had not interpreted the crystallography structure right . . . as Wlodawer later proved."[40] Three months later, Roche chemists synthesized Ro31-8959, which would become known as saquinavir.

The initial results with the drug were encouraging. It was extraordinarily potent in the test tube. But the euphoria quickly faded as company scientists faced two major problems. The drug was difficult to make, requiring twenty-three separate steps. Roberts checked with company chemists. They assured him they could make it in sufficient quantities and a low enough cost to ensure its commercial viability. "They turned out to be completely right," Roberts later said. "We've had no problem making this in bulk.[41]

The second problem was more difficult to resolve. Keith Bragman, a cancer doctor in Bristol-Myers's European operations, joined the company that fall to run clinical trials on saquinavir. He would oversee the clinical development of the drug all the way through its European and FDA licensing in December 1995. In mid-1990, Bragman arranged with doctors in France, Italy, and the United Kingdom to begin human testing. Those tests were designed to determine how much drug could be administered before provoking unacceptable side effects and how much had to be administered to get enough into the bloodstream to have an antiviral effect.

The initial reports were devastating. While the drug was sufficiently nontoxic for further human trials, only 4 percent of the administered dose got into the bloodstream. Patients took eighteen hard capsules a day, but the dose had a minimal effect against the virus. Bragman and Roberts were desperate to get a better drug. They went to top management to get authorization for company chemists to pursue an analogue of saquinavir that would be more easily absorbed into the bloodstream. Or, barring that new expense, they wanted to start a new clinical test with higher dosing.

By mid-1991 AIDS had already become a terrifying epidemic with global implications. Yet efforts to find treatments for HIV were no more than a blip on the radar screens of top managers at Roche. They still perceived it as an orphan disease without much economic potential. Research spending on AIDS at the closely held firm didn't exceed more than 5 percent of the total research budget.[42] Even the ddC program, which by 1991 was in the final stages of government-funded clinical trials and less than a year away from licensing, was perceived as "sort of a side venture," according to Miklos Salgo, who came to Roche in 1989 to direct the ddC clinical trials. He saw his first AIDS patients in 1982 at Bellevue Hospital while a medical student at New York University and completed his medical training at Albert Einstein Medical School at Montefiore Hospital in the Bronx. "How could you not pay attention to the biggest epidemic taking place in our times," he recalled a female co-worker telling him as they labored long into the night to treat the steady stream of AIDS victims from the South Bronx.[43]

That attitude wasn't shared by the managers contemplating the Bragman and Roberts request. More than a decade later, now a top official at the firm, Salgo recalled their decision with some hesitancy. "It was only after we got Hivid [the trade name for ddC] licensed that [they realized] the extent of the epidemic and accepted that this was a field that pharmaceutical companies could make . . ." He paused and then clarified, ". . . be productive in and be worthwhile to enter."[44]

Management turned down Bragman's requests to go hunting for an analogue of saquinavir with superior bioavailability. Jürgen Drews, then president of global research for Roche, was a key member of the senior management committee that vetoed new funds to continue searching for a better protease inhibitor candidate. The committee also turned down Bragman's request for new first-stage clinical trials at higher doses. In his 1998 book, *In Quest of Tomorrow's Medicines*, Drews described how "one pharmaceutical company developing the first protease inhibitor against AIDS questioned whether an economically feasible synthesis would ever be developed."[45]

Roberts and his chemists, who were certain saquinavir could be manufactured at a reasonable cost, weren't invited to the meeting and thus couldn't counter the argument. Neither was Bragman, who wanted to initiate new clinical trials at higher doses. "Concern about the economic viability of this medicine reached the point where a highly placed employee of the firm attempted to forbid the use of high dosages in the clinical trials, though from a scientific standpoint these were deemed absolutely essential," Drews wrote. "He was convinced that this medicine would forever remain unprofitable. 'How effective it is at higher dosages I have absolutely no desire to know,' he declared."[46]

A decade later, the scientists involved in developing saquinavir would look back on that decision as a dreadful mistake. But they would largely blame it on the external political environment, not top management. Roche was under intense pressure to offer ddC, then in late-stage trials to AIDS patients under a compassionate use program. Under the rubric of compassionate use, doctors with desperately ill patients, often near death, can ask companies for drugs that are still in clinical trials, even though they have not yet been proven effective. Companies believe compassionate use programs hinder them from recruiting patients for double-blind, placebo-controlled clinical trials, which are the gold standard of the drug industry and preferred by regulators. But desperate

AIDS patients rebelled against what they called "dead body" trials. One of the more famous placards held by AIDS activists as they marched outside FDA headquarters in the late 1980s read, "I died on a placebo." Compassionate use for drugs in clinical trials, or expanded access, as the AIDS activists preferred to call it, was one of their main demands. Roche, unaccustomed to hearing from patients, much less accepting criticism from them, was unwilling to change its research procedures to accommodate their demands.

The company's top managers were also rattled by the ongoing controversy over price, which was again in the headlines. NCI's ddI, which the government had licensed to Bristol-Myers Squibb, had just been approved by the FDA. Its hefty price tag, coming on top of the price of AZT, had restoked the anger of the AIDS community and the Democrats who controlled Congress. Public Citizen, which had been created by Ralph Nader in 1971 to fight abusive corporate practices, filed suit to cancel Burroughs Wellcome's AZT patent. The government intervened on Barr Laboratories' behalf when the generic drug manufacturer sought to void Burroughs Wellcome's exclusive manufacturing rights. The firm wanted NIH named as coinventor of the drug so that it could be licensed to generic manufacturers like Barr.

"This was a conservative Swiss company dealing with some difficult characters," Bragman recalled a decade later. "For Hoffmann–La Roche, money [for additional research] would not have been the issue. This was an extraordinarily hot political area to work in. We had [a protease inhibitor] that was well tolerated, that had activity, that was comparable to AZT. Why don't we just develop it and get it on the market? You can understand how the company might say let's not make our lives more difficult than they already are."[47]

Yet Drews learned a very different lesson from the experience. "As long as the search for new drugs, and above all, their development, is almost exclusively the province of profit-oriented enterprises, it will be impossible to untangle the relationship between economic calculation and the needs of medicine."[48] Bragman never got a better molecule.

5

The Divorce

offmann–La Roche's AIDS scientists weren't alone in dealing with executive suite problems. As the winter of 1991 melted into a typically slushy Chicago spring, the handful of researchers working on Abbott Laboratories' protease inhibitor project suddenly found themselves operating in an environment dominated by corporate scandal.

Abbott, one of the largest employers in the suburbs north of the city, took pride in its conservative ways. Its sprawling Abbott Park campus had expanded steadily in the postwar years, fueled more by marketing acumen than a drive to produce medicine. The company traced its origins to a family-run pharmacy started by Wallace Calvin Abbott on the north side of Chicago. A physician who had migrated to the Windy City from Michigan, Abbott began mixing his own medicines after becoming frustrated by the poor quality of the available supplies of morphine, quinine, and strychnine that were the mainstays of his turn-of-the-century medical practice. He soon began peddling his concoctions to fellow physicians.

His big breakthrough came during World War I and ushered in the company's long history of involvement with government programs. The war disrupted trade between the United States and Germany, then the undisputed leader in pharmaceutical development. To provide the latest painkillers to American soldiers wounded at the front, the United States seized the German patents on novocaine and barbital and awarded them to Abbott as a wartime emergency measure. Abbott asked University of Illinois chemists to develop a process for making the painkillers in bulk. The company rapidly expanded through wartime contracts.

Shortly after the war, one of the young doctoral candidates who had worked on the project, Ernest H. Volwiler, joined the company. Volwiler went on to become research director and president. Under his direction Abbott emerged as a leading manufacturer of anesthetics and was best known for developing sodium pentothal, the so-called truth serum. The company also bought out the nonprofit Dermatological Research Laboratories of Philadelphia, which during World War I had been awarded the nationalized patent for Paul Ehrlich's process for making arsphenamine, the first cure for syphilis.

World War II gave the company another financial shot in the arm. It won a government contract to make penicillin and worked closely with the Agriculture Department's new research lab in Peoria to develop the process. Ten days after Pearl Harbor, Robert Coghill, chief of the fermentation division at Peoria, briefed the chief executives and research directors of Merck, Squibb, Pfizer Inc., and Lederle about the breakthrough processes developed in his lab. They, like Abbott, became penicillin suppliers. After the war, Abbott recruited Coghill to run its research division, where he stayed until 1957, when he returned to the government to run the National Cancer Institute's chemotherapy program.[1]

Though its roots were in pharmaceuticals, the company never developed a full range of drug products that might have made it a major player in the field. During the booming postwar years, it chose instead to diversify into other lines of business. In 1964, it purchased Ross Laboratories, which had developed the first infant formula. With Abbott's marketing savvy, Similac became the leader in its field, and the nutritionals division became Abbott's biggest money maker. The company also expanded into hospital supplies such as intravenous feeding systems and disease diagnostic kits. Its AIDS test, licensed from the National Institutes of Health (NIH) in the mid-1980s, was one of dozens in its salespersons' bags. When John Erickson began pushing the company to jump into AIDS drug discovery, pharmaceuticals represented less than one-fifth of company sales.

During the business-friendly 1980s, the company was run by Robert A. Schoellhorn, who had joined the firm in 1973 after a twenty-six-year career with chemical maker American Cyanamid. Abbott's bottom-line oriented board recruited Schoellhorn because of his reputation as a tough manager. But to their consternation, he became better known as an overbearing manager with a lavish corporate lifestyle. Schoellhorn's tenure was marked by a steady exodus of executive talent as frustrated potential successors abandoned ship. The nation's biotechnology industry in its start-up years used Abbott's executive suite like a minor league farm team: James L. Vincent left in 1980 to become chairman of Biogen, George Rathmann left that same year to become chairman of Amgen, and G. Kirk Raab left in 1985 to become president of Genentech.

While strife-torn Abbott came up with a handful of new prescription medicines in the 1980s, its research efforts were puny and ineffective compared to industry giants like Roche, Pfizer, and Merck. Like many companies with unproductive research staffs, Abbott went shopping for promising drug candidates. But unlike firms that look to Wall Street for buyout targets, Abbott under Schoellhorn took what at the time was the unprecedented step of looking abroad. In 1988, the company entered into a joint venture with Takeda Chemical Industries to test and market drugs developed by Japan's largest pharmaceutical manufacturer. The joint venture, dubbed TAP Pharmaceuticals, ignored the rising national concern about U.S. competitiveness vis-à-vis Japan, which was then at the height of its financial bubble. If you can't beat them, join them, Schoellhorn seemed to be saying as he jetted around the world. Indeed, at the same time that he was slashing domestic research-and-development budgets to meet his profit targets, he ordered a new $25-million Gulfstream, complete with custom-made seats.

The final straw for the board of directors came in August 1989, when Schoellhorn pushed out Jack W. Schuler, a highly touted Stanford Business School graduate who had been hired as the combative chief executive officer's third chief operating officer. The move triggered a slew of hostile articles in the financial press. "Schoellhorn rarely brooks dissent and bridles when a talented manager gets too close to the seat of power," *Business Week* concluded after interviewing a score of former and current top officers. "Schuler never cared much for Schoellhorn's rigid 15-percent-profit target and argued against cutting research-and-development spending."[2]

Schuler left his mark on the firm, though. One of his last moves was recruiting Ferid Murad from Stanford, his alma mater. Murad, a noted academic researcher who would eventually win the 1998 Nobel Prize for medicine, was a physician by training. He was born in 1934 to an Albanian immigrant who ran an all-night restaurant in the shadows of the

Standard Oil refinery in Whiting, Indiana, which is just outside Chicago. Looking for a profession where he wouldn't have to work as hard as his father, he chose medicine and enrolled in Cleveland's Western Reserve University (now Case Western Reserve). His father's work ethic stuck, however, and his medical school performance earned Murad a prestigious internship at Massachusetts General Hospital, where he studied under, among others, Edward Scolnick, who would go on to NIH before becoming Merck's top scientist. Murad soon followed Scolnick to Bethesda for a postdoctoral fellowship at the National Heart Institute. The stint taught him how to navigate the grant-making politics of NIH, leading the University of Virginia to recruit him in 1970 to launch a clinical pharmacology program.

Murad did his most significant scientific work while at Virginia, identifying how nitric oxide acted as a cell signaling mechanism for the cardiovascular system. The Nobel-quality science laid the intellectual groundwork for the development of erectile dysfunction drugs like Viagra. He moved on to Stanford and was continuing that research when Schuler made what seemed at the time to be a very attractive offer. "I enjoyed the access to all of Abbott's resources, scientific staff, instrumentation, and what initially seemed like an unlimited research budget," Murad wrote in his Nobel autobiography. "I eventually learned that one can never have enough resources when one looks for novel therapies of major diseases."[3]

It didn't take long for Murad to bump into the glass walls of the corporate fishbowl he had jumped into. Within months of his arrival, Schuler, the man who had brought him to Abbott, was gone and the company was wracked by high-level intrigue among a board of directors intent on ousting Schoellhorn. Murad had to devise a strategy to avoid being pulled under by the tempest. His solution was simple. He kept his more controversial programs—like the AIDS program that Erickson, the academically inclined X-ray crystallographer, was just getting underway—under the radar screen of top management. When Erickson came to him with his early models of the HIV protease and a strategy for going after drugs to inhibit its action, Murad said, "Fine, but let's not make a big deal out of it." He later described Abbott as "a very conservative place. There were several projects I thought important [but] they didn't want to pursue. They were not very excited about the HIV program initially, and that's why we didn't talk about it."[4]

Murad dubbed the protease inhibitor program a pilot project and encouraged Erickson to pursue an NIH grant to hire postdoctoral researchers to supplement the meager bench support he could offer the young scientist. Murad won similar grants for a number of Abbott drug development programs. At the peak of the program in the early 1990s, Abbott had thirty-five NIH-funded researchers on staff. The cooperative research programs ended shortly after Murad's departure in 1993.

Shortly after the first government-funded postdocs came on board in the fall of 1988, Dale Kempf and his small chemistry team began making progress in the search for a protease inhibitor. He rejected suggestions from higher-ups that he blindly test chemicals that had been synthesized as potential renin inhibitors against the HIV enzyme. All the major companies that had renin inhibitor programs would be using the same strategy, Kempf figured. Moreover, they had far more chemists and resources than Abbott was ever going to give him. A colleague stopped him in the halls one afternoon and put an arm on his shoulder. "My condolences, Dale, I hear Merck has thirty chemists on its HIV project."[5] He had only three.

Instead of screening, Kempf looked to Erickson's evolving model of the clamshell-like protease for guidance. He designed symmetric chemicals that in theory would bind to both sides of the enzyme and thereby gum up the works. (Kempf calls protease inhibitors "molecular peanut butter," a phrase suggested to him by a fourth grader during one of the many grade school presentations he makes about his work.) Whenever his team came up with a chemical that succeeding in binding to the cloned protease, Erickson shipped it off in the overnight mail to the NCI lab in Bethesda, where Hiroaki Mitsuya tested it for activity against HIV in his assays. There was nobody better in the country at conducting such tests since Mitsuya had polished his skills during the cancer agency's successful hunt for the first generation of AIDS drugs.

Within a few months they hit pay dirt. Unfortunately, Abbott's first protease inhibitor presented its inventors with huge problems. The molecule was so large that it couldn't be tested for safety, even in animals. It was simply too big to be safely injected into mammals. A dejected Kempf continued looking for a more soluble protease inhibitor. In the spring of 1990, the Erickson-Kempf team came up with one that they thought was worth sending to human clinical trials. Abbott filed its first protease inhibitor patent in May 1990.

A-77003 (each drug company has its own system for numbering and naming its synthetic chemicals, usually using the first letters of the company's name with a number) was itself almost useless as a drug candidate. The large molecule was rapidly digested in the gut, meaning it could never be manufactured in pill form. Erickson and Kempf knew they were going to need a better drug, one that wouldn't have to be injected intravenously. But to come up with something better, they needed to throw more chemists at the task. And to convince top management that it was worth ramping up the program, they had to show that a protease inhibitor—any protease inhibitor—would eventually be a viable alternative to AZT as an AIDS drug. At that point, no protease inhibitor had ever been successfully tested in humans.

Erickson again turned to the government for help. In the fall of 1990, he set up a meeting between his Abbott team and every top official at NIH involved in the fight against AIDS. Anthony Fauci, who had primary responsibility as head of the National Institute for Allergies and Infectious Diseases (NIAID), was there; so was Broder, chief of NCI; Dan Hoth, head of the AIDS Clinical Trials Group (ACTG); and Bruce Chabner, who was heading the drug discovery unit at NCI. "Abbott won't develop this drug as an intravenous agent, but I need to know if it will work," Erickson told the small crowd. His plan was simple. He wanted the government to subsidize the cost of testing the drug for its pharmacological activity in animals. He also needed help in developing it into a form that could be injected into humans. With those two steps out of the way, he would then have the results needed to convince Abbott's top management to fund the scale-up and production of the drug to do the initial testing in humans to prove the concept. "It would save us all a lot of grief if the protease turns out not to be a very good target," he told them.[6]

The government scientists were more than happy to perform the tests for Abbott. From a scientific perspective, it was an extraordinary opportunity to test the first of a new class of drugs that had been specifically designed to combat AIDS. They also thought they had every right to be part of the trials. Abbott's protease inhibitor had been developed with the help of federal grants. "We wanted to collaborate on clinical trials," Hoth said. "We thought they had good science and a promising drug. Their research people were outstanding." The result of the meeting was an agreement to let NCI do the initial animal testing on Abbott's new drug.[7]

Murad and Erickson were overjoyed. The agreement allowed them to pursue their exciting discovery while maintaining the program's low profile inside the firm. But their glee would be short lived. A few months after Schuler's departure, the company's board of directors, fed up with Schoellhorn's constant upheavals, stripped him of day-to-day responsibilities and installed Duane Burnham, the chief financial officer, as chief executive. Schoellhorn wasn't one to accept public humiliation without a fight. Throughout 1990, the board and its former chief executive officer engaged in a high-profile court battle. Schoellhorn accused the board of acting like a "rogue committee," while the board lawyers suggested he had "repeatedly misappropriated the company assets," including the installation of company-owned artwork in his home. The board's new man, Burnham, was a bean counter through and through, and a micromanager to boot. Besides limiting the ostentatious expenditures of the Schoellhorn reign, he began scaling back the aggressive moves Schuler had made in research and development.[8]

Erickson saw the handwriting on the wall. A company that for a few years under Schuler and Murad had allowed him to move unimpeded through the wilds of early-stage drug research was now going to concentrate on bringing the few drugs in its pipeline to market. Erickson's future at the firm would be managing those projects toward completion, not cutting-edge drug design. During one of his frequent trips to Bethesda, he voiced his concerns to the senior scientists at NCI. They suggested an alternative. Why not join NCI to set up a government-run X-ray crystallography department?

The top scientists at NCI were excited at the prospect of snaring Erickson. It would bring the government agency one of the nation's top scientists in X-ray crystallography, a man who also had industrial experience designing drugs with the latest technologies. Broder got directly involved in recruiting Erickson. A few months earlier, he had convinced several top cancer researchers to return to the government fold after short stints in industry. It was part of the NCI chief's high-profile campaign to reverse the brain drain that usually saw scientists leave NIH for better-paying industry jobs. "We still have considerable difficulty in recruiting senior-level scientists and clinical researchers," Broder said. "Government service as a calling just doesn't seem to have the same force that it might have had in another era."[9] He wasn't just concerned about rebuilding the government's public health service. Broder was still seething over Burroughs Wellcome's snub of NCI's contributions to developing AZT. His response was to plunge deeper into drug development.

Word of Erickson's imminent defection soon trickled back to Murad, who had his own contacts in NIH. He implored Erickson to stay. The bearded scientist said he wanted the company to commit some chemists to the purely scientific side of his research. Erickson wasn't interested in just designing drugs, he wanted to perfect his ability to model proteins on his computers. Murad, a brilliant research scientist himself, understood the instinct, but there was no money in his budget for that kind of pure science endeavor, he told Erickson. In January 1991, the crystallographer left Abbott to join NCI.

By itself, the defection of one high-level scientist in its AIDS research and development department might not have set off alarm bells, especially at a company preoccupied with dumping its chief executive officer. But Abbott's North Shore soap opera was about to take a more ominous turn. In February, local police arrested Seymour Schlager, a physician earning $140,000 a year as head of Abbott's AIDS clinical research, for attempted murder after he tried to smother his wife with a plastic-encased pillow in his spacious Highland Park home. She escaped and ran screaming down the quiet residential street of their tony suburb. Within days the local papers' gossip columns were filled with tales of Schlager's affair with his twenty-four-year-old assistant. His lawyers would later claim job stress led to a mental breakdown. An unsympathetic judge eventually sentenced him to thirteen years in prison.

Schlager was indeed in a stressful position in the early months of 1991. He had been overseeing the testing of clarithromycin, an experimental antibiotic that top company officials hoped to turn into a blockbuster drug. Abbott researchers had been testing the drug against a range of serious respiratory infections. One of those infections was mycobacterium avium complex, or MAC, which struck down more than half of AIDS patients after their immune systems collapsed. Clinical trials in Europe had already documented clarithromycin's value in combating MAC. However, trials in the United States were moving slowly because Abbott was aiming for much wider labeling for the drug than just its AIDS-related use. Radical AIDS activist groups were outraged that the company put its sales strategy ahead of the well-being of people who were dying. They demanded that the company immediately make the drug available even though it was still in clinical trials. Schlager was the company's point man in that controversy. A few weeks after his arrest for attempted murder, activists belonging to the AIDS Coalition to Unleash Power, or ACT UP—the most militant of the AIDS groups—began picketing the company's offices in San Francisco. Their demand: immediate access to clarithromycin.

Once the controversy hit the newspapers, Abbott's top management and its corporate public relations staff got involved. The company issued a press release offering to make the experimental drug available to very sick patients in an expanded access program, but only after it had obtained more data from studies that were then underway at Johns Hopkins University under the auspices of the government's ACTG program. Outraged AIDS activists in Los Angeles, New York, and San Francisco began organizing patients into so-called buyers clubs. The clubs smuggled Abbott's most promising new drug into the United States from Europe, where it was not only available, but sold for far less than what the company planned to sell it for in the domestic market. If Abbott's top officials hadn't been paying close attention to what was going on in their AIDS program before, they certainly were now.[10]

Andre Pernet, a career manager at the firm with a background in chemistry and chemical engineering, was brought in to begin sifting through Abbott's AIDS programs. What he found didn't please him. The ACTG, increasingly sympathetic to the AIDS activists, was pushing the clarithromycin trials in directions the company didn't want to go. Furthermore, tests on the most promising new class of drugs to combat AIDS to come along in years—represented by their first protease inhibitor, A-77003—were being performed in government labs.

Throughout 1991, NCI scientists in Bethesda conducted the experiments on A-77003 that Erickson had requested during his last months at the firm. They developed an intravenous formulation, tested it on mice and rats for toxicity, and then used those tests to establish a range of potentially appropriate doses for humans. Meanwhile Kempf and his team continued looking for better versions of the molecule. In the fall he came up with one. But he needed more chemists to perfect it as well as to make sufficient quantities of the first one for the upcoming clinical trial designed to prove that a protease inhibitor—any protease inhibitor—could work in humans. From research's point of view, everything was coming up roses. Pernet's review—conducted over the same months—reached a similar conclusion. Abbott's protease inhibitor search was about to turn into a major program. The last thing Pernet wanted was the government's fingerprints all over the company's new drug.

The government, in industry's eyes, had become an unreliable partner. By mid-1991, AIDS activists' outrage over the price of AZT was at a fever pitch. To industry executives, it seemed like NCI scientists had intervened on the activists' side by insisting on proper credit for their role in discovering the drug. In July, Bernadine Healy, who had just been named director of NIH after a research career at the Cleveland Clinic, threw the weight of the federal agency behind the activists. She granted generic manufacturer Barr Laboratories a conditional license to manufacture and market AZT. The only caveat was that the license depended on Barr making the government a coowner of Burroughs Wellcome's patent, which the company was pursuing in court.

Healy's decision on AZT reflected national concerns about the rising cost of health care. The Democratic-controlled Congress that summer jumped on the issue of skyrocketing prescription drug prices with highly publicized hearings on the price of Taxol, a cancer-fighting extract from the bark of the Pacific Yew tree. The drug was one of the great success stories of NCI's long-standing program for screening natural products from around the world for their anticancer properties. But once government researchers discovered Taxol and turned it over to Bristol-Myers Squibb for marketing, the company charged a fantastic markup for the extract. Congressional Democrats, who planned to make high drug prices a major campaign issue in the 1992 elections, argued that a so-called reasonable pricing clause that had been inserted in the contract the government signed with Bristol-Myers Squibb gave it the right to reduce the high price placed on the drug. NIH had begun inserting such clauses in its contracts with industry in 1989 in response to the public outcry over the cost of AZT.

The Taxol and AZT debates set off alarm bells in drug company boardrooms across the United States. Pernet called NCI's Chabner, who was overseeing the animal tests on Abbott's experimental protease inhibitor. He demanded a meeting in Bethesda to discuss the terms of the company's arrangement with the government. The meeting took place in November 1991.

Abbott brought out the big guns. While Pernet and Murad were present, Paul Clark, president of the pharmaceutical division, ran the show. He brought along the company's chief corporate counsel for legal support. Chabner and Hoth, representing the clinical testing wings of NCI and NIAID, respectively, were stunned by the presentation. "It was Clark's meeting," recalled Hoth. "The legal counsel advised that this was a risk. They could invest in all this research, and the government could march in. Clark said, 'We can't afford to take that risk.'"[11]

The company team informed the government scientists that Abbott planned to go abroad to test its new drug and wanted all tests done at Abbott expense. "The evolution of industry/government relationship and the decision at Abbott to initiate a global development have forced us to consider a new basis for the relationship," Pernet said in a follow-up letter. The company would allow a joint scientific development board to oversee testing. But that board would have an Abbott scientist as its head, and he would have to sign off on any clinical protocols. The first tests would be done abroad because government authorities in some European countries didn't require government filings for first-stage clinical trials. If NCI conducted any studies that eventually wound up in an application to the FDA, Abbott would reimburse NCI for all expenses. "My only purpose is to direct a concerted worldwide effort that can be executed in a record time and to be sure that Abbott is clearly seen as having funded and executed the development of the drug," Pernet wrote.[12]

The company talked about speed. But the issue was price. In 1987, Burroughs Wellcome brought the first AIDS drug to market at a price to patients (or, more typically, insurers and government welfare agencies) of ten thousand dollars a year. But after four years of public protests, the company had been forced to cut its price in half. Coupled with a growing recognition that less could be used to gain the same effect, the company was now realizing less than twenty-six hundred dollars a year from AIDS patients. Abbott wanted to avoid similar meddling with the future price of protease inhibitors. It was bad enough that Abbott's protease inhibitor patents had to include a clause that stated the government had helped develop the technology and therefore retained "certain rights" over its eventual use. To most corporate officials that meant only one thing: The government might one day step in and set the drug's price.

There has never been a case where the government has actually marched in and set prices on inventions produced at public expense. Yet the debate over that prerogative has a long and contentious history and became a headline issue after the sea change in U.S. industrial policy that took place in the 1980s as the nation sought to deal with its declining industrial competitiveness.[13] The Bayh-Dole University and Small Business Patent Act and the Stevenson-Wydler Technology Innovation Act—both passed in the waning days of the Carter administration—and the Federal Technology Transfer Act of 1986 established a new paradigm for the transfer of government-funded technology from federal labs and nonprofit institutions to industry. The debate over reasonable pricing of government-funded inventions followed in those bills' legislative wake.

During the 1970s, the U.S. economy suffered its worst economic performance since the Great Depression. Two recessions triggered by oil shortages hammered U.S. industry. Productivity growth rates, which had been better than 2 percent a year throughout the 1950s and 1960s, slipped to just over 1 percent. The economic woes of slow growth and rising unemployment were exacerbated by high and persistent inflation.

A new word—*stagflation*—entered the economic lexicon. Year after year, U.S. companies lost ground to their Japanese and German competitors in markets where Americans had once been preeminent, including automobiles, steel, machine tools, and electronics. Vast swaths of the major cities and towns of the Northeast and Midwest became deindustrialized wastelands. Factories shut down, and their workers were permanently laid off.

Competitiveness gurus in business-oriented think tanks and business schools believed a solution for industry's waning skills lay in the nation's universities and federal labs. The United States had the best scientists and technology in the world, they lamented, but their output was left sitting on the shelf because companies had few incentives to commercialize it. The Kennedy administration had created an open-door technology-transfer policy. In 1963, it stipulated that the government would freely license any invention to all comers if it was going to be used by the general public or if the invention involved the public health or welfare. Though President Nixon tweaked the regulations slightly more in industry's favor, open licensing resulted in most federally funded inventions remaining unused. One study in the late 1970s showed that less than 5 percent of the government's twenty-eight thousand patents had been licensed. Why would a company spend the money to commercialize a scientific invention if any company could rush in and get a similar license once it became a proven success in the marketplace?

As the stagflation decade neared its end, the political will to change the technology transfer landscape cut across party lines. On October 31, 1979, President Carter called for change in a major address to Congress. Soon after, Senators Birch Bayh, a Democrat from Indiana, and Robert Dole, the Kansas Republican, cosponsored a bill designed to encourage commercialization of inventions made by government-funded researchers. Universities and small businesses would be given the patents to discoveries made on government grants, which they could then commercialize as long as the licensing and royalty revenue were shared with the inventor and the university used its share of the proceeds to further research and education. The proposed law also gave federal agencies that held patents the right to offer industry exclusive licenses on their inventions. The Stevenson-Wydler Act gave the same rights to federal labs run by private contractors.

The bills passed, but not before serious qualms were raised by influential voices in and out of Congress. Admiral Hyman Rickover, the straight-talking commander of the nation's nuclear submarine fleet, complained that the legislation would benefit large corporations at the expense of small business. Rep. Jack Brooks, a Democrat from Texas, wanted the patents put out for competitive bid. Senator Russell Long, a Louisiana Democrat and the last of a long line of populists from his state, stated the opposition in its boldest terms: There is "absolutely no reason why the taxpayer should be forced to subsidize a private monopoly and have to pay twice: first for the research and development and then through monopoly prices."

Some protections were built into the bill to assuage the critics. The government retained the right to seize the patent and issue a compulsory license to other manufacturers if it was "necessary to alleviate health or safety needs which are not reasonable satisfied" by the original patent holder. In other words, failure to commercialize an important invention after it had been licensed gave the government the right to "march in" and put it to public use. The law also said that any government-funded invention should be made "available to the public on reasonable terms." In 1989, with the uproar over the price of AZT and Taxol rising, NIH would interpret these clauses as giving the government the right to set prices on drugs developed by the government or on government grants. It began inserting reasonable pricing clauses in all cooperative research and development agreements with industry, which had been authorized by the Federal Technology Transfer Act.[14]

The original public debate over the Bayh-Dole Act swirled around competitiveness issues in basic U.S. industries like machine tools, electronics, and autos. The health of the pharmaceutical and nascent biotechnology industries rarely entered into the discussion, even though NIH had long been one of the major agencies involved in technology transfer. Yet in the wake of the bill's passage, no industries benefited more from the conveyor belt that was set up to move federally funded research from laboratory to industry. The gene-splicing revolution set off an explosion of entrepreneurial activity in the life science departments of the nation's universities and medical schools. The commercialization orgy transformed their institutional culture. For many researchers, the eureka moment no longer came when they discovered a medical breakthrough. Rather, pay dirt was defined as the moment the scientist issued public stock in the company he had set up to commercialize his NIH-funded discovery.

There were some institutional qualms in the early days of the biotechnology-pharmaceutical entrepreneurial revolution, but they didn't last long. Stanford professor Paul Berg, a gene-cloning pioneer, initially criticized UCSF professor Herb Boyer's decision to form Genentech. Yet a few years later he formed his own firm. Walter Gilbert, the Nobel Prize–winning biologist at Harvard, raised a firestorm of criticism when he quit his prestigious post to run Biogen. He retorted: "One half of my colleagues at Harvard are involved in companies in one form or another."[15]

Over the years, numerous university officials, bioethicists, and scientists have complained that the gold-rush mentality inevitably riddled academic medicine with conflicts of interest and threatened the independence of basic research. But those voices went largely unheeded. The system of encouraging commercialization of government-funded inventions has now become thoroughly institutionalized. A survey by the Association of University Technology Managers found that institutions of higher education generated $1.26 billion from licensing revenue in 2000, and university technology transfer officers said most of that came from pharmaceutical and biotechnology firms. Government licensing followed a similar pattern. In 1999, a Government Accounting Office survey of the six major federal agencies with substantial licensing activity found NIH with 990 active licenses, or 71 percent of the total. The public health agency generated fully 95 percent of $107 million in royalties the government received from industry that year.[16] Despite the fears of Abbott and other pharmaceutical firms that licensed those inventions, the government has never exercised the rights enumerated in the patents issued for all those taxpayer-financed inventions.

Abbott's plan to distance its protease inhibitor project from its government roots didn't sit well in Bethesda. Yet NCI's Chabner, in a letter sent back in early January 1992, agreed to the new terms "in the interest of bringing this promising agent to the clinic as rapidly as possible." But he put his own twist on the meeting. NCI would continue to collaborate with Abbott under the new circumstances. Abbott could reimburse NCI for the preclinical expenses already incurred if it liked, but it was Chabner's understanding that future studies would be joint endeavors and that "NCI scientists will direct and monitor these studies as usual." Abbott could go elsewhere for additional studies, but the joint scientific board proposed by Abbott "will have the opportunity to review all preclinical protocols."[17]

In March Abbott brought in a new man to run the clinical side of its antiviral team. John Leonard, who had worked for a small contract research house before coming to Abbott, was under strict marching orders. "We had a decree from our CEO that we would accept no government funding for our work," he said.[18] In one of his initial briefings about the program, Leonard heard stunning news from Kempf, who, with Erickson gone, was heading the science team. Kempf's chemists had synthesized a third potential inhibitor, a chemical cousin of the first two drugs. But this molecule was small enough to take in pill form. It would eventually be called ritonavir. Keeping the news about the better drug strictly in-house, Leonard began working on its intravenous predecessor to prove the new class would work. He decided to ignore the joint advisory committee that had been set up during the November meeting. He asked Sven Danner, an Amsterdam physician whom he knew from work with his previous employer, to conduct the first clinical trials for Abbott's intravenously administered protease inhibitor in Europe.

Word soon got back to Hoth and Chabner, who fired off angry letters to Leonard. "I am dismayed to learn that the NCI was not adequately included in the discussions to initiate clinical trials," Chabner wrote on May 13, 1992. "Based on our written agreement, we expected to be included as a full partner in the efforts to bring this drug to the clinic and were surprised to learn of your plan to delay entry of the drug into testing in the United States." Chabner reminded Leonard of the studies already conducted by government scientists to bring the drug to that point. "Since government funding was used to conduct the majority of the toxicology and pharmacology studies on this drug, we feel that the AIDS patients in the United States have a right to treatment as rapidly as possible." He then cut to the chase. "I realize that Abbott has agreed to reimburse NCI for these studies and hope that a suitable mechanism can be developed to accomplish this stated goal. It was not our intention, however, at the start of this 'collaboration' to act as a contractor for Abbott. Reimbursement would not eliminate the fact that NCI personnel conceived, monitored, and executed these studies over the last year." The angry NCI director fired off copies to the top leaders of both organizations: Broder and Fauci at NIH, and Burnham and Clark at Abbott. He didn't help his cause when he addressed the Abbott chief executive officer as "Dwayne Burham," misspelling both of his names.[19]

A month later Leonard fired back. With first-phase safety tests unregulated in Europe, it would be easier to get studies underway there. "This approach will benefit all HIV-infected patients regardless of their nationality," he wrote. He offered Hoth "a formal line of communication" by allowing an ACTG-affiliated doctor to sit on an advisory committee, but he wouldn't allow official government representation. "You express that NCI should be a full partner in the development of HIV protease inhibitors based on funding provided to Abbott," he wrote. "I must emphasize that [A-77003] was discovered by Abbott and is owned by Abbott. The government funding received by Abbott was and will continue to be a small part of the total development costs." A few weeks later, Abbott sent NCI a check for more than nine hundred thousand dollars to reimburse the government for its expenses for the preclinical work and animal trials.[20]

With the Abbott-NIH dispute at a fever pitch, NIAID director Anthony Fauci trekked to Capitol Hill to defend the Bush administration's 1993 fiscal budget request for AIDS research. At the hearing of the House Commerce Committee's health subcommittee on February 24, 1992, longtime drug industry critic Rep. Henry Waxman, a Democrat from California, wanted to know how much of the $232 million earmarked for government-run clinical trials was going toward combination therapy trials, which he viewed as the most pressing item on the AIDS agenda. Waxman wanted to know if a combination of the anti-HIV drugs that had already been approved by the FDA would be any better for patients than taking just one of the drugs alone. "Was industry a willing participant in those trials?" he asked.

In the early days of AIDS research, it wasn't obvious that it was going to take a combination of drugs to tame the disease. While there was precedent for combination therapies conquering an infectious disease— tuberculosis was the most famous example—the dream of discovering a magic bullet that would take out HIV lived on, especially inside drug companies.

That wasn't Hoth's mindset, though, and he was running the ACTG. The physician-researcher brought years of experience running cancer clinical trials at NCI. "Cancer is all about combination therapy," he said later after moving on to a biotechnology firm on the West Coast. "One of the things I learned at NCI is that there is a difference between a drug focus and a disease focus. At NCI we had one group focused on drugs and one on the disease, and we'd get together on a regular basis to integrate the two. The ultimate benefit is the merger of those two things," he explained. "Early on I created that dual focus in the AIDS division. We needed people who didn't have an allegiance to any particular drug."[21]

In mid-1991, the second NCI-discovered nucleoside reverse transcriptase inhibitor—Bristol-Myers Squibb's ddI—was approved by the FDA. More were on the way. There was also a non-nucleoside reverse transcriptase inhibitor (NNRTI) in the drug approval pipeline. Progress was being made on the protease inhibitor front. To Broder and his colleagues at NCI, the future seemed clear. Writing in the *Journal of the Federation of American Societies for Experimental Biology,* they predicted, "Before long, combination therapies using multiple antiretroviral drugs will be available. Such therapies will exert major effects against the morbidity and mortality caused by HIV."[22]

Indeed, the first combination trials were already underway under ACTG auspices. As early as June 1990 at the sixth International AIDS Conference in San Francisco, Margaret Fischl of the University of Miami and Douglas Richman of the University of California at San Diego had presented preliminary data from ACTG 106. The study was designed to come up with proper dosing when combining AZT and ddC, which NCI had just licensed to Roche for clinical trials. The early results were heartening. Not only was the combination safe enough to take, it appeared to increase the number of infection-fighting white blood cells (scientifically known as CD4 lymphocytes) in the fifty-six patients in the test. The researchers began enrolling patients for a much larger study, ACTG 155, designed to prove once and for all that two drugs were better than one.

Waxman, with the backing of the AIDS lobby, wanted the ACTG to do more. He grilled Fauci at the 1992 hearing. "Is it your professional judgment, then, that if we don't fund this work of combinations to see how well they work that the private sector will not take up that slack?" Fauci had years of experience trekking up to the wood-paneled hearing rooms of the Rayburn Building to parry questions from politicians who almost always had less than perfect information. He was a master of employing the Beltway dodge, especially when a clear-cut answer would offend some powerful special interest. But his recent experiences with the pharmaceutical industry had left a sour taste in his mouth, and his answer that day was more straightforward than usual. "It has generally been our impression that drug companies and pharmaceutical corporations are less likely to want to push or support a trial that compares one drug with another, one of which is theirs and another of which is not theirs," he responded. "And that's one of the reasons and the rationale for the AIDS Clinical Trials Group to study combinations as well as study those kinds of drugs that may not necessarily be of great commercial interest to a company but would be of some public health impact on the disease."

Unlike Abbott and Roche, which were attempting to get by on shoestrings, Merck was pouring substantial resources into the AIDS fight.

After its first protease inhibitor proved toxic, the company's research team began focusing on NNRTIs. Scientists knew why nucleosides worked. They bound to the last link on HIV's DNA chain as it reproduced and brought the additive process to a crashing halt. But no one knew how or why non-nucleosides worked. As a result, all the companies pursuing NNRTIs had to use traditional medicinal-chemistry means to come up with drug candidates—in other words, massive screening. It was labor intensive work, and at Merck it was run by Emilio Emini at the company's sprawling research and manufacturing complex in West Point, Pennsylvania. Spurred on by top management's desire to do something about this dread disease, they hired more people and then hired some more. They expanded the existing containment lab, and when that filled up they built a new building. In the early 1990s, Merck had sixty chemists working on AIDS research and three times that number of support staff. "We were into hundreds of people by that stage," Emini recalled.[23]

The company screened an estimated twenty-three thousand compounds in pursuit of the elusive NNRTI, finally coming up with one in early 1991 that inhibited viral replication. The company's chemistry team made four analogues of the compound and, contrary to customary Merck policy, sent them all into first-stage clinical trials, which are designed to establish safety and a proper dosing level. Early safety trials also determine whether there is enough evidence of efficacy to justify further testing. Though chief executive officer Vagelos and research director Scolnick, both veterans of NIH, were firm believers in keeping the government at arm's length from their chemistry labs, they had no problem cooperating with the ACTG when it came to clinical trials. Trials on L-661 (the most promising NNRTI candidate) were conducted at NIH and at the University of Alabama in Birmingham, a major ACTG site. The company also had trial sites in Brussels, Amsterdam, and Frankfurt.[24]

The firm had another partner in the process: the AIDS activist community. While most drug companies involved in AIDS research found themselves at one time or another in nasty confrontations with the activists, Merck from the outset tried to assuage the industry outsiders. Responding to repeated demands for information about their research, Merck top officials instructed their government and public relations officers to keep the activists informed. What they got in return was a steady stream of desperate applicants anxious to participate in their trials, and advice in designing those trials. "We developed a substantial amount of respect for each other," Emini said.[25]

In early November, Emini and the company's top clinicians met with

AIDS activists to share the results of the first NNRTI tests. The curly haired scientist, an eternal optimist, visibly sagged as he presented the data. The virus quickly mutated around Merck's NNRTI. They would continue one test where L-661 was being used in combination with AZT, but they weren't hopeful. One of the AIDS activists present put an arm around his shoulder and advised him to take two weeks off before getting back to work. The company paid a price for its openness. Within days, articles appeared in the *Wall Street Journal,* the *San Francisco Chronicle,* and the *Philadelphia Inquirer* announcing to the world that Merck's AIDS scientists had come up with another disappointment.[26]

Desperate after four years of AIDS research that had yet to turn up a viable drug candidate, Merck returned to the hunt for a protease inhibitor. While development had continued during the time when NNRTI was in trials, it clearly had been de-emphasized. Now it was their last hope of coming up with a drug to fight the disease. They decided to return to one of the original strategies employed by Irving Sigal, who had died in the crash of Pam Am 103. They deployed X-ray crystallographers to help their chemists design drugs that might work. One of them called Erickson, who was now at NCI, to get his data as they raced to catch up with others in the field.[27] The Merck scientists also borrowed from their competitors. They reproduced Roche's saquinavir, which that company had sent to the patent office in November 1990 and subsequently shared at scientific meetings and "learned that while it was a very potent inhibitor, it had very limited bioavailability."[28] But by combining elements of the Roche compound with elements of their earlier failed protease inhibitor, they came up with a new molecular entity that had spectacular results in the test tube. By August it had been moved into first-stage clinical trials.

To Merck's top brass, the drug candidate called L-735,524, later indinavir, looked like a winner. Its bioavailability and potency seemed vastly superior to either of the two known rivals at Roche and Abbott. Other potential competitors seemed far behind. Coverage of AIDS research in the financial press routinely suggested a dozen companies were working on protease inhibitors. But precious little had emerged at scientific meetings. Biotech companies such as Vertex and Agouron—both firms had been created to pursue rational drug design—had developed a top-flight capability of grabbing headlines. But there was still no evidence that either had gotten anything to work in a test tube, much less move a drug candidate into a clinical setting.

And the people who run clinical trials—largely academic researchers affiliated with university medical complexes in the United States and Europe—do like to talk. By the fall of 1992, Abbott and Roche had their protease inhibitor candidates in first-stage trials in Europe. But management pressure to hold down costs had forced Roche's Bragman to initiate talks with the University of Washington's Ann Collier, a member of the ACTG network, about starting a second-stage trial in the United States. These early trials allowed Merck officials to keep a close eye on the competition. Emini recalled the optimistic mood inside the firm. "Saquinavir [Roche's drug] barely worked. It is not a drug we would ever develop. Ritonavir [Abbott's drug] had several metabolic and drug interaction problems. We would never have developed that either. Ours was potent. It was active," he said.[29]

In May 1993, the company began enrolling patients who had never taken AIDS drugs before for a first-stage test of indinavir's safety and tolerability and to get an initial estimation of its antiviral effect. The trials took place at Thomas Jefferson University Hospital in Philadelphia. Although the company didn't talk about it at the July Berlin conference, indinavir was already well into its first major clinical trial.

The news from the ninth International AIDS Conference in Berlin cast a pall over the entire field of AIDS research. It was especially disheartening for those who believed the key to taming the disease lay in combination therapy. Those hopes had soared earlier in the year when a medical student at Massachusetts General Hospital in Boston had reported that he may have found the "Achilles' heel of HIV." Taiwan-born Yung-Kang Chow had combined three reverse transcriptase inhibitors in a test tube—AZT, ddI, and nevirapine, which was an experimental NNRTI that had been discovered by Boehringer Ingelheim, a German firm whose U.S. operations were based in Ridgefield, Connecticut. Chow's paper in *Nature* suggested the combination eliminated the virus from human cells entirely.[30] It was a remarkable coup for a medical student. While a front-page story in the *New York Times* cautioned that the drug combination was only at the earliest stages of human testing and there was the potential for adverse drug reactions, most readers saw only the "Achilles' heel" statement. Hope in the beleaguered AIDS patient community soared. The ACTG, under pressure from AIDS activists, threw the three-drug combination into a four-hundred-person clinical trial, twice the size of the trial originally sought by Martin Hirsch, who was Chow's supervisor at Harvard Medical School and a leading member of the ACTG network.

By the end of July, the hope that combination therapy would cure AIDS patients was, if not defeated, in full retreat. The European Concorde trial's preliminary results had shown that early use of AZT did not prolong life any longer than waiting until the disease had manifested itself. The study results, when first reported in the British biomedical journal *Lancet* in April, had sent Burroughs Wellcome's stock plunging.[31] In desperation, many dying patients began using AZT in combination with one of the other two nucleosides that had been approved, ddC and ddI. The FDA, in granting their approvals, had suggested they be used in combination with AZT since neither by itself had been shown to be more effective than the first AIDS drug. The combinations worked better, the agency seemed to be saying.

But in Berlin, the University of Miami's Margaret Fischl reported the long-awaited results of ACTG 155, the trial that combined AZT and ddC. The definitive study showed that taking the two together was no better than taking each one separately. The original studies for AZT had shown that while the drug was effective in slowing the progression of disease, the virus mutated, and within a year almost half of the patients were once again being ravaged by opportunistic infections as their immune systems deteriorated. ACTG 155, which had followed patients for up to three years, showed that 42 percent of patients taking AZT became seriously ill or died, as did 43 percent on ddC and 39 percent on the combination, a statistically insignificant difference. The only positive result was that those patients who entered the trial with higher CD4 counts did somewhat better, suggesting early treatment might improve an HIV carrier's long-term prospects. Fischl emphasized that relatively minor point in her presentation to the meeting, which infuriated the AIDS activists present. David Barr, a New York City lawyer and ACT UP member, stepped to one of the floor microphones. "The answer to the study you designed is that the study shows no difference between combo and monotherapy," he shouted. "You have staked your career on these drugs. I have staked my life."[32]

Combination therapy suffered another setback in late July when Harvard Medical School announced that Chow's original test-tube study on the three-drug cocktail was flawed. Scientists at the Wellcome Research Laboratories in England and the Pasteur Institute in France had challenged the study. Hirsch and Chow, forced to retest their samples, sheepishly admitted that mutant HIV did in fact eventually overwhelm the combination. Lawrence Altman, the physician-journalist who covered

AIDS for the *New York Times*, wrote a scathing attack on the govern-ment-funded research establishment. "It points up the risks run by sci-entists and federal health officials when they rush into clinical trials on the grounds that a lethal disease justifies greater speed," he wrote. "AIDS scientists work in the hope that their findings may stop a major scourge as well as bring personal glory."[33]

Altman hedged his comments deeper in the article by reporting many experts still believed the desperate situation with AIDS justified testing drugs in combination or in sequence. "Other evidence, in addition to the now-flawed theory, supports the triple-drug therapy," he wrote.[34] But the drug companies developing the next generation of AIDS drugs weren't listening.

6

Breakthrough!

Combination therapy wasn't on the minds of Abbott, Hoffman–La Roche, or Merck as they moved their most promising protease inhibitor candidates into full-scale clinical trials. They wanted blockbusters, a billion-dollar seller. For AIDS, where the ultimate market size was thought to be limited, that meant monotherapy.

By the summer of 1993, Abbott Laboratories had already dropped its intravenously administered protease inhibitor that European physicians had presented in Berlin. Earlier that year, Kempf and his small chemistry team had come up with an analogue of the huge molecule that passed its initial test-tube experiments. Leonard quickly approved it for clinical trials. Its chief attraction was that it could be administered orally. While European clinics began testing this second candidate in patients, Kempf continued cooking up new possibilities.

Shortly after Labor Day, Kempf cautiously advised Leonard that his group had come up with a third protease inhibitor candidate. The senior official gathered the small group of Abbott scientists working on AIDS in a conference room to showcase the molecule. An air of expectancy filled the room. Kempf, a quiet, self-effacing bench scientist, rarely spoke up during their regularly scheduled brainstorming sessions. Asking for time on the agenda meant he was onto something.

Deploying a series of overhead slides, Kempf showed how he had re-configured one side of his original symmetrical molecule to make it eas-ier to absorb through the gut. The change had not knocked out its effec-tiveness in blocking protease action in the test tube. Best of all, Kempf's preliminary tests in animals showed one of the analogues of this new molecule stayed in the bloodstream for hours rather than being quickly metabolized by the liver and excreted. "I want that drug," Leonard said. A-87538, later known as ritonavir, moved almost immediately into human trials. The patent application, filed September 14, 1993, still con-tained the government rights clause since work on the molecule was completed while the company was still receiving government money. The five-year government research grant, which Abbott had used to provide support for Kempf, expired two weeks before the patent application.[1]

While Abbott had relied on European physicians to test its two previ-ous candidates, Leonard was now prepared to return to the United States for clinical trials. His way was eased by the close relationship that Kempf had forged with David Ho, the director of the Aaron Diamond AIDS Research Center in New York City.

Kempf first met Ho in late 1991 at a Florida conference that brought together several hundred of the world's leading AIDS researchers. Ho, an ambitious virologist, was eager to learn more about Abbott's protease inhibitor project, which was revealed for the first time at the conference. Philanthropist Irene Diamond had shocked the AIDS research world when she chose Ho to run her well-endowed new center, and two years later he was still scrambling to establish its program. The two men struck up a conversation after bumping into each other in a car rental checkout line. Ho offered to run tests on Kempf's newly synthesized chemicals for their antiretroviral activity. His offer was timely. Kempf's superiors had just cut the firm's ties to the National Cancer Institute (NCI) article, which had previously done those tests. Kempf needed a new partner. "They didn't have a lot of virology in-house," Ho recalled.[2] Kempf be-gan sending his drug candidates to New York instead of Bethesda.

Ho's relationship with Abbott would eventually lead to the central theoretical breakthrough that underpinned the emergence of triple-cocktail therapy. The contribution would later earn Ho worldwide fame as *Time* magazine's 1996 "Man of the Year," even though George Shaw of the University of Alabama at Birmingham shares the credit in the sci-entific literature. For Ho, the breakthrough brought together the threads of his entire career and would not have been possible without crucial support from Los Alamos National Laboratory.

Born in mainland China in 1952, Ho was raised in the United States and graduated from the Massachusetts Institute of Technology and Harvard Medical School. He was a medical resident at UCLA's Cedars-Sinai Medical Center in 1981 when doctors there reported the world's first known AIDS cases. The budding virologist immediately gravitated to the new field. In 1982, Ho accepted a postdoctoral fellowship in Martin Hirsch's lab at Massachusetts General Hospital, where he raced to become the first to discover the virus that caused AIDS. He lost that battle, but through his daily contact with AIDS patients he gleaned crucial insights into the dynamics of the disease. In 1985 he coauthored a paper that first described the flulike symptoms that accompanied a person's initial HIV infection.[3] But it would take the emergence of protease inhibitors nearly a decade later before he learned the deeper significance of his own observations. At the time, he, like most AIDS researchers, believed infected individuals built up antibodies to knock down the initial infection, and those antibodies kept the retrovirus in a near dormant state for years before losing their potency.

He carried those beliefs with him when he moved from Boston to the new Aaron Diamond Center, which provided the young scientist with an ideal setting for pursuing intriguing avenues of research. Irene Diamond, the wife of a wealthy New York real estate developer who was devoted to medical research and the arts, believed the city that was an epicenter of the AIDS epidemic needed to do more to combat the disease. Forging a partnership with the New York City Department of Health, her foundation created the specialized center in 1988 and pledged $220 million over the next ten years for its support. The center officially opened next door to Bellevue Hospital in 1991.

Often overlooked in policy debates, nonprofit institutions like the Aaron Diamond Center have long been major players in biomedical research. The Howard Hughes Medical Institute, for instance, which was endowed by the reclusive billionaire's fortune and is located around the corner from NIH headquarters, pours more than a half billion dollars a year into basic and applied medical research. The research arm of the practice-oriented Mayo Clinic, which is headquartered in Rochester, Minnesota, spends more than $125 million a year of its own resources on applied research. Like most nonprofits, even the best endowed, the Aaron Diamond Center's permanent staff also competes for government funds. Ho and his colleagues received major AIDS-related grants from both NIH and New York City. Coupled with the Diamond family's generous bequest, Ho had the wherewithal to forge an independent relationship with drug companies that were looking for help in testing their new drugs but wanted to steer clear of the government's AIDS Clinical Trials Group (ACTG).

In early 1994, Ho's relationship with Kempf at Abbott blossomed. Leonard included the Aaron Diamond Center on his short list of clinics testing the company's latest and most promising protease inhibitor. Ho and his colleague Martin Markowitz began testing ritonavir in twenty AIDS patients. In designing the trial, they relied on a brief first trial that had been conducted in Europe. Like all first trials, the drug had been tested alone to determine its safety and an appropriate dose. How much can be given before intolerable side effects kicked in? How much needed to be taken to have an effect on the virus? How often must it be taken to maintain an appropriate level in the blood throughout the day? Most early protease inhibitors had to be taken in large amounts two or three times a day because they were cleared by the liver soon after entering the bloodstream.

The patients in the second-stage trial at Aaron Diamond were given fairly high doses of ritonavir. A few months into the trial, the clinicians began pouring over the data to get the first hints of the drug's effectiveness. They were aided by the recent arrival of the first tests that could measure the amount of HIV in the blood. Previous tests to gauge the progression of the disease had measured either the level of disease-fighting white blood cells or the antibodies that fought HIV. Now scientists could actually measure viral load.

The results from that first U.S. trial for ritonavir stunned Ho and his colleagues. None of the earlier AIDS drugs had shown such rapid and dramatic ability to clear the virus. "[Of] the first twenty patients we treated, each one had their viral load drop fifty to one-hundred-fold in the first two weeks," he recalled. "That was a crucial moment for us in this whole field because it showed how potent protease inhibitors could be."[4] Abbott also tested ritonavir at the University of Alabama at Birmingham, where Shaw was turning up similar results. Danner in Amsterdam also participated. By April, the data were streaming into Abbott Park. The drug worked—spectacularly so. But hidden in the data were hints of disaster. Patients rapidly developed resistance to ritonavir, just as they had to AZT and the other nucleosides before it.

While Abbott massaged its data, Ho and his colleagues pondered the implications of their limited test results. Markowitz's test-tube experiments on ritonavir had shown that HIV was capable of mutating around the protease inhibitor. Though it required several simultaneous mutations along the protease's genome before it escaped the drug's blocking action, it happened relatively quickly, the test-tube results showed. The Aaron Diamond Center team wasn't surprised when the same thing happened in humans. What did surprise them was the rapid escalation in the levels of HIV in the blood once the mutant strain emerged. For years, scientists had believed the AIDS retrovirus hid in the bloodstream and the lymph nodes at fairly low levels until it somehow broke out and overwhelmed the immune system. But the rapid reemergence of HIV after an initial knockout punch delivered by the protease inhibitor suggested a very different scenario.

Ho, never a math whiz, sent his data to Alan Perelson, a biophysicist at Los Alamos in New Mexico. Ho had gotten his name from a scientist in his lab who had met Perelson at a scientific meeting, one of the chance encounters that often start significant scientific collaborations. After crunching Ho's numbers on a spreadsheet, Perelson delivered his verdict. HIV-infected cells weren't part of a guerrilla army hiding in the hills. They were waging a Gallipoli-style campaign in the bloodstream, sending wave after wave of the proliferating retrovirus against the immune system. Perelson estimated that HIV reproduced at a rate of 680 million viral particles a day.

The finding had two major implications. First, the immune systems of HIV-infected individuals waged a valiant and largely successful fight to clear the virus that went on for years. It was only when the immune system gave up the fight (for as yet unexplained reasons) that the HIV army overwhelmed the carrier. Second, since the virus was reproducing so quickly, drug-resistant strains were bound to emerge. Indeed, given HIV's replication rate, they would emerge very quickly. Scientists studying the process of genetic transcription during reproduction have known since the early 1970s that every time a genome reproduces, the offspring has at least one mutation somewhere along the strand of chemical base pairs that makes up its genetic code. Most are benign since they either do not affect a gene's function or occur at places on the genome that don't have a function. But the HIV genome was only ten thousand base pairs long. With 680 million new viral particles entering the bloodstream every day (a number since raised to more than a billion), Perelson believed every base pair on the HIV genome was mistakenly transcribed not just once, but thousands of times a day. That meant that a mutant that could escape a single drug's action and still maintain its essential function was almost a certainty. Indeed, it probably happened within hours of the drug's introduction into the bloodstream.[5]

That summer, Ho attended another of the many annual scientific conferences aimed at AIDS researchers, this one in Seattle. Over a dinner arranged by Dani Bolognesi, a senior researcher at Duke University who had helped Burroughs Wellcome conduct the first trials on AZT in the mid-1980s, Ho and Shaw of Alabama compared notes on their single-drug trials. "We looked at each other and realized we had made the same observation," Ho recalled. The retrovirus reproduced so fast and mutated so often that it was going to take a number of drugs to knock it out. A single drug aimed at a single target was doomed to failure. But hitting it with drugs that effectively blocked a number of targets simultaneously would make mutant survival extremely difficult. Indeed, according to Perelson's computers, it was almost a mathematical impossibility. "The odds of making five or six mutations simultaneously are one in a trillion," Ho said. "Those are odds we like." [6]

Their job now was to tell the world. In the fall of 1994, the Interscience Conference on Antimicrobial Agents and Chemotherapy, the major annual conference of the American Society for Microbiology, gathered in Orlando, Florida. Ho and Shaw were both slated to give major addresses to a plenary session on emerging AIDS therapies, and both wanted to release their latest data. Abbott's Pernet and Leonard flew in from Chicago. Ho asked if he could present his findings. Leonard hesitated. Abbott was still debating how to move forward with the final clinical trials needed for Food and Drug Administration (FDA) approval. The senior company scientist still wanted to know if ritonavir could work as monotherapy if given at a higher dose. Ho said no. "Everybody was looking for a home run, but we didn't put a lot of stock in that," Ho recalled. Abbott gave the go-ahead to release the study data at the meeting and began laying plans for ritonavir's final clinical trials.

Companies with promising new drugs had one obvious incentive for working with the ACTG on clinical trials. It saved them a lot of money. In an ACTG trial, the company often did little more than supply the drug. The government-funded clinicians at academic medical centers recruited the patients, paid for their care and blood tests, and kept track of the records. These clinical tasks were by far the costliest component of clinical trials, and the AIDS program of the National Institute for Allergies and Infectious Diseases (NIAID) spent hundreds of millions of dollars a year supporting them. However, there were trade-offs for pharmaceutical firms that chose to cooperate with the government, which took place at both ends of the experiment. On the front end, the company didn't have the final say in designing the trial (although as a practical matter, academic researchers worked closely with company doctors on trial design because they wanted to maintain good relations for future access to drug candidates coming out of their labs). On the back end, the company had no control over the release of a study's conclusions.

Hoffman–La Roche's clinicians gladly accepted those limitations, given top management's decision to veto more money on the search for a better protease inhibitor candidate or new trials that might escalate the acceptable dose of their poorly absorbed drug, saquinavir. Indeed, by the time saquinavir entered clinical trials through the ACTG in 1993, the company had several years' experience working with government-funded clinicians. Between 1990 and 1992, the ACTG conducted Roche's trials for ddC, the nucleoside reverse transcriptase inhibitor that the company had licensed from NCI.

Those trials took place in an environment that had been radically transformed by nearly six years of AIDS activism, which dated from playwright Larry Kramer's fiery speech in a Greenwich Village church in March 1987. Over those six years, angry AIDS activists had forced the most dramatic liberalization in FDA rules in the agency's history. Most of these changes were welcomed by the drug industry since they hastened approval of new drugs. But liberalization had unwanted side effects. The activists simultaneously blasted open the opaque process for designing ACTG trials, won expanded access to drugs while in clinical trials, and held up every corporate decision that might affect the health of AIDS patients to public scrutiny. Those were changes the industry could do without.

As early as June 1987, FDA commissioner Frank Young had unveiled new regulations in direct response to the exploding AIDS crisis and the fact that dying AIDS patients across the country were clamoring to get into the recently concluded AZT trials. Young's new rules encouraged companies that were testing experimental AIDS drugs to give them to the doctors of desperately sick patients who weren't lucky enough to be part of the trials. The policy became known as compassionate use or expanded access and set off grumbling among traditionalists within the agency and outside safety advocates. Both groups feared that unproven and potentially deadly drugs would be unleashed on a population that was willing to swallow almost anything to stay alive.

Sixteen months later the agency loosened its rules another notch. When evaluating new drugs that tackled life-threatening diseases like AIDS, the FDA would grant so-called accelerated approval if a company presented positive results from a limited set of first- and second-stage trials. The only quid pro quo for a company seeking accelerated approval was a promise to conduct postapproval studies to document the drug's impact once in general use.

The first ddC trial, headed by Margaret Fischl at the University of Miami and Douglas Richman at the University of California at San Diego, threw a third liberalization into the mix. ACTG 106, which was conducted during 1989 and 1990, was designed as an early-stage study to determine what doses to use when combining ddC with AZT. AIDS patients, especially those who had been on AZT and were failing, were exhilarated by early results from that trial, which were unveiled in San Francisco in June 1990. Patients on the two-drug combination who had entered the trial with severely compromised immune systems saw their count of infection-fighting CD4 cells double within days. John James, writing in *AIDS Treatment News,* an activist newsletter, noted that the trial "had established a de facto standard of care among many of the best-informed patients and physicians."[7]

The problem from the FDA's point of view was that measuring surrogate markers like CD4 cells didn't tell the agency anything about the long-term effectiveness of the drug being tested. Did it delay death? Did it delay the onset of opportunistic infections? Surrogate markers were used elsewhere in medicine. Drugs that lowered blood pressure or cholesterol to reduce the risk of heart disease had been approved on that basis. But their approvals were based on long, costly trials that established the connection between the surrogate marker and the progression of the disease. Many AIDS activists wanted approval for ddC and ddI, Bristol-Myers Squibb's nucleoside that was moving through the approval process at about the same time, based only on the improvement in the CD4 cell marker. Their position was endorsed by NIAID in February 1991 and given regulatory sanction that summer when the FDA, now under David Kessler, approved ddI for use after a divisive public hearing of the agency's Antiviral Advisory Committee.

A year later the FDA approved Roche's ddC using just surrogate marker data. However, the FDA overruled the company's request that the new drug be approved for monotherapy, which Roche had requested. Roche failed to show that using it alone was any more effective than AZT alone. Still, the transformation of the drug approval landscape was complete. In late 1992, the FDA codified final accelerated approval regulations in the federal register. The rules stated a drug could be approved based on surrogate marker data (for AIDS drugs, the best surrogate marker at that time was the CD4 changes) if it was "reasonably likely" the changes would predict clinical benefit. "We cannot wait for all the evidence to come in when people are suffering and dying from these devastating diseases," Kessler said.[8]

While activists were pushing the FDA to loosen its drug approval criteria, they were also attacking the NIAID and the ACTG for failing to get more drugs into the pipeline. Their repeated protests outside NIH headquarters in Bethesda convinced Fauci and Hoth to open up their grants process. In the early days of the AIDS fight, the ACTG had followed the traditional NIH pattern in approving new trials. Investigators proposed studies, and secret panels made up of their peers approved their funding. But in late 1989, Fauci agreed to open all ACTG meetings to the general public and put several AIDS activists, including Mark Harrington of the Treatment Access Group, a spin-off from the New York chapter of ACT UP, on the governing board. By the time Keith Bragman and Miklos Salgo of Roche approached the ACTG to conduct a second-stage trial on saquinavir, Harrington had emerged as the AIDS community's most trenchant critic of drug companies' efforts to manipulate the new rules to their own advantage. The Harvard-educated freelance scriptwriter, who was HIV-positive, had also learned enough science to become an astute observer of the medical implications of clinical trial design.

The Roche team faced an impossible situation as it entered negotiations with the ACTG for testing saquinavir. The first-stage studies in Europe had not established a maximum tolerated dose for the drug because Roche's top management had cut off funding for further tests. Patients in those early trials were already taking eighteen capsules a day, yet the drug's level in the blood remained low because of its poor absorption, estimated to be about 4 percent. Could patients tolerate even higher doses without crippling side effects? No one knew. It wasn't a minor question. Giving someone a suboptimal dose of the drug might allow the rapid emergence of resistance. Nevertheless, the company proposed studying the new drug in combination with AZT and in combination with AZT and ddC, which by the fall of 1992 were the generally accepted standards of care for advanced AIDS patients.

The ACTG committee that approved clinical trials met in mid-1992 to discuss the proposed trial, which became known as ACTG 229. Harrington immediately began raising questions about the design of the study. Why was the dose so low? Would a patient who failed a therapy regimen containing saquinavir have bred a virus in his or her body that would be resistant to other protease inhibitors when they came along? The University of Washington's Collier, who was the study's principal investigator, briefly left the room with the Roche representative to discuss the company's earlier European studies, whose results had not been fully released to the committee.[9] "We wanted to make sure there's an effective dose, shown to have activity," said Collier. "A small group of leaders of the ACTG were shown confidential data that proved we had an adequate dose that had activity. In the end, there is a limit to the number of pills any one person can take. The dose was subjected to a lot of scrutiny—by me, by the ACTG, and by Roche itself."[10]

The committee voted to allow ACTG 229 to move forward. Collier and her colleagues enrolled 302 patients between March and July 1993 for a twenty-four-week trial that used surrogate markers to evaluate the various drug regimens. New tests that had recently come on the market allowed the clinicians to measure not only the level of CD4 cells in the blood, but the patient's level of HIV. These viral load tests, as they became known, were considered a superior indicator. The preliminary results weren't released until May 1994 and showed slightly better results in the three-drug combination than with either AZT alone or in combination with ddC. "While the results weren't fabulous compared to what came later, it was clearly better than we had at the time," Collier later said.

Roche management's failure to fund tests of higher doses of the drug may have saved the company money in the short run, but its long-term costs were enormous. Because ACTG 229 used a suboptimal dose of saquinavir, the scientific community lost a golden opportunity to obtain early knowledge of the potential effectiveness of triple-combination therapy.

It wasn't just bad science, it was bad business since the company lost its first-mover advantage. In the drug industry, the first company to develop an entry for a new class of drugs—assuming its entry is effective—almost always gains the lion's share of the market. But as subsequent tests would show, saquinavir in its original formulation was not a very effective drug because of its poor bioavailability.

Fearing Roche would use ACTG 229 to pursue accelerated approval at the FDA, a coalition of AIDS activist groups centered on the East Coast asked the agency to hold off on rapid approval for saquinavir. "We feel that such an approval would penalize people with AIDS/HIV by setting an inappropriately low standard of evidential requirements that would govern the regulation of this entire class of therapies," they wrote in a joint letter to Kessler. Pointing to Roche's failure to conduct follow-up studies on ddC after its rapid approval in 1992, the activists complained that "we have learned through difficult experience that we cannot depend on the goodwill of pharmaceutical industry sponsors to produce the information that is necessary to make life-or-death treatment decisions."[11]

The letter set off a firestorm of controversy within the AIDS activist community, stoked in part by Roche's decision to fax copies of the letter to other AIDS groups across the country. West Coast activists in particular accused the Treatment Access Group and its allies of denying life-saving medications to people with AIDS, who were clamoring to get their hands on the new drug. The FDA, accustomed to vilification for going too slowly, was stunned by the opposite charge, especially after a headline appeared over an August 1994 cover story in *Barron's* magazine asking, "Do We Have Too Many Drugs for AIDS?" The agency held a two-day hearing that fall, giving industry officials and anxious AIDS activists a chance to attack Harrington and his allies publicly. There would be no change in the FDA's policy of accepting surrogate markers when approving new drugs for AIDS.

Kessler's decision was defensible at the time and later proven scientifically correct. But politics played a huge role in the decision. That fall the American political scene underwent an upheaval the likes of which hadn't been seen in several generations. Republicans led by Rep. Newt Gingrich of Georgia won control of the House of Representatives. One of the core planks in their "Contract with America" called for dismantling the regulatory burdens on business. The drug industry played a key role in fueling those changes. Its famous Harry and Louise ads—"Keep the government out of our medicine chest"—had helped turn public opinion against the Clinton administration's health care plan, which included elements designed to control the rising cost of drugs.

The industry also engaged that fall in a massive lobbying campaign to convince NIH to eliminate its reasonable pricing clause on therapies developed with government funds. Academic researchers complained they were being cut off from the most promising new drugs being developed in industry's laboratories. Responding to their pleas, a new NIH director, Harold Varmus, held two hearings on the subject in the second half of 1994. Industry representatives crowded the docket with testimony suggesting the mere threat of price controls was keeping its scientists from cooperating with their government-funded counterparts at NIH.

In April 1995, Varmus ordered his technology transfer office to eliminate all references to reasonable pricing in future NIH agreements with the pharmaceutical industry. "The pricing clause has driven industry away from potentially beneficial scientific collaborations with Public Health Service scientists," Varmus said in a prepared statement. "One has to have a product to price before one can worry about how to price it." Democrats decried a move they said would open the floodgates to price gouging. But there was nothing they could do about it. "No one is oblivious to the political climate," commented Senator Ron Wyden, a Democrat from Orgeon.[12]

But the change came too late to corral Roche back into the government program. In the summer of 1994, after consulting with the FDA about the results from ACTG 229 and realizing it wasn't going to get accelerated approval, the company began planning for the final third-stage trials. In two trials in the United States and Europe, company-paid physicians recruited more than four thousand AIDS patients for a final study of saquinavir's efficacy. Patients in just one of the studies' seven arms received three anti-AIDS drugs. By early 1995 the tests were under-way. To assuage its critics in the AIDS community, the company agreed to a generous expanded access program, offering the drug to an additional four thousand patients through a lottery. "There have been improvements in the manufacturing and the number of steps required [has been re-duced]," Jürgen Drews, Roche's president of research, told the editors of Gay Men's Health Crisis' *Treatment Issues*. "We now think we can pro-duce the drug in sufficient quantities and at a price that is feasible."[13]

The company presented its preliminary results at the FDA's antiviral advisory committee meeting on November 7, 1995. By this time, the AIDS field was well aware how quickly resistance could emerge when patients were treated with a single drug. Ho and Shaw had presented their data on viral replication at a major conference in Washington early in the year. Martin Markowitz of the Aaron Diamond Center presented data from his ritonavir trials showing the rapid emergence of resistance to the drug in monotherapy and, alarmingly, those strains' widespread cross-resistance to other protease inhibitors then in development. The answer was plain: The drug had to be used in combination with other drugs. "One drug won't work. Two drugs won't work. Three drugs might work. Four drugs can cure," Markowitz reported.[14]

To counter the mounting evidence against monotherapy, Roche began releasing information from its ongoing follow-up studies with patients in its earlier trials. At a July conference in Sardinia, Italy, a company physi-cian suggested to AIDS activists that saquinavir did not cause resistance for at least a year after beginning monotherapy or in combination with other drugs, and those new strains of HIV were not cross-resistant to other protease inhibitors.[15] Indeed, when the company went before the FDA advisory committee in early November, it did not present any data from its ongoing triple-combination study. It relied instead on the smaller of its two third-stage trials, which tested saquinavir as monotherapy and in combination with ddC, the company's other AIDS drug. The company's application asked for approval as either a monotherapy or in combination with other already approved anti-HIV drugs. "It was the first HIV protease inhibitor," said Bragman. "It was the first of a new class of drugs. We really had no idea what was going to happen in that hearing."[16] The committee recommended against monotherapy.

On December 7, the FDA approved saquinavir, a little over three months after Roche had submitted its new drug application. It was the fastest turnaround in the agency's history. But the agency, following its usual custom of hewing closely to the advisory committee's advice, turned down Roche's request for monotherapy. The approved label said the drug should only be used with one or more already approved nucleosides and preferably ones that a patient had never used before.

FDA's interactions with pharmaceutical companies during a drug's development are not public records since companies demand privacy to keep their test results hidden from potential competitors (and the prying eyes of Wall Street if tests go poorly). But drug approval letters often contain a review of their developmental history. The FDA reviewer of saquinavir dated the agency's concern about the drug's poor bioavailability from the initiation of human trials. The reviewer recalled how the agency had suggested that Roche try saquinavir at higher doses, which would probably require a new formulation. Roche had rejected those pleas as it moved into its final clinical trials. It told the federal agency that it was "not feasible to either commercialize or study greater doses" because of "manufacturing limitations."[17]

Roche's official comments to the FDA were radically at odds with its public posture. At the same time that it was kicking off those trials, Drews was telling AIDS activists that the company had overcome the manufacturing problems. And during 1995, the year of the final trials, the company had enough capsules of its drug to expand access to more than four thousand patients.

Technical difficulties and the cost of manufacturing had indeed been a major issue for drug companies when they started their research programs on protease inhibitors. The drugs are large, complicated mole-

cules. But the companies rapidly mastered the art of how to produce protease inhibitors in large quantities and at reasonable costs. That there are
no inherent difficulties in manufacturing the drug would be proven in the
late 1990s when Cipla, a drug manufacturer in India, began producing its
version of Merck's indinavir for less than one thousand dollars a year.[18]

Yet those facts remained hidden from public view when Roche got its
FDA approval letter for saquinavir. The next day, the company began
wholesaling the drug at a price of $5,800 per year per patient. Martin
Delaney, the head of San Francisco's Project Inform, the AIDS activist
group with much closer ties to the drug industry than its East Coast
counterparts, told the *Wall Street Journal* he was "appalled" by Roche's
price, which was three times higher than any AIDS medicine then on the
market.[19]

As it launched its final round of trials on ritonavir, Abbott continued to
steer clear of the ACTG. It also refused to cooperate with other drug
companies. In mid-1993, a consortium of drug companies pursuing
AIDS-related research launched the Intercompany Collaboration (ICC).
The idea was to test combinations of AIDS drugs. Sixteen drug companies eventually joined the group. Though it received a lot of press attention when launched, the ICC never made a significant contribution to the
field. Neither Abbott's nor Merck's protease inhibitors were included in
the ICC's first major test, which was initiated in June 1994. Instead, the
intercompany collaborators used the same inadequate dose of Roche's
saquinavir that was used in the triple-combination arm of Roche's own
trial.

The research officials at the companies involved in AIDS research
were publicly committed to the idea that an effective AIDS regimen
would require cooperation. But their competitive instincts and the internal imperative to pursue big-selling drugs (or turn every drug under
development into a big seller) precluded meaningful collaboration. "That
was an organization where pharmaceutical companies could look like
they were collaborating because it looked like AIDS required collaboration," Abbott's Leonard said much later. "But people didn't share the
information that mattered because people are highly competitive. I never
went to an ICC meeting. People who went from other companies told me
it was a huge waste of time."[20]

Instead, Abbott ran its independent third-stage ritonavir trials in various clinics around the world. The dose-ranging studies conducted in
Europe during late 1994 had shown the drug had impressive antiviral

activity. But three to four months after the onset of monotherapy, the viral loads in patients returned to their original levels, which suggested the virus had mutated around the drug. Despite those results, only Ho's admonitions finally convinced the company it had to pursue combination therapy in addition to its preferred monotherapy trials.

The company's final two trials tested nearly fifteen hundred patients with either ritonavir alone or in combination with the patient's existing therapy, which for most meant AZT. The company also initiated a third study in France to test ritonavir in combination with two nucleosides, AZT and ddC. But they enrolled just thirty-two patients. This small trial provided the company, and eventually the world, with the first dramatic evidence of the success of triple combination therapy.

The company presented its preliminary results for the tiny French trial at the Interscience Conference on Antimicrobial Agents and Chemotherapy (ICAAC) meeting in San Francisco in the fall of 1995. The results wowed the AIDS activists who attended the meeting. The company that had broken free of the government and then labored in secrecy for more than two years went public with the most startling results in AIDS therapy to date. Daniel Norbeck, then only thirty-seven years old, presented the data. Norbeck, who had received his undergraduate chemistry degree from Wheaton College, an evangelical Christian school in the western suburbs of Chicago, before earning his doctorate from the California Institute of Technology, reported that more than half the patients in the trial had cleared 99.9 percent of the virus from their bloodstreams. "The reservoirs of virus are emptying," Norbeck declared. The reaction among activists was a mixture of joy and disbelief. "It is debatable whether Dr. Norbeck can claim such success on the basis of one small study," one activist said.[21]

Norbeck, who several years later would become head of Abbott's pharmaceutical research division, had other good news for the meeting. What had been considered a major flaw in ritonavir—its propensity to impede the liver's ability to clear many drugs from the body—actually might turn out to be a major plus. When mixed with saquinavir, a small amount of ritonavir (eventually given the trade name Norvir to honor Norbeck's role in the latter stages of its development) kept the Roche drug in the bloodstream of rats long enough for it to have its potent antiviral effect. The company announced plans to begin testing the combination in humans immediately.

While that testing would eventually prove a boon to the marketing of ritonavir, it wouldn't be part of the data that Abbott presented to the

FDA's antiviral advisory committee on the last day of February 1996. The pivotal trial presented to the committee added either ritonavir or a placebo to patients already on drug therapy. That was either AZT alone or AZT and ddC. The company did not report on the subgroup on triple-combination therapy. After twenty-four weeks, the death rate and onset of opportunistic infections among those patients given ritonavir alone was half that of the placebo group, Abbott officials told the federal reviewers. The second trial presented to the reviewers, which did not contain any patients on triple combination, had peculiar results. Patients on ritonavir alone did better than those taking both AZT and ritonavir. Abbott admitted that "patients on combination therapy may have been less compliant with their drug regimen," the FDA's reviewer wrote. "This may have explained the poorer performance of combination treatment in this study."[22]

The next day, the FDA granted Abbott a license to sell ritonavir. The agency's approved label said the drug could be given either as monotherapy or in combination with existing antiretrovirals. Two days later, Abbott began shipping the drug to pharmacies across the country. It cost sixty-five hundred dollars for a year's supply. The retail price hit a stunning eight thousand dollars a year—a price not seen on a single AIDS drug since the early days of AZT. Combination therapy, the new coin of the AIDS therapy realm, soared to nearly fifteen thousand dollars a year.[23]

The dream of a monotherapy knockout punch died hard at Merck, too. The initial reports on indinavir's first clinical trials, which took place in late 1993, sent hopes soaring at the company's research headquarters in West Point, Pennsylvania. The drug had a "marked antiviral effect in monotherapy." Its ability to lower viral loads immediately and its bioavailability suggested indinavir was going to be a superior drug to the competitive products being cooked up by Abbott and Roche. "We were delirious," research director Edward Scolnick later noted. "We absolutely thought we had the cure for AIDS: monotherapy."[24]

But through the early months of 1994, the handful of patients who were on indinavir began exhibiting the same pattern that had affected every AIDS drug that came before. A few months into therapy, viral loads began creeping back up to where they had been before the drug treatments began. Emini and Jeffrey Chodakewitz, the Merck physician in charge of clinical trials, suspected that the AIDS virus had once again figured out a way to mutate around the best efforts of scientists to control it. Yet there was one mysterious patient, dubbed patient 142, a "wise-cracking, forty-one-year-old law student from Philadelphia," whose viral load had gone down and stayed down.[25] Perhaps his story contained the key to understanding how indinavir knocked out the AIDS virus. Merck needed to keep the tests going.

Late one evening, just as Scolnick was sitting down to dinner with his wife, Emini called him with the bad news–good news story. The virus appeared to be mutating around their new drug. But one patient seemed to be doing well. Scolnick heard only the first part of the message. His dinner ruined, Scolnick immediately went over his own scientists' heads to get a second opinion. He called Anthony Fauci, the head of the NIAID and the government's leading AIDS expert. After explaining their results, Fauci confirmed the bad news. "Ed, you've got resistance," he said.[26] Merck's research team once again faced the prospect that it had come up empty.

For weeks Merck scientists batted ideas back and forth about how to keep the protease inhibitor project moving forward. The fact that one patient was improving on indinavir alone suggested to some that the dose may not have been high enough. Although they didn't have access to David Ho's data, Merck scientists also realized that the rapid emergence of resistance meant the virus was reproducing at an extraordinarily fast rate. Perhaps, they finally admitted, they should hit it with two or more drugs at once. They won management approval for a second set of clinical trials to test the drug at higher doses and in combination with other antiretrovirals. "Because of 142, some of us argued that [indinavir] was doing something right," Emini later told the *Wall Street Journal*. "We finally decided to go forward, to try some new things, to up the dosage and combine [indinavir] with other drugs. If not for 142, it's possible we might have ditched the whole thing."[27]

These second-stage trials began recruiting patients at nine sites around the United States in mid-1994. Company officials met with AIDS activists that summer to bring them up to date on the program. Merck sent a clear signal at the meeting that they now had modest hopes for the drug. The company revealed it wouldn't pursue accelerated approval under the new FDA guidelines. They also rejected pleas for an expanded access program for desperately ill patients. "The company's position is that, at this time, [indinavir's] potential does not appear great enough to merit what it claims is the substantial investment in rapidly expanding production," an activist newsletter reported.[28]

Merck was a company in transition by the time these second-stage trials got underway. Roy Vagelos, who had spent a decade at NIH and in academia before moving to Merck, was slated to step down from his chief executive post in June. Research director Scolnick would soon be reporting to a new man.

Fears swept through the AIDS activist community that the company with a social conscience—the one that had been the most open to their incessant demands for access and information—would soon be cutting back on its research programs as a result of the changeover. In April, outgoing chief executive officer Vagelos gave an exclusive interview to Gay Men's Health Crisis' newsletter to diffuse the issue. The mixed early results from the indinavir studies must have weighed heavily on his mind. The company had gotten involved in AIDS research in 1987 with a promise to develop a breakthrough within five years, he said. Yet here it was, seven years later, and the company still had nothing to show for the "several hundreds of millions of dollars" invested in AIDS research. But that didn't matter. "Our company is dedicated to it. It doesn't matter who succeeds me," he told the newsletter editors. "We don't like to quit just because things aren't going well."[29]

His replacement, Raymond V. Gilmartin, would make the critical "go/no-go" decision on indinavir. Gilmartin, an engineer with a master's of business administration from Harvard, joined Merck after a successful career guiding Becton Dickinson to the top of the medical supply industry. The board of directors hired him for his reputation as a brilliant business strategist and because he was a professional manager who could keep an eye on the company's stock price at the same time it pursued global markets, a new emphasis at the firm. Compared to his predecessors at the nation's most admired drug company, he knew almost nothing about the intricacies of pharmaceutical research. What he did know about was pricing and profits, and like the rest of the drug industry, Merck's officialdom was embroiled in 1994 in the ongoing war with the Clinton administration over health care cost containment. The pause in economic growth that spread across the economy that year had also slowed the growth of company sales. The company's stock price was half of what it had been just two years earlier.

Fortunately for the AIDS research team, by the time Gilmartin began focusing on its project, Scolnick had better news to report. The early results from the two-drug combination showed 40 percent of patients had lowered their viral load below the level of detection. While this was nowhere near the results that would later be shown with triple-combination therapy, it was good enough to encourage the research staff to press for third-stage trials. These were the large-scale tests, often involving a few thousand patients, that when successful led to FDA approval. Few companies undertake third-stage trials unless they have a pretty good indication from earlier tests that larger trials will be successful.

Merck had its own approach to third-stage trials. The firm almost never launched one without building the facilities needed to produce the drug in bulk. Their reasoning—some called it arrogance—was that nothing they took that far would fail, so they might as well be prepared to hit the ground running when they got final approval. Merck engineers estimated costs would run anywhere from $100 million to $200 million to build the facilities needed to synthesize indinavir in bulk. Chodakewitz, the physician in charge of the clinical trials, presented the data from the second-stage trial at a January 1995 meeting that reassured the company's top officials that the money wouldn't be wasted. Gilmartin, who attended, gave the nod to move forward, both with the final trials and production of a new plant in Elkton, Virginia.

Between April and December 1995, Merck enrolled just ninety-seven patients in what turned out to be its crucial clinical trial. A few months earlier, Ho and Shaw, who were working with Abbott's ritonavir, had stunned the AIDS research world with their findings about viral replication and its implications for combination therapy. Merck scientists, who claim they independently came to the same conclusion, designed the critical trial to evaluate indinavir alone against the most popular two-drug combination at the time—AZT and 3TC. It also added a wing to the trial that tested all three together. Dying AIDS patients across the country clamored to get into the trial, dubbed Merck 035. Barring that, they wanted access to the drug. The company, fearing it wouldn't have enough of the drug for its other trials, which included a thousand-patient indinavir-AZT trial being conducted in Brazil, initially resisted. It invited AIDS activists to a presentation at its corporate headquarters, where they detailed their production concerns. But as the new plant got up to speed, those concerns melted away. By late summer, more than two thousand AIDS patients were taking the drug.

Merck, still pursuing traditional FDA approval, anticipated a long, leisurely rollout of the new drug. Their original target date was late 1996. The company knew its drug was vastly superior to the poorly absorbed saquinavir, and the early reports of toxicities and drug interactions from Abbott's ritonavir led them to believe it wouldn't be a serious contender. More important, the initial reports on Merck 035 suggested the nearly ten years that Merck scientists had spent on AIDS research had paid off in spectacular fashion. The patients in the triple-combination therapy wing of the trial had nearly undetectable viral load counts. Merck scientists left the meetings where the preliminary results were unveiled in tears. Some compared the moment to Merck's famous triple-therapy trials in the late 1940s that had provided the first breakthrough against tuberculosis.[30]

It took outsiders to shake Merck out of its complacency. In the middle of September, Abbott went public with the stunning results from its triple-combination study. Abbott also indicated at the San Francisco ICAAC meeting that it would soon seek accelerated approval for ritonavir. Two months later, an FDA official asked Merck's chief of regulatory affairs, "What are you guys waiting for?"[31] Merck filed for accelerated approval for indinavir on January 31, 1996.

The day after filing, Emini gave the leadoff presentation to the annual conference devoted to the latest in AIDS research. He called for a "new paradigm" for treating the disease. Shutting down HIV replication could eliminate or delay the accumulation of mutations leading to drug resistance, he said, and three-drug combinations that included indinavir had succeeded in lowering viral loads below the level of detection. The FDA advisory committee meeting in early March was a mere formality. The company received its license to begin selling the drug on March 13. It was the fastest approval in agency history.

Though clinical tests showed Merck had the most effective drug with the least side effects, it had the disadvantage of being the third entrant into the protease marketplace. The company established its initial price below its rivals—around six thousand dollars per year retail. The company put a humanitarian spin on its pricing strategy. "We saw what Roche and Abbott did with pricing, and we felt that we had to do something different," a public relations official said. "We had to make a statement that we recognized that access is an issue."[32]

The next year reshaped the AIDS treatment landscape in ways unimaginable only a few short months before. The new drugs transformed the number-one killer of young male adults in America into a manageable disease. *Time* and *Newsweek* magazine covers heralded the end of the AIDS plague. The nation's airwaves crackled with miraculous recovery stories, where young men that only a few months earlier had been on the brink of death were shown pumping iron to rebuild their once-wasted bodies.

The media lavished most of its praise for the breakthrough on the pharmaceutical companies that brought the new drugs to market. Michael Waldholz, the Pulitzer Prize–winning reporter for the *Wall Street Journal* who had followed the AIDS story longer and more closely than any reporter in the United States, set the tone. His front-page story in June 1996 emphasized the corporate mad dash to the finish line after "a decade of disappointment and frustration, unexpected product failures, intense corporate rivalries, and secrecy." His account made no mention of the government's significant scientific and financial contributions to basic and applied research that took place from the early 1980s through 1992, nor of its support for many of the clinical trials that took place in the two years leading up to the drugs' approvals.[33]

The alleged cost of private industry's research investment mushroomed almost as quickly as media's coverage of the amazing breakthrough. Two years after Merck's chairman had spoken about spending "several hundreds of millions" on all AIDS research, a *Wall Street Journal* reporter led a story about the marketing of indinavir by claiming the company spent more than $1 billion to develop the drug.[34] The *Washington Post Magazine* a few months later raised the financial stakes even higher when it declared the protease inhibitor "drama was a decade-long, multibillion-dollar race pitting the world's top drug companies against AIDS and one another—arguably the most time, money, and scientific manpower ever focused on a single medicinal target."[35]

Large pharmaceutical companies do not report their research and development costs by individual drugs. They do not even break them down into areas of research, like, say, AIDS or cancer or heart disease. But the Merck example is instructive since it had by far the most comprehensive research program on HIV- and AIDS-related diseases and its officials have not been shy about releasing data about their expenditures. The company began a multifaceted research program on AIDS in the mid-1980s, which pursued vaccines, non-nucleoside reverse transcriptase inhibitors (NNRTIs), protease inhibitors, as well as novel pathways for attacking the virus. The company conducted a number of early-stage clinical trials on possible drug candidates and by 1995 had pushed indinavir to the point where it was ready for a final, multicenter clinical trial involving at least a thousand patients. The company also deployed its renowned vaccine research expertise against HIV. It is fair to say that no company devoted more of its resources to the fight against AIDS, and it is likely that no other company spent even half of Merck's total.

Business historian Louis Galambos of Johns Hopkins University, who had access to internal Merck memos and interviewed all its key players for an in-house history of indinavir's development, wrote that officials told him that Merck had spent $400 million on all of its AIDS research programs by early 1995. This was not just for the development of indinavir. It was for all of its research and development into AIDS: drugs, both the one that worked and the several that failed; vaccines; and the manufacturing facilities for the drugs sent into clinical trials. At that point they finally had a drug—indinavir—ready for its final clinical trials, and they were faced with the "go/no-go" decision on building a $200-million plant to produce the new drug in sufficient quantities for both the trials and its eventual marketing. It got built. They also began their final clinical trials.

Clinical trial costs have been well documented, both by the government, which ran the ACTG, and by outside groups, who are interested in promoting research into new drugs to combat the diseases devastating the developing world. The Global Alliance for TB Drug Development, which operates on major grants from the Rockefeller Foundation and the Bill and Melinda Gates Foundation, during 2000 asked consultants from private industry to put together a study on the cost to develop new drugs to combat the disease. The Global Alliance sponsors research into new drugs to fight virulent strains of drug-resistant tuberculosis that have emerged in many parts of the world, since the pharmaceutical industry has abandoned the field. Their report, issued in October 2001, estimated that all phases of clinical research for a new drug cost about $26.6 million, with the lion's share of that—$22.6 million—coming in the third and final set of trials.[36]

By taking the final clinical trial-stage estimate—$22.6 million, as of 2000—and adding that to Merck's total expenditures up to the time it entered the final stages of testing indinavir, one can arrive at a ballpark estimate for Merck's total AIDS research and development investment before the company succeeded in bringing one antiviral drug to market. That total would have been about $623 million.

As the preceding chapters showed, Merck spent far more than any other drug company in its efforts to combat AIDS. Indeed, Merck spent more than twice as much as any other company involved in the hunt. Abbott consciously operated its program on a shoestring. Its one reported comment on costs came in early 1997, when John Leonard told the *Washington Post* that by late 1993 the company had spent $75 million on its AIDS program.[37] Given that the company at that point was entering its major clinical trial phase, it is unlikely the company spent much more than $100 million on AIDS-related research by the time its successful product—ritonavir—entered the marketplace. Roche, which sharply curtailed its AIDS-related research program in 1993, probably spent about the same amount.

There is another way to estimate the typical research budget for a company investigating AIDS-related drugs. Within three years of the first three protease inhibitors entering the marketplace, the two biotechnology companies whose efforts received significant press coverage over the preceding decade succeeded in getting their drugs approved by the FDA. Unlike the major drug companies, the research and development efforts of these firms are easily documented.

Agouron Pharmaceuticals Inc. was launched in the mid-1980s in La Jolla, California, for the express purpose of using X-ray crystallography and structure-based drug design techniques to develop drugs. It focused the company's limited staff on two major programs. One was an experimental drug that might inhibit the HIV protease. The other was a chemical agent designed to inhibit solid, malignant tumors in several major cancers. Its protease inhibitor, generically known as nelfinavir, gained FDA approval in March 1997. Its annual Securities and Exchange Commission (SEC) report, filed four months later, showed the firm through June of that year had spent $299 million on all research-and-development projects since its inception. Since both of its major programs had drugs in clinical trials, it is reasonable to assume the company spent about half that, or $150 million, on AIDS-related research to bring nelfinavir to market.

A year later, Agouron told the SEC that during its first year on the market, about 85,000 people in the United States and 120,000 worldwide were taking nelfinavir (the trade name is Viracept). Those AIDS patients generated $358 million in sales for the company. A year later, Pfizer Inc. bought the biotech firm, and separate reports for its research-and-development budgets ceased. But based on the earlier filings, it is safe to assume that Agouron spent less than $200 million on research and development for a drug that in its first year on the market generated nearly twice that in sales, of which more than half (57 percent) was profit.[38] In other words, the company earned back its research investment in the first year.

Vertex Pharmaceuticals Inc., the Cambridge-based biotech company headed by Merck exile Joshua Boger, received more journalistic attention during the protease inhibitor hunt than any other firm except Merck. It finally brought a successful product to market in April 1999. The company licensed it to GlaxoSmithKline (the product of several mergers), which began selling it under the trade name Agenerase. Vertex, which ignored HIV research during its formative years and didn't return to it until the early 1990s, went public in 1992. From 1992 to 1999, the company spent $328.2 million on all its drug research projects, which included major investments not just in AIDS-related drugs but in drugs to combat multidrug resistant cancers, rheumatoid arthritis, and psoriasis.[39] It is reasonable to assume that Vertex—like Agouron—spent less than $200 million on developing Agenerase, a total that included the final clinical trials.

A number of companies entered the hunt for a protease inhibitor but dropped out along the way. Only G. D. Searle, later a unit of Monsanto, got far enough along in its program that its drug candidate entered second-stage human trials. But even if a half dozen companies spent $100 million each on protease inhibitor programs, every company directly involved in searching for what turned out to be the breakthrough product that turned AIDS into a manageable disease spent a combined total of less than $2 billion.

It is almost impossible to calculate a grand total for all AIDS-related research by private pharmaceutical and biotechnology firms. But it is reasonable to assume—based on estimates by Merck, which was the outlier in the industry—that the total through the end of 1996 was significantly less than $5 billion. The government, by comparison, spent a shade under $10 billion on AIDS-related research in the decade leading up to the breakthrough discovery. Taxpayer-financed projects ranged from pure science to drug discovery to clinical trials. NIH bureaucrats and university-based peer review panels undoubtedly wasted some of that money—as press accounts based on the angry protests of AIDS activists would occasionally point out. But there can be no doubt that the government program was the driving force behind the private sector's eventual development of a treatment for the disease.

Was the investment worth it for the drug companies? Did the risk of getting involved in the fight against a seemingly intractable disease require the high prices that the successful companies ultimately set on their drugs? The emergence of protease inhibitors in 1996 ended the era where HIV treatment was a desperate attempt to extend life for a few months or years at the end of the tragic course of AIDS. Triple-drug therapy enabled the majority of people with AIDS to live relatively normal and productive lives as long as they took their medicine regularly. As the annual death toll plunged, the number of people taking HIV antivirals soared, reaching more than a half million by the end of the 1990s.

Not only did sales for protease inhibitors soar, but so did the sales of the existing drugs on the market, whose efficacy had been wondrously enhanced by the addition of the new class of drugs. A successful therapy turned AIDS into a chronic disease and created a permanent market. All the drugs in the cocktail saw their sales soar. By 2000, the protease inhibitor market in the United States was a shade under $1 billion a year, according to IMS Health, the market research firm that closely tracks sales of prescription drugs in the United States. The total market for antivirals reached nearly $3 billion a year. Worldwide sales of protease inhibitors totaled about $2.2 billion, which was again about a third of what had become a $6.5-billion market for anti-HIV drugs.

Profits from selling HIV drugs are easily derived since there are several small biotechnology companies that generate most of their sales from those drugs. If the profit margins of the major companies are the same as the biotech firm whose only sales come from selling HIV drugs, substantially more than half of those total sales fell to the bottom line as profit. In other words, the drug industry each and every year earns before taxes nearly as much as it invested in all of its anti-AIDS research in all of the years leading up to the major breakthrough.

FDA approval of the first three protease inhibitors did not end the fight against AIDS. The HIV strain inside a small fraction of patients remained resistant to the drugs, and over time that fraction was growing. Once again, the wily virus was outwitting the best efforts of medical science to stamp it out.

Doctors recognized several patterns among these therapy resistant patients. Some HIV carriers who did not respond to triple-cocktail therapy had been on single- or double-drug therapies in the mid-1990s. By the time the protease inhibitors came along, they had already developed viral strains inside their bodies that were resistant to the reverse transcriptase inhibiting drugs in the cocktail.

But the biggest part of the problem came from poor patient adherence to the complicated pill-popping regimens associated with the new drugs. In some manufacturers' formulations, rows of pills had to be taken three times a day, and some people had violent gastrointestinal reactions after taking them. Yet anything less than 95 percent fealty to the regimen allowed mutant strains of the rapidly multiplying virus to emerge.

Alarmingly, these new strains not only resisted the action of the protease inhibitor they had been subjected to, but they were resistant to all the protease inhibitors on the market. A government study released in December 2001 estimated nearly half of all HIV carriers had drug-resistant strains inside their bodies.[40]

John Erickson, who had left Abbott in 1991 to join NCI in Frederick, Maryland, decided to devote his government X-ray crystallography lab to this resistance problem. He had collaborated with his former colleagues at Abbott until management cut the ties. He then stayed in touch with their program by talking to the physicians at the Aaron Diamond Center, who were doing the initial resistance studies on ritonavir. "I knew from the beginning, resistance was going to be a big problem from these drugs," he told me over a cup of coffee at his home in the Catoctin foothills outside Frederick, Maryland. "I didn't know the extent to how complex it was going to be. You struggle for years to develop a drug candidate, and the virus mutates around it within days. It was humbling."

The mild-mannered researcher resumed probing of the scissors mechanism of the HIV protease, looking for the key to the resistance problem. During viral replication, the enzyme cut the long protein chain produced by the HIV genome into small pieces, which would eventually make up the new virus. Protease inhibitors blocked that scissors action by fitting themselves into the folds of the enzyme where the cutting took place. Yet mutant strains emerged that still got the job done. There must be a part of mutant protease that was common to every protease—the fragment that actually did the work. If he could only find that common component, Erickson reasoned, he might be able to design a drug that blocked the protease action in all strains of HIV.

Throughout the mid-1990s, Erickson's lab at NCI worked with chemists at the University of Illinois at Chicago to synthesize new compounds capable of jamming up the scissors in all strains of the HIV protease enzyme. In December 1994, they came up with their first molecule that worked against every test-tube strain of the virus they had. After filing a patent, they turned to the NIH's Office of Technology Transfer, whose job under the 1980 Bayh-Dole Act was to move government-discovered technologies from the laboratory to the private sector. Tibotec, a Belgian biotechnology company that was later bought by Johnson and Johnson, was interested in conducting the human trials. After a year of negotiations, NIH licensed Erickson's invention to the European start-up. And in mid-1998, Erickson went with it, moving his entire lab to Tibotec.

The results of the first human trials on what Tibotec called TMC 126 were released at the eighth annual Retrovirus Conference held in Chicago in early February 2001. Erickson called a press conference to describe his new discovery. He glowingly described how his flexible molecule could jam up the mechanism of mutant protease scissors by bending to fit into the new shape of the active part of the enzyme, no matter what shape it took. He called the molecule "resistance repellant." His longtime colleague at the Aaron Diamond Center agreed. "We have for the first time a very, very powerful protease inhibitor that could suppress resistant virus," said David Ho. "That's pretty impressive."[41]

But by the following summer, Erickson was not a happy man. As he paced the kitchen of his modest home, he said he couldn't talk about his experiences with Tibotec. The company had just shut down his lab, laying him off, along with the two dozen colleagues that had moved with him from NCI. The company kept his equipment, his lab notes, and his molecule, the products of a decade and a half of methodical work that had brought him to the brink of his second major triumph. "They had to cut costs to keep the drug development going, so they cut early-stage drug development," he told me dejectedly. Erickson, the idealist who has now twice failed to find a congenial home in the private sector, said he hoped to reconstitute his lab, perhaps as a nonprofit, where he could research new molecular entities to combat drug-resistant strains of tropical diseases ravaging the developing world.[42]

His departure did not stop Tibotec from pursuing his drug. At the December 2001 ICAAC Conference in Chicago, Tibotec reported on its latest trials. But TMC 126 was no longer in the picture. Using Erickson's original molecule, company chemists synthesized seven hundred analogues and used an automated screening system to pick a more promising drug candidate, which they dubbed TMC 114. "Single doses of this novel candidate protease inhibitor were safe and well tolerated at all tested dosage levels," a company spokeswoman said. It would soon move into second-stage clinical trials. Nowhere in the accompanying press release did the company as much as hint that TMC 114 was the direct descendant of a drug that had been invented in a government-funded lab.

7

The Failed Crusade?

f the government's role in reducing AIDS mortality represents a great victory for the idea that directed research campaigns can substantially affect the history of an epidemic, the war on cancer is an entirely different matter. For more than half a century, all the weapons of directed medical research—extramural grants to academic researchers, intramural programs of research and drug development, public-private partnerships, and outright support of industry—have been deployed against cancer with far less satisfactory results.

It has been more than three decades since President Nixon signed the National Cancer Act. The government over those years spent more than $50 billion combating what one social historian called "the dread disease." The National Cancer Institute (NCI), the largest arm of the National Institutes of Health (NIH), created and financed a nationwide academic research establishment dedicated to understanding the biochemistry of cancer. It also devoted a sizable fraction of its resources to a wide-ranging hunt for drugs.

Those efforts transformed the commercial landscape. At the campaign's outset, the pharmaceutical industry for the most part ignored cancer. But by the early twenty-first century there were dozens of firms pursuing more than four hundred potential cancer drug candidates.

Why? NCI-funded basic science had created a multitude of potential drug targets. And the chemotherapies that emerged from the government's half-century hunt for drugs, licensed at no cost to industry, created a market where none existed before.

But selling drugs is not the same as curing disease. Any objective survey of the most recent statistics would show that cancer as a public health problem has not changed much over the years. Cancer—a catchall term for a class of more than 110 separate malignancies—claimed the lives of more than 555,000 Americans in 2002, leaving it the nation's number-two killer, a position it has held since the early 1930s.

There were tentative signs of progress in the 1990s in the long-running campaign against the disease. The rate at which cancer killed fell gradually after decades of increases and by 2000 was 11 percent below its peak. However, the biggest factor behind the decline had nothing to do with medical intervention. The falling cancer mortality rate was largely driven by the public health campaign that convinced many people to stop smoking in the 1970s and 1980s, which led to a falling incidence of lung cancer in the 1990s. There were also small reductions in the death rates for colon, breast, and prostate cancers, which have been attributed to improved treatments and early screening techniques like mammograms, although that assertion has been challenged.[1] But those improvements have been modest at best. After it had been adjusted for the age at which people contract cancer, the cancer death rate stood at 203 per 100,000 persons in 1999, slightly worse than 199 per 100,000 persons in 1975, which in turn was slightly worse than the 195 cancer deaths per 100,000 persons recorded in 1950.

The chances of surviving cancer are certainly better than they were a generation ago. Six in ten cancer patients survived at least five years after a diagnosis of cancer by the late 1990s, compared to a shade less than five in ten in the mid-1970s. But those gains were offset by cancer incidence rates that were still rising, especially among the elderly. As people lived longer by surviving infectious diseases, heart attacks, strokes, and the complications of diabetes, they increased their risk of contracting and eventually dying of cancer.

Cancer incidence among the middle-aged went up compared to three decades earlier (with slight declines in the past decade in some cancers). But it was among these younger cancer patients that oncologists registered their greatest treatment gains. Every age group under sixty-five years posted declines in cancer mortality rates between 1973 and 1999, with the biggest gains among the very young, as clinicians deployed improved treatments for childhood cancers like leukemia and some solid tumors.

The population that contracts cancer has also shifted. In the nineteenth and early twentieth centuries, cancer was considered a woman's disease. Cancers of the breasts and uterus were observable, while many cancers of internal organs, whether they killed women or men, went undiagnosed. As late as 1950, the cancer mortality rate was higher among women than men. But as tobacco began taking its terrible toll on the American people, the demographics of cancer changed dramatically. Lung cancer rates among men soared in the 1950s and 1960s as the direct result of the marketing and glamorization of cigarette smoking that had begun three decades earlier. By midcentury, women's smoking rates began to catch up to men's with predictable results. Virginia Slim, meet the Marlboro Man. During the 1980s and 1990s, the rates at which women contracted lung cancer rose sharply. With lung cancer accounting for nearly one in three cancer deaths, the cancer gender gap began to shrink.[2]

One would think these unyielding statistics and the grim prognosis for nearly half the people diagnosed with cancer would dampen enthusiasm for cancer war stories in the popular press. But in their frequent updates from the frontlines of research, editors and reporters remained invariably upbeat, with their enthusiastic embrace of the latest laboratory discoveries often bordering on the deliberately misleading. A *New York Times* story splashed across the top of the paper's Sunday front page in 1998 was typical of the genre. Gina Kolata, an experienced medical writer, set off a media frenzy when she published an article proclaiming, "Hope in the Lab: A Cautious Awe Greets Drugs That Eradicate Tumors in Mice." Judah Folkman, an NIH-funded researcher at Children's Hospital in Boston, had come up with experimental drugs that cut off blood flow to rodent tumors. No less an authority than James Watson, codiscoverer of the DNA double helix, anointed Folkman the next Charles Darwin. Richard Klausner, the head of NCI, called his work "the single most exciting thing on the horizon" and the data "very compelling," although he did mention "the big ifs" when talking about a drug that had never been tried in humans. The stock of EntreMed, the company Folkman worked with, soared. Book contracts got signed. (A few days after the story broke and controversy about its overhyped nature emerged, editors at the *New York Times* advised Kolata to reject her multimillion-dollar offer.) Over the next few years, the drugs quietly disappeared from view as the company began the long slog toward proving their usefulness against several rare forms of cancer.[3]

Cancer therapy for most patients had changed over the decades because the government had poured enormous resources into understanding the basic biology of the disease and developing drugs for treating it. But most oncologists still prescribed some combination of surgery, radiation, and chemotherapy—"slash, burn, and poison," in one deflating description.[4] In recent years, the surgery had become less invasive, the radiation better targeted, and the newer chemotherapy agents slightly more effective. The new drugs also had fewer side effects, or other drugs were developed to offset their toxicities. But in the end, patients on chemotherapy were still left praying that the cancer hadn't metastasized to some hidden corner of the body, which, alas, for many it had. The cure for nearly half of cancer patients turned out to be nothing more than a temporary respite from the ravages of the disease, therapy's success measured by a few, often miserable, months or years of life.

To the extent that drug treatment options have improved, the government played the central role in bringing them about. The Food and Drug Administration (FDA) approved fifty-eight cancer drugs between 1955, when NCI launched its cancer drug development program, and 2001. NCI played the lead role in the development of fifty of those cases. It found the molecule, assisted in late-stage preclinical studies, or directly sponsored the clinical trials. In some cases, it did all three. Even in the post-1980 era, when the number of private firms involved in cancer therapy research expanded rapidly, more than 70 percent of all new cancer drugs approved by the FDA had at least some government involvement.[5]

Is it fair to say then, as many observers have, that the government's war on cancer is a failure? Does its performance call into question all public sector attempts to solve pressing medical problems through targeted programs of applied research? Jerome Groopman, the respected AIDS oncologist and medical journalist, concluded the government would have been better off focusing exclusively on basic research during its long war on cancer rather than supporting research into new drugs. In a provocative essay published in *New Yorker* magazine on the thirtieth anniversary of the Cancer Act, the Harvard Medical School professor noted the recent round of ebullient press accounts praising the latest targeted cancer drugs. Groopman allowed that "the current atmosphere of hope is not without foundation." But he went on to say that "it is not without precedent, either. Ever since 1971, when President Nixon declared war on cancer, oncologists and cancer patients have been caught in a cycle of euphoria and despair as the prospect of new treatments has given way to their sober realities. The war on cancer turned out to be profoundly misconceived—both in its rhetoric and in its execution."[6]

A closer examination of the history and accomplishments of the war on cancer would suggest that a blanket condemnation of the government's directed research program is far too harsh. The government never ignored basic scientific inquiry into the biochemical and biomolecular processes behind cancer. Far from it. From the cancer war's outset (which actually dates back to the late 1930s), the leadership of academic medicine and nonprofit research institutes insisted that autonomous, peer-reviewed researchers and their proposals occupy a central role in the campaign. At the end of the century, basic research still consumed more than three-quarters of NCI's resources. Indeed, as Groopman admitted, the most recent drugs emerging from industry's labs owed their existence to the understanding of the basic biology of the disease derived from the previous thirty years of government-funded basic research.

However, the public, speaking through its representatives in Congress, would have never supported that vast expansion of basic science unless it was coupled with the simultaneous search for cures. In the late 1960s Mary Lasker, a key member of the American Cancer Society's board and a longtime booster of NIH, recruited elite financiers to her Citizens Committee for the Conquest of Cancer with the promise that increased science funding would be linked to a "moon shot" to cure cancer. Liberal Howard Metzenbaum, a retired parking-lot magnate from Cleveland who would soon become a senator, served as Lasker's cochair. He got his start in politics by championing the targeted research approach. Senator Edward Kennedy, new to the Senate and heir to his family's liberal legacy, introduced the bill in the upper chamber.

The pharmaceutical industry also jumped on the applied research bandwagon in the person of Elmer H. Bobst, the retired president of U.S. operations for Hoffmann–La Roche. Bobst, a longtime member of the American Cancer Society board, used his close friendship with President Nixon to push for an autonomous NCI and "subject it to a carefully considered program of directed research in the most promising areas."[7] They got what they wanted, but not as a substitute for basic scientific inquiry into the biology of the disease. The war on cancer vastly expanded both realms.

If there was any misconception at the outset of Nixon's war on cancer, it was in the academic- and institute-based scientists' narrow definition of basic research. They focused resources almost exclusively on microbiology, biochemistry, and genetics, the fields they knew best.

Great academic empires and eventually even large fortunes were built on the foundations laid by NCI-funded research. Unfortunately, these same scientists, whose administrators controlled the panels that oversaw grants, gave much shorter shrift to in-depth investigations into the environmental and social roots of the disease. Nor did they emphasize public health prevention strategies for curbing its incidence since to do so would have brought them into conflict with some of the same powerful economic interests whose representatives were championing a strictly clinical approach to combating the disease.

The cancer crusade did not begin with President Nixon's proclamation in 1971. By the late 1920s, rising cancer rates had prompted Senator Matthew Neely of West Virginia to seek a special appropriation of one hundred thousand dollars to study the disease. Speaking on the floor of the Republican-controlled Senate, the Democrat Neely called cancer "humanity's greatest scourge," a "monster that is more insatiable than the guillotine," and a force "more destructive to life and health than the mightiest army." He warned his colleagues that "if the rapid increase in cancer fatalities should persist in the future, the cancer curse would in a few centuries depopulate the earth."[8]

Neely's overwrought rhetoric set off a debate whose parameters echo to this day. One senator wondered if the increasing cancer rates had more to do with better diagnostics than a rising tide of tumors. Others spoke for a large portion of the public who preferred to put their faith in religion, quacks, and patent medicines, which, as cancer historian James Patterson has noted, were part of "a very diffuse but stubbornly persistent cancer counterculture, one of the many constants in the modern social history of cancer in the United States." Neely's rhetorical flourishes won support from his colleagues in the Senate, but the legislation died in the House.[9]

By 1937, the nation's mood had shifted. The Depression and Franklin Delano Roosevelt's New Deal awakened Americans to the possibilities of government solving its most pressing economic and social problems, including the fight against disease. Surgeon General Thomas Parran, whose wife died of cancer in 1929, spearheaded a coalition that made curing cancer a central thrust of the U.S. Public Health Service's new National Institute of Health.

The coalition was a classic example of the divergent interests that sometimes come together to grow a new public policy in the Washington petri dish. It was led by the American Society for the Control of Cancer

(ASCC, later the American Cancer Society) and its Women's Field Army, whose door-to-door fundraising and early detection public awareness campaigns had become a fixture in many middle-class communities. Senator Homer Bone, a Democrat from the state of Washington, championed their cause in the belief that cancer especially hurt the poor, who couldn't afford the doctor visits that might enable them to catch cancer in its early stages, while it was still treatable. They were joined by a growing research community, led by a frustrated physician from San Antonio named Dudley Jackson. His anger grew out of the fact his cancer-related research proposals had been turned down by the fledgling NIH.

This disparate coalition was joined by a new and rising cancer establishment in which the ASCC played a leading but far from exclusive role. Shortly after the turn of the century, John D. Rockefeller had endowed the Rockefeller Institute for Medical Research in New York City. By the mid-1930s, its prestigious faculty had turned to cancer research as one of its major activities. In 1936, the oil tycoon gave another $4 million to build the world's most modern facility dedicated to cancer treatment—Memorial Hospital. In the postwar years, the hospital would merge with the Sloan-Kettering Institute, which was endowed by General Motors industrialists Alfred P. Sloan and Charles F. Kettering. Also in 1936, the wife of Starling Childs, who made his millions in New York utilities, died of cancer. Childs gave $10 million to the Yale University to study the disease—at the time the largest ever bequest for medical research. These endorsements of cancer research by leading philanthropists and one of the nation's top medical schools helped the field emerge from its quack-ridden roots and emboldened politicians to authorize the government to play a bigger role in combating the disease.[10]

By the late 1930s, Congress was well along the path toward giving government a role in medical research. In 1930, responding to complaints that the private sector's investment in medical science was far from adequate, it created NIH from the Public Health Service's Hygienic Laboratory, which had been founded in the 1880s to study infectious diseases. But in expanding the agency, Congress limited it to basic research. The original authorizing legislation established its purpose as the "study, investigation, and research in the fundamental problems of the diseases of man."[11]

The new NIH was swamped with proposals from outside researchers. Dudley Jackson, who would play the key role in getting the NCI legislation passed in the House, was a surgeon who saw how the disease ravaged his mostly poor clientele. Jackson asked NIH for money to study carbohydrate metabolism in dogs in order to gain insights into the fundamental causes of cancer. The agency repeatedly turned down his requests. If their goal was to drum up hinterland support for more funding for the agency, they picked the right man to ignore. Angered by what he saw as the tunnel vision of bureaucrats in Washington, Jackson convinced his powerful cousin, Rep. Maury Maverick of Texas, to sponsor a bill creating a separate cancer institute. He then traveled to the Capitol to drum up support.

Creation of the new agency was never in doubt. But the debate over the legislation sparked heated arguments about who should control the institute and what it should fund. Surgeon General Parran was convinced that a powerful central authority should play the lead role in tackling the disease. "Whatever path we take," he said, "inevitably will conform to the governmental framework." But Peyton Rous, the Rockefeller Institute researcher who had created a stir in 1911 when he discovered a virus that caused tumors in chickens (he would champion the mistaken viral transmission theory of the disease until his death in 1970), expressed the concerns of many scientists who feared government control of science. It would lead to "regimented direction," he wrote to a friend. The American Medical Association also warned against government control of medical research but did not actively oppose the bill, preferring to save its political capital for what it considered to be a more important battle—the fight against national health insurance.[12]

The 1937 law passed easily. It gave the new institute broad authority to fund "researches, investigations, experiments, and studies relating to the cause, prevention, and methods of diagnosis and treatment of cancer."[13] In short, its job was to cure cancer, not just study it. But in its early years, virtually all of its limited funding went to basic research. While the blue ribbon advisory panel set up under the law was dominated by leading anticancer figures of the day, it included prominent academicians such as Harvard University president James Conant, for whom the autonomy of science was sacrosanct.

The panel left treatment to the doctors and public education about early detection to the ASCC. It rejected an emphasis on prevention. Instead, the new NCI set up a small in-house research staff to focus on basic biology and established a peer-review system for screening and approving outside grant proposals. The system would become the model for all of NIH when dozens of new institutes were added to its roster in the two decades after World War II.

The advisory panel was far less democratic than Dudley Jackson would have liked. It concentrated the majority of its grants in the leading research institutions, whose heads took turns sitting on the board. Jackson dealt with his new problem by lobbying the Texas legislature to create what is now the M. D. Anderson Cancer Center at the University of Texas in Houston, today the second largest cancer research institution in the United States.[14] "The scientists, taking firm command of the anti-cancer alliance, then implemented the law in ways that advanced their own laboratory research and institutional interests and that mainly dismissed preventive approaches," wrote Patterson. The cancer lobby was born.

The battle over the program's direction was renewed in the immediate postwar years. Despite fealty by men at the top of NCI to Vannevar Bush's vision of concentrating on basic research, powerful forces gathering outside the agency began demanding a more practical approach. Early detection and surgery had been the primary method of treating cancer since the late nineteenth century. Radiation took its place alongside surgery in the early 1900s in Europe and won a wide following among American physicians after Nobel Prize winner Marie Curie toured the United States to tout the process in 1921. In those early years of cancer treatment, people who peddled medicinal cures were considered quacks.[15]

The image began to change during World War II in the wake of a tragic wartime incident. In December 1943, German bombers launched a surprise attack on Allied shipping in Bari Harbor on the Italian coast. One vessel that sank, the USS *John Harvey*, was carrying mustard gas, a weapon banned after World War I. President Roosevelt had ordered it stockpiled just in case Hitler decided to use it. The contents leaked into the harbor, mixed with the burning oil, and vaporized. Hundreds of sailors, fishermen, and other local civilians died, their skin covered with welts and their lungs filled with blood. Autopsies later showed that the victims' white blood cells had been wiped out by the gas.

Several physicians in the army's Chemical Warfare Division, headed by Memorial Hospital chief Cornelius "Dusty" Rhoads, speculated that minute amounts of mustard derivatives might prove useful in treating leukemia and other fast-growing cancers of the blood. The government's Wartime Office of Medical Research began testing the proposition at Yale, the University of Chicago, and other top-secret labs around the country. Rhoads continued that research when he returned to his post at the merged Memorial Sloan-Kettering Hospital after the war.[16]

Rhoads was driven by two central beliefs. First, he saw cancer as primarily a disease of cells. Instead of surgery or radiation, which eliminated the tumor mass, he wanted to focus on finding chemotherapy agents that would stop cancer cells from dividing. His second basic principle was based on advice from the industrialists who sat on his board. They wanted to model Sloan-Kettering after the leading industrial labs of the day, like Bell Labs, which married efficiency and high throughput to scientific inquiry.[17] Rhoads implemented their vision. Between 1946 and 1950, scientists at Memorial Sloan-Kettering synthesized and tested fifteen hundred derivatives of nitrogen mustard gas for their cancer-fighting properties. In 1949, the FDA made mechlorethamine (Mustargen) the first government-approved cancer chemotherapy agent (in those days, one only had to prove it was safe, not effective, to get FDA approval).

Though the treatment was hardly curative, *Time* hailed the discovery. The magazine featured a confident, crew-cut Rhoads on its cover clad in a white lab coat with the symbol of the American Cancer Society—a sword smashing through a crab—in the background. "Some authorities think that we cannot solve the cancer problem until we have made a great, basic, unexpected discovery, perhaps in some apparently unrelated field. I disagree," Rhoads was quoted as saying. "I think we know enough to go ahead now and make a frontal attack with all our forces."[18]

He wasn't the only clinician-scientist pushing NCI to pay closer attention to the treatment mandate in its authorizing legislation. Shortly after the war ended, Sidney Farber, the scientific director of the Children's Cancer Research Foundation in Boston and a member of the faculty at Harvard Medical School, began experimenting with chemical blockers of folic acid, which is needed for DNA replication. His target was acute leukemia in children. A prodigious fundraiser with good connections to many leading politicians, Farber scored the first major success of the chemotherapy era when he came up with the antimetabolite compound methotrexate, which produced remissions in some leukemia patients. Farber began pushing for government funds to expand his experiments. Over the next two decades Farber would serve as the chief advocate for more money to develop new cancer chemotherapies.

Responding to pressure from key opinion leaders like Rhoads and Farber, NCI in 1955 launched the Cancer Chemotherapy National Service Center, a formal effort to develop new drugs. Many top scientists at the agency, including its director Kenneth Endicott, were appalled. "I thought it was inopportune, that we really didn't have the necessary information to engineer a program, that it was premature, and well, it just had no intellectual appeal to me whatever," he said a decade later.[19] But researcher-activists like Farber ran roughshod over those objections. Within two years, nearly half the agency's budget was going toward drug development.

By 1970, the year before the government officially declared war on cancer, the NCI drug development program had already screened more than four hundred thousand chemicals for their cancer-fighting potential. Some were obtained from academic investigators, others from industry, and still others were manufactured in-house. NCI scoured the world for exotic microbes, plants, and marine organisms to test in its labs. Taxol, a derivative of the Pacific Yew tree, whose chemical equivalent remains one of the more successful chemotherapy agents on the market to this day, was a product of those efforts.

The agency took on all the functions of a private drug company. It designed screening assays for testing compounds for their anticancer potential. It learned how to perform preclinical tests for determining toxicity and proper dosing. It recruited a nationwide network of academic oncologists capable of conducting clinical trials. It hired contractors that could mass produce the handful of drugs that slowed the progression of the disease in early clinical testing. "In many respects, the program operates in a fashion similar to that of a pharmaceutical company," one NCI staffer noted in the mid-1980s, on the thirtieth anniversary of the drug development program. There was one big difference, however. "There is no consideration of profit, although cost-benefit considerations obviously play an important role in the choice of drugs to pursue or problems to investigate."[20]

The other half of the budget went to basic scientists, who grouped themselves around two competing theories of cancer causation, although there was no grand design fashioning their academic proposals. The minority school followed in the footsteps of Percivall Potts, the eighteenth-century British physician and epidemiologist who had first noted the high incidence of testicular cancer among British chimney sweeps. The young Brits failed to bathe at the end of their daily labors and as a result developed cancer in the most sensitive area, where the soot and tar came to rest. Relying on similar epidemiological studies, the environmental school of thought believed cancer was caused by exposure to toxic substances. Limit those exposures, it argued, and you limit cancer.

Inside NCI, its cause was championed by Wilhelm C. Hueper, who ran the agency's Environmental Cancer Section from its founding in 1948 to his retirement in 1964. Hueper, a German immigrant, was fired from his job as an industrial hygienist by DuPont de Niemours and Company in 1937 after concluding that the high incidence of bladder cancer among workers in its dye factories was caused by exposure to chemicals used in the manufacturing process. Over the next five years, while working for a small chemical company, he wrote an eight-hundred-page textbook entitled *Occupational Tumors and Allied Diseases*. After being turned down by Yale University Press, he raised three thousand dollars to self-publish the tome. His persistence was rewarded in 1962 when Rachel Carson drew heavily from his obscure work to produce her classic *Silent Spring*. Carson's book inspired the movements that led to passage of the Clean Air and Clean Water acts and the creation of the Environmental Protection Agency and the Occupational Safety and Health Administration.[21]

The chemical carcinogenesis crowd's cause was bolstered by the growing body of research connecting cigarette smoking to lung cancer. During the 1940s, lung cancer rates grew at five times the rate of other forms of cancer. To many hypothesizers, the obvious suspects behind the plague were cigarette smoke and the increasingly visible air pollution of major cities. The former was easier to document. On May 27, 1950, the *Journal of the American Medical Association* published the first articles tying tobacco to elevated incidence of the disease.

One article was written by Ernst L. Wynder, a German Jew who had fled Nazi Germany with his parents. During the war years, he studied medicine at Washington University Medical School in St. Louis and did summer hospital internships at New York University, where he had studied as an undergraduate. One wartime summer, he began questioning the widows of lung cancer victims, virtually all of whom told him their husbands had been heavy smokers. When he returned to St. Louis, he asked his anatomy professor, the well-regarded thoracic surgeon Evarts Graham, if he could systematically question lung cancer patients who entered his clinic for surgery. Graham was a heavy smoker and extremely skeptical about Wynder's hypothesis. But his scientific curiosity prevailed and he gave Wynder permission to travel the country to scour medical records and conduct interviews with lung cancer patients or their survivors. The article that eventually appeared under both of their signatures, "Tobacco Smoking as a Possible Etiologic Factor in Bronchiogenic Carcinoma: A Study of 684 Proved Cases," was the first epidemiological evidence tying heavy smoking to lung cancer. Four months later, a similar article by Richard Doll, a leading British epidemiologist, and his colleague, A. Bradford Hill, appeared in the *British Medical Journal*. A follow-up study by Wynder in 1953 convinced the editors of the *Journal of the American Medical Association* to stop taking cigarette ads. The war on smoking had begun.[22]

Over the next decade, the tobacco industry fought a dissembling campaign against the mounting evidence. Its chief spokesman was renegade researcher Clarence Cook "Pete" Little, who had once headed the American Society for the Control of Cancer. A direct descendant of Paul Revere, Little was a Harvard-trained biologist who harbored huge ambitions in both science and academic administration. In 1922, at age thirty-four, he became the youngest president of the University of Maine and three years later repeated the trick at the University of Michigan. He was fired from that post, though, after being accused of conducting an adulterous affair. But by 1929 he had already raised enough money from a wealthy auto executive to open a genetics research institute in Bar Harbor, Maine, which he would run for the next twenty-five years.

Shortly after moving back to his native state to run the new institute, he was asked by the physicians who ran the ASCC to head up its shoe-string operation. He commuted two days a week to its New York offices to spread its main message that early detection was the best hope for beating cancer. (Celsus, Roman physician in the first century A.D., was the first to offer this enduring insight.) The organization stagnated under his command, and in 1944, Mary Lasker, whose husband Albert, an advertising man, had coined the slogan "Lucky Strikes Means Fine Tobacco," engineered his ouster. A highly refined socialite whose close friends included many of the leading industrialists and financiers of New York City, she was upset, according to at least one account, by an attitude that she felt was both patronizing and predatory toward women.[23]

Little, a "self conscious big shot" without a wider stage, returned to Bar Harbor. In 1954, with retirement looming and his financial prospects dim, he accepted a position as scientific director of the newly established Tobacco Industry Research Committee, which had been set up by the tobacco industry to question reports linking smoking to cancer. For the next two decades he would be the industry's main spokesman debunking the smoking-cancer connection. He consistently raised questions about the data behind the studies that showed they were linked. His efforts became the model for other industry trade groups that wanted to counter epidemiological studies showing the carcinogenic properties of their products.[24]

The Surgeon General's report of 1964, warning that cigarette smoking was hazardous to health, coupled with the growing movement against industrial pollution, seemed to vindicate the epidemiologists' approach to cancer. But to the growing ranks of geneticists, cell biologists, molecular biologists, and virologists studying the disease, the epidemiologist road led nowhere. How did those chemicals turn the body's cells into out-of-control mutants? How did one account for the majority of cancers that seemingly had no environmental cause? One could spend an entire career giving mice cancer by exposing them to carcinogens. How would this knowledge help cure someone who already had the disease? "By the 1960s, the wider scientific community . . . became dismissive, viewing the research on chemical carcinogenesis as an intellectually bankrupt enterprise—nothing more than a mountain of facts with few good ideas propelling it forward," Robert A. Weinberg, one of the nation's leading research scientists, wrote in his chronicle of the scientific history of the war on cancer.[25]

Virologists, cellular biologists, and geneticists rushed in to fill the void. The viral theory of cancer, first enunciated by Peyton Rous in 1911, had virtually disappeared from scientific discussion by the 1930s. But in the late 1950s, it was resuscitated by Sarah Stewart and Bernice Eddy, longtime researchers at the NIH labs in Bethesda. They discovered a virus that induced tumors when injected in mice. They dubbed it the polyoma because the cancers included solid tumors as well as tumors of the blood. The discovery created a stir among the growing number of geneticists interested in the cancer problem, including genomics pioneer James Watson, who referred to the NIH scientists as "two old ladies" in a talk he gave at his Long Island laboratories to spread the news to a wider audience. Viruses were the smallest known organisms and had very short genetic sequences, Watson noted. If they caused cancer, the number of genes in the host cell that were affected by the virus also must be quite small and were therefore identifiable.[26]

Other scientists began replicating and expanding the Stewart-Eddy work. In 1962 virologists in Houston found that the human adenovirus, which causes common respiratory infections, induced tumors in hamsters. Two years later, British virologists discovered virus particles in cells of lymphoma patients in Africa. The cancer-virus connection also began gaining treatment adherents. In the late 1950s, scientists working in France had identified an antiviral protein given off by cells when they were attacked by viruses. They dubbed it interferon. It would be nearly two decades before interferon could be isolated and produced through biotechnology means. But in those early days, a number of researchers began to believe that if viruses caused cancer, then interferon might prevent or cure it through its antiviral activity.[27]

A 1964 *New York Times Magazine* article pulled together the straws in the wind. "A new stage in the struggle against cancer cannot be more than months or at most a year or two away," it gushed. The attention prompted Congress to appropriate $10 million in 1965 for a Special Virus Cancer Program (SVCP). The government hunt for the viral causes of cancer was on. By the end of the decade, it had grown to a $30-million-a-year program.[28]

But how did these cancer viruses do their dirty work? Conventional viruses like the polio virus killed cells by entering them and destroying their reproductive machinery. But cancer cells weren't dying. They were living long, hostile lives and proliferating wildly. Howard Temin of the University of Wisconsin and David Baltimore at the Massachusetts Institute of Technology solved the mystery. Their intellectual spadework prepared the ground for a rapid expansion of the SVCP once the 1971 National Cancer Act passed.

The Watson-Crick DNA double-helix model, sometimes referred to as the central dogma of cell biology, postulated that cell reproduction always proceeded through DNA replication and division. Most viral researchers therefore assumed that viruses like polio and Rous sarcoma, which were made up of RNA, or messenger genetic material, operated in a similar fashion. The only difference was that their RNA reproduced. Working separately in labs hundreds of miles apart, Temin and Baltimore showed that the Rous sarcoma virus replicated by producing a DNA template of itself after it infected a host cell, which then became part of the cell's normal DNA machinery. They were called retroviruses. Temin and Baltimore won the Nobel Prize in 1975 for discovering the enzyme that facilitated the process, which they called reverse transcriptase. Not only did scientists now have a theory for how cancer evolved inside the body, they had a plausible model for how it happened.

Although these stirrings in the world of basic science encouraged advocates to push Congress for a broader war on cancer, they played a secondary role in the debate. When Lasker began lining up political support for bigger anticancer budgets, she turned primarily to the already well-established network active in the search for medicinal cures. She leaned heavily on Farber, the aging patriarch of cancer research. He told Congress that more money and a federally directed battle plan would get the job done. "Based on the new insights with which I am familiar there is no question in my mind that if we make this effort today, and if we plan it, organize it, and fund it correctly, we will in a relatively short period of time make vast inroads in the cancer problem," Farber testified in support of the legislation. "Everything that we have said finally must be directed and pointed to clearly for the benefit of the patient with cancer and all of the basic research and the great expansion of clinical investigation which we have recommended will be the surest way of bringing that about." The rhetoric of the day called for curing cancer by the nation's bicentennial, a scant six years off.[29]

Champions of basic science fought back, led by Francis Moore, a professor of surgery at Harvard Medical School and chief surgeon at Boston's Peter Bent Brigham Hospital. Moore argued that a government-run institute would never have funded German scientist Paul Langerhans, who in 1889 discovered the cells in the pancreas that, when damaged, led to diabetes. Nor would it have funded Frederick Grant Banting and Charles Herbert Best, who discovered insulin in 1921 at the University of Toronto (they patented their method for purifying it from livestock headed for slaughter and licensed it for one dollar to any drug company that wanted to produce it). Moore argued that discoveries almost inevitably came from "young people, often unheard of people" housed in universities. His testimony bolstered those in the House who wanted to keep the beefed up NCI underneath the NIH umbrella and maintain its system of peer-reviewed science.[30]

In the end, the heated arguments that pitted advocates of basic science against applied researchers didn't matter much. NCI budgets quintupled over the next decade to nearly a billion dollars a year. It was enough money for the agency to support a massive expansion of every program in its purview. Basic research grants; a far-reaching hunt for new drugs; the nationwide network of academic clinicians willing to test them— everyone got a piece of the growing pie.

On the basic science front, tens of millions of dollars poured into the SVCP. Far larger amounts went for related basic science research at the nation's universities. It eventually bore fruit. In 1976, two virus hunters, Michael Bishop at the University of California at San Francisco and his ambitious young postdoc, Harold Varmus, who would go on to become head of NIH and Memorial Sloan-Kettering, discovered something that suggested a very different theory of cancer causation. They found a gene inside cells for regulating cell growth that, when mutated, made those cells cancerous. They called the healthy version a proto-oncogene, and its mutated version an oncogene. Their Nobel Prize–winning discovery opened the floodgates for other researchers, who within a few years identified a number of proto-oncogenes—given names like *erb, ras, myb,* and *src*—whose mutations led to cancer.

Ironically, the discovery of oncogenes provided a temporary opening for the chemical carcinogenesis theorists. If a virus could transform a tiny stretch of cellular DNA and make a cell cancerous, then it stood to reason that a constant assault on cells by mutagenic external agents would do the same thing. Their cause got a major boost from Bruce Ames, chairman of the biochemistry department of the University of California at Berkeley. In the mid-1970s Ames developed a simple way to test the mutagenic properties of chemicals. Previously, chemicals had to be tested on rats or mice to see if they caused cancer, an expensive, time-consuming process. By combining human liver extract with fast-growing bacteria, Ames created an assay that rapidly revealed the mutagenic properties of any given chemical. He gained national attention for his test in 1977 when he showed that a popular flame retardant used in children's pajamas was a carcinogen. Overnight, regulators began using the Ames test on industrially and commercially available chemicals to determine their carcinogenic properties.[31]

The following year, the anticarcinogen movement reached its apogee when NCI, the National Institute of Environmental Health Sciences, and the National Institute for Occupational Safety and Health published a paper that estimated that anywhere from 20 to 40 percent of all cancers were environmentally induced. The paper has been called the most radical environmental document ever produced by the U.S. government. Joseph Califano, secretary of Health, Education, and Welfare, gave a rousing speech to the nation's labor leaders at an annual meeting of the AFL-CIO charging that as much as 40 percent of all cancers were caused by six commonly used industrial chemicals.

The study closely paralleled the work of physician and epidemiologist Samuel S. Epstein, who in 1978 published his encyclopedic *The Politics of Cancer*. Epstein accused industry of hiding data that showed many of its products and chemical intermediates caused cancer. He attacked NCI for focusing almost exclusively on the mechanisms of cancer while ignoring its causes. "Billions for cures, barely a cent to prevent," Epstein summed up in an environmentalist newsletter.[32]

Rival epidemiologists immediately began poking holes in the Epstein thesis. In 1981, Oxford University's Richard Doll, who had helped put cigarettes in the dock during the 1950s, and his protégé Richard Peto, conducted a study for the U.S. Office of Technology Assessment that suggested two-thirds of all cancers were caused either by smoking (30 percent) or diet. Cancers caused by either occupational exposures or exposure by the general population to industrially generated chemicals accounted for just 6 percent of cases, they said. Industrial trade groups began echoing those findings by funding a host of scientists willing to raise doubts about the chemical carcinogenesis thesis.

The election of Ronald Reagan in 1980 signaled a shift in the nation's mood, and the antienvironmentalist message began falling on receptive ears. Even Ames switched sides. He used his test to show that many common foods and plants were also mutagens, a natural defense against animal predators developed over many eons in the wilds. By the late 1980s, the general consensus among scientists was that environmental exposures other than cigarette smoke were only minor contributors to the overall cancer burden, representing somewhere between 2 and 6 percent of all cases. A 1988 broadcast of ABC-TV's 20/20 featured Ames and declared that "for two decades now, we of the media have brought story after story where experts warn of links between all kinds of pollutants and cancer. But tonight a distinguished research scientist makes a case that many of the warnings we hear are unnecessary, that all the concern about this toxin, that pesticide, is 'Much Ado about Nothing.' Wouldn't it be nice if he was right?"[33] By the early 1990s, journalistic explorations of the link between environmental toxins and cancer had largely disappeared from the mainstream media. The ranks of academic scientists interested in the topic began to shrink.

The backlash against the environmentalist lobby and the changing politics of the nation created an environment where NCI could largely ignore the links between toxics, the environment, diet, and cancer. Investigators who wanted to explore questions about the concentration of certain cancers among subgroups like blue-collar workers and minorities, or clustered in certain parts of the country, were rarely funded. The results of the few studies that did get done were poorly disseminated. Few researchers focused on the social support needed to get people to stop smoking or the economic and advertising forces that encouraged people to eat unhealthy diets. The billions spent on cancer research largely excluded social scientists who might have provided both the public and policy makers with road maps for reducing the incidence of cancer in American society.

NCI's basic science budget after 1980 concentrated on delineating the biological mechanisms of various cancers. By the early 1980s, the cancer virus hunt had been shelved. A decade had turned up only two or three minor cancers that were related to viruses, leading some cancer researchers to brand the SVCP "a profligate waste, a major boondoggle."[34] But in fact, the SVCP had created a corps of scientists who thoroughly understood the anatomy of retroviruses. When HIV arrived on the U.S. scene in the early 1980s, those scientists were able to identify the retrovirus rapidly, understand its inner workings, and target its cellular weak spots (see chapter 4).

The SVCP also prompted scientists to begin looking inside the living cancer cell, work that exploded in the early 1980s. By the end of that decade, nearly 80 percent of NCI's budget was going for basic research and the agency was funding more than half of all microbiology work in the world.[35] Working from insights gained from the discovery of oncogenes, scientists began exploring the ways those genes worked. Edward Scolnick, who worked at NCI before going to Merck to run its research labs, conducted pioneering research into the on/off switch in cells that gets locked in the on position when oncogenes go bad. Other scientists focused on the signaling mechanisms on the surface and inside cells. These enzymes, called kinases, ran wild in cancer cells. There are hundreds of them in the body. When a particular kinase associated with a particular cancer was identified, researchers began searching for a drug or a biotechnology-derived monoclonal antibody that might block its action and slow and possibly stop the cancer's growth.

In the late 1980s, scientists working under Bert Vogelstein at Johns Hopkins University identified the so-called tumor suppressor gene, the body's natural mechanism for correcting the inevitable mistakes that occur during the ten thousand trillion (that's ten with fifteen zeroes after it) cell divisions that take place during the average person's lifetime. Using biotechnology techniques, which by the mid-1980s were readily available in both academic and industrial labs, scientists isolated these genes and their proteins and expressed them in bulk so they could be studied for potential clues as to how they might be manipulated to arrest cancer. "Most every significant basic research project we fund is seeking to characterize the genes that turn tumor growth on and off," Richard Klausner, head of NCI from 1995 to 2001, said in the mid-1990s. "That represents a major shift in the direction of cancer research over the past few years. It's becoming pretty clear that the 1990s will be seen as a time when scientists finally uncovered the strategies that will be the foundation for every future research effort to eventually conquer cancer."[36]

Another strain of basic research projects focused on the genetic anomalies or family predispositions to developing cancer. Mary-Clair King began her work life as one of Ralph Nader's raiders before gravitating to genetic research as an outlet for her social activism. In October 1990 she shocked the annual meeting of the American Society of Human Genetics when she reported that her small lab at the University of California at Berkeley (she later moved to the University of Washington) had found a gene responsible for breast cancers that ran in families.[37] The news electrified the gene-hunting world, which was just beginning its geometric growth with the money pouring out of the federally funded Human Genome Project (see chapter 3). Within a few years, scientists had identified genes connected to heritable forms of colon cancer and prostate cancer and created tests that could screen people to see who carried the mutations.

However, the hoopla surrounding the gene hunters (*Wall Street Journal* reporter Michael Waldholz called his 1997 book documenting their exploits *Curing Cancer*) overshadowed the fact that inheritance—like toxic exposures—plays only a minor role in cancer causation. Women who carry the breast cancer gene account for just one in twenty cases of the disease. Just one in ten men with prostate cancer carries a gene that predisposes him to developing the condition. From an epidemiological point of view, neither is any more significant than environmental toxins as a cause of cancer. Yet gene seekers fervently believe that identifying the genetic flaw associated with some cancer cases will one day help scientists come up with drugs that will mitigate the effects of the flawed genes and perhaps shed light on other forms of the disease. "Do I think all this will some day lead to a cure?" King said. "You bet I do."[38]

The drug developers inside NCI plugged away amid this explosion of knowledge about the biochemistry of cancer. In 1979, Tadatsugu Taniguchi of the nonprofit Japanese Cancer Research Institute cloned an interferon gene. Within a few years, more than twenty interferon genes had been identified, mostly by university scientists who immediately transferred the results of their research to biotechnology start-ups. During the 1970s and early 1980s, interferon research was pushed by the American Cancer Society and Mathilde Krim, a geneticist at Memorial Sloan-Kettering who was married to Arthur Krim, former chairman of United Artists who contributed heavily to the Democratic Party. At their urging, the government invested heavily in dozens of new companies' work on interferon therapies.[39] Little came of it. In the middle of the 1980s, similar attention was lavished on interleukin, an immune system booster. Again, this early fruit from the biotechnology revolution generated government grants, venture capital from Wall Street, hope for patients, and intense media scrutiny. But in the end, it had little impact on improving cancer therapy.

The success stories in NCI's drug development program came from its massive screening efforts. Only after bicyclist Lance Armstrong won his first Tour de France in 1996 did the general public learn about the extraordinary advances that had been made against testicular cancer, which strikes about eight thousand young men between the ages of fifteen and thirty-five every year. By the time the twenty-seven-year-old cyclist sought treatment for one testicle swollen to twice its normal size ("I'm an athlete, I always have little aches and pains," he told one reporter), the cancer had spread to his lungs and brain. He eventually wound up in the hands of Lawrence Einhorn, a physician at the Indiana University Medical Center who more than any individual had been responsible for the advances in testicular cancer therapy over the previous quarter-century.

Early chemotherapy regimens thrown against testicular cancer in the 1950s had achieved anywhere from a 10- to 20-percent remission rate, with about half those patients ultimately cured. NCI-funded tests at the M. D. Anderson Cancer Center in the 1960s used newer chemotherapy agents, upping the disease-free survival rate to 25 percent. In the mid-1970s, Einhorn, an inquisitive and innovative clinician, began adding cisplatin, a platinum-based compound, to the regimen.

Cisplatin had been discovered in the mid-1960s by Barnett Rosenberg, a biophysicist at Michigan State University studying the effects of electric currents on E. coli bacteria growth. To Rosenberg's surprise, the bacteria stopped reproducing because of exposure to a compound generated on the platinum electrode. He published his findings in *Nature* in 1965.[40] Alerted to a potential anticancer agent, NCI researchers began testing it against various cancers. But the heavy metal's severe side effects (it causes horrible nausea and damages the kidneys) led most oncologists to dismiss platinum's potential in cancer chemotherapy.

Those early experiments would bear fruit a few years later when Einhorn, a testicular cancer specialist, learned from the early literature on cisplatin that the drug had achieved remissions in a few patients with germ cell tumors. Since fast-growing germ cells are precursors to sperm cells, he decided to test it on his patients. He was amazed to see that their tumors "melted away." Einhorn, thinking he had achieved the major breakthrough that the government's cancer warriors so desperately desired in the bicentennial year, nervously reported his findings to the May 1976 meeting of the American Society of Clinical Oncology (ASCO).

For a brief moment, optimism that the war on cancer had found its magic bullet flourished. But those hopes quickly dissolved. No one knew how cisplatin worked, and it had only limited effects on other tumors. Germ cells, it turns out, are particularly susceptible to chemotherapy, and the human immune system is more resilient in the face of testicular cancer than most other cancers.

Still, it was a near cure for one cancer and a major victory for the government program. Michigan State licensed its method-of-use patent on cisplatin (the molecule itself was a very old and well-known compound) to Bristol-Myers, which marketed the highly effective agent. By the time Armstrong had his bout with the disease, ongoing trials by Einhorn and others had raised the cure rate to 95 percent. Cisplatin was also found useful against several other cancers and for many years was the first line of defense against ovarian cancer until it was replaced by Taxol in 1998.[41]

Taxol was the most significant victory for the government's thirty-year screening program. The long and convoluted tale of its development is worth reviewing in depth since the resolution of the controversies surrounding its eventual licensing to Bristol-Myers, its pricing, and its post-approval marketing helps explain the private sector's growing interest in the 1990s and early twenty-first century in pursuing cancer therapies.

NCI began scouring the natural world for potential cancer drugs in the mid-1950s. The agency was inspired in part by Eli Lilly's success in developing vinblastine and vincristine, alkaloid extracts of rosy periwinkle. The company's botanists had been led to the low-growing tropical plant's enticing pink blossoms by folk doctors in Madagascar. Every human society uses plants as medicine, and their use in cancer treatment is part of the folklore of virtually every culture. The Madagascar medicine men were onto something. By extracting the active ingredients from the blossoms, Eli Lilly's scientists were able to trigger remissions in some patients with Hodgkin's lymphoma and childhood leukemia.

Jonathan Hartwell, the overseer of the government's new natural products drug screening program, would not have had much to do if he waited for leads provided by shamans and folklorists. So between 1958 and 1982 (when the program was temporarily suspended), the agency collected and tested more than 180,000 microbe-derived, 16,000 marine organism-derived, and 114,000 plant-derived extracts to test for their anticancer potential. It was a mammoth government undertaking, one that would have made industrialists Sloan and Kettering proud. One botanist estimated nearly 6 percent of the world's plant species passed through NCI's screens. But in the end, only 4 percent of those extracts displayed any activity against cancer in test tubes or mice, and only a half dozen would ever make it into advanced clinical trials.

In 1962, U.S. Department of Agriculture botanists, working on a contract from NCI, tested *Taxus brevifolia*, an extract from the bark of the Pacific Yew tree. It was one of those rare hits, active against the cancer cells in one of NCI's early screens. It soon found its way to the laboratories of Monroe Wall at the Research Triangle Institute in North Carolina. Wall, a former Agriculture Department biochemist who had honed his fractionating skills in the government's hunt for natural sources of cortisone in the 1950s, initially ignored the Yew extract, focusing instead on a rare Chinese tree called *Camptotheca acuminata* (derivatives of its active ingredient, camptothecin, were later developed at Johns Hopkins and Smith Kline on NCI grants and eventually led to three drugs, including Topotecan, which extends life briefly in lung cancer patients who have failed other therapies). A few years later, Wall finally turned his attention to the bark of *Taxus brevifolia*, and in June 1967 isolated its active ingredient, an alcohol he named Taxol. "It had a nice ring to it," he later said. He spent the next four years elucidating its chemical structure and developing methods for its large-scale extraction.[42]

For half a decade, Taxol languished in NCI's labs. It was only mildly active against leukemia, a major focus of researchers in those years. It wasn't until it got into the hands of Susan Horwitz, a molecular pharmacologist at Albert Einstein College of Medicine in New York, that scientists began to recognize its potential. She studied microtubules, a kind of scaffolding that cells temporarily erect when they divide. Peering through her electron microscope, Horwitz saw that Taxol froze the microtubules in place, thus preventing cell division. After publishing her findings in *Nature* in 1979, interest in Taxol took off.[43]

Over the next few years, NCI scientists showed Taxol was active against colon and mammary cancers in mice (by the early 1980s, NCI's skill at breeding mice with various cancers had become a high art and a subject of derision to outsiders who referred to the agency's scientists as mouse doctors). It took several more years to figure out how to suspend the toxic chemical in a solution so that humans could tolerate it. It wasn't until April 1984 that the first cancer patients received intravenous infusions of Taxol. It took another year for physicians at seven oncology centers to figure out proper dosing, and even then there was strong opposition to continuing with the experiments since nearly a fifth of patients had strong allergic reactions to the drug. More important, there was no evidence that it shrank tumors. But with NCI's blessing, oncologists at Johns Hopkins, Albert Einstein, and teaching hospitals grouped into the Eastern Cooperative Oncology Group proceeded with a second round of clinical trials.

By the end of 1986, only the Johns Hopkins group, led by William McGuire, had anything positive to report. Two of his seven patients with ovarian cancer who had failed other therapies showed a partial response, and one showed a marginal response. Word began getting out there was a new treatment for women dying of ovarian cancer, and they flocked to McGuire's clinic. In May 1988, he reported to ASCO that 30 percent of his refractory ovarian cancer patients (refractory means their cancer had returned or had been unresponsive to earlier treatments) had responded to Taxol therapy. Their tumors had shrunk by at least half and in some cases had disappeared entirely.[44]

Before proceeding to the third and final stage of clinical trials needed to gain FDA approval, NCI had to confront the major issue that had dogged it throughout its initial decade of experimentation—the problem of Taxol supply. The Pacific Yew is a slow-growing evergreen found in the Pacific Coast range from Northern California to Alaska. Even after 125 years, the tree grows to only thirty feet in height with a diameter of less than a foot. The bark from several trees that size produce enough Taxol to treat only a single patient. For decades, timber companies operating on public lands had treated the trees like trash, burning them after they had taken out the surrounding giants in clear cuts. Now they were a valuable resource.

During the 1980s, NCI hired contractors to harvest the trees and a chemical company to extract the bark's Taxol. As experimental demand for the drug expanded, so did the number of foresters making a living from harvesting Pacific Yew bark. Some timber companies, such as Weyerhaeuser, became interested in developing the technology after making a strategic decision to add high-value products to their basic logging operations. In terms of value, nothing is higher on the industrial food chain than pharmaceuticals.

But environmentalists soon jumped into the fray. Some saw mass Taxol extraction as a small price to pay for developing an alternative economic engine for a region that depended on clear-cutting the forests of the Pacific Northwest. Others hugged every tree. "This is the ultimate confrontation between medicine and the environment," said Bruce Chabner, chief of the investigational drugs branch at NCI. "It's the spotted owl versus people. I love the spotted owl. But I love people more."[45]

NCI officials had foreseen the problem. In mid-1988, as it was preparing to move Taxol into third-stage clinical trials, NCI began looking for industrial partners to take over the final stages of developing the drug. The 1986 Federal Technology Transfer Act, designed to expedite the movement of government-owned inventions to the private sector, had established a new mechanism, the Cooperative Research and Development Agreement (CRADA), to facilitate the process. The new CRADA arrangement allowed NCI to spell out its goals when it advertised for a Taxol partner in early 1989. The industrial partner chosen to develop the drug would have to do more than just support the third-stage trials, the CRADA proposal said. It would be responsible for sharing the costs of collecting bark and purifying the drug. The agreement included the government rights clause, which bound the company to establish a "just and reasonable price" once it was on the market and to assure access for all patients who needed the drug, whatever their financial status. The original draft of the CRADA even included a clause asserting the government "will receive a reasonable share of income once the drug is marketed for general use." That clause was eliminated in the final draft.

Only four companies responded to the request for proposals, which Bristol-Myers won over Rhône-Poulenc and two small companies.[46] The lack of interest didn't surprise officials at NCI. Previous drugs tested by the agency had either been licensed directly to private firms or developed in informal collaborations. No company benefited more from this arrangement than Bristol-Myers. It licensed its first NCI-developed drug in 1972 and by the late 1980s had more than a dozen oncology drugs in its portfolio. "They never invented anything themselves but they were great developers," recalled Joseph Rubinfeld, who ran Bristol-Myers's oncology division from 1968 to 1980. "They took the jobs that somebody else had done, especially NCI, and commercialized them."[47] The company bolstered its cancer expertise via the revolving door at NCI. Top agency officials who went to work for the firm included Stephen Carter, who was at NCI until 1975; John Douros, who had been chief of the natural products branch in the mid-1980s; and Robert Wittes, a drug development program specialist who would return to NCI in 1990 as its chief clinician after two years at Bristol-Myers.

Rep. Ron Wyden, a Democrat from Oregon, challenged the ethical implications of the government's dealings with the firm during hearings in 1991 and 1992, after public interest groups branded the Taxol CRADA a giveaway of taxpayer-funded research. By that time, the drug's success in the clinic suggested it might become cancer's first blockbuster. Before

Taxol, cancer was not a lucrative market, and few drug companies even bothered with the disease. At the time of the NCI and Bristol-Myers CRADA, anticancer drugs accounted for less than 3 percent of pharmaceutical sales.

But Taxol was about to transform the commercial landscape. During the first two years of the CRADA, NCI and Bristol-Myers cosponsored the major third-stage trial on women with advanced ovarian cancer. They also conducted smaller, early-stage trials that tested the drug against breast, colon, gastric, head and neck, prostate, cervical, and lung cancers. The government agency organized and paid for the trials while the company provided the drug. In July 1992, the company submitted data supporting a new drug application to the FDA. Patients given Taxol who had failed previous therapies lived on average almost a year longer than patients without the drug. The FDA approved the drug after just five months of deliberations. In 1994, the agency gave the green light for relapsed breast cancer patients to take Taxol. In that trial, one in four patients saw their tumors shrink more than 50 percent. Their life expectancy increased by nearly a year.

It had taken more than thirty years to bring Taxol from its initial discovery to a government-approved drug. Like most chemotherapy agents, Taxol was no cure. It depleted white blood cells and left patients prone to infection. Their hair fell out and they lost feeling in their fingers and toes. But it extended life in some patients. And in the world of cancer therapy, that was progress.

Bristol-Myers still had to deal with the long-term supply problem. In the late 1980s, NCI had recognized that bark processing would remain an expensive and controversial process. It began funneling millions of dollars to academic chemists to develop a synthetic method of producing Taxol. More than two dozen investigators eventually worked on the problem, including Robert Holton of Florida State University. In 1990 he patented a semisynthetic process that started with the renewable leaves and twigs of Yew trees. Bristol-Myers licensed his invention.

The stage was now set for a company bombshell. In January 1993, with Bill Clinton newly arrived in the White House and rising health care costs high on the Democratic Party's agenda, Wyden held a hearing of his small business subcommittee to question Taxol's price and the cozy relationship between NCI and the one pharmaceutical firm that had consistently shown interest in commercializing its products. Bristol-Myers had set its initial Taxol price eight times higher than the price NCI had paid to its contractors to produce the drug. A typical course of therapy would cost patients or their insurers more than ten thousand dollars. Ralph Nader and James Love of the Consumer Project on Technology demanded the government exercise its "march in" rights and establish a reasonable price for the drug. Wyden was listening.

At the public hearing, the Oregon representative, whose constituents had jobs because of this new use of its forest products, read a letter from NCI director Sam Broder. It reviewed the history of Taxol, which showed NCI had not only been instrumental in its development but had been alone nearly every step of the way. "There are limits to what Americans ought to pay for drugs developed through billions of dollars of federal research and federal tax credits," Wyden complained. "Americans should not be held hostage to drug companies who threaten to walk away from cures if the Congress requires reasonable price justification."[48]

Bruce Chabner, the director of NCI's cancer treatment division, defended the company. The price was in the midrange of cancer drugs, he suggested, and the agency had ensured that poor and uninsured patients would get access to the drug. He then addressed the issue that was at the heart of NCI's fear of getting involved in drug pricing. Alluding to his recent experiences with Abbott Laboratories (see chapter 5), he said several companies had recently stopped participating in a government program to develop a novel anti-AIDS drug because of the "reasonable pricing" clause. Other potential collaborators had rejected the pricing clause outright. "There is no doubt that companies will not accept the risk of investing large sums in the development of a government product if their freedom to realize a profit is severely compromised," he said.[49]

Finally, Zola Horovitz, a vice president at Bristol-Myers, took the microphone. He ignored the price issue and made headlines by declaring the Taxol supply fears were over. The drug would be available to every woman in the United States who needed it. Moreover, the company would no longer harvest the Pacific Yew tree for its bark. By 1994, the company would rely exclusively on synthesized Taxol manufactured through the Holton process. He made only one oblique reference to the controversies swirling around the price of Taxol. "Substantial financial incentives are necessary to justify an enormous investment, sometimes measured in hundreds of millions of dollars, required for the rapid development of new pharmaceutical products," he said. "Any attempt to regulate prices will destroy the financial incentives necessary to attract private companies to these important collaborative research projects."[50]

Bristol-Myers, the major beneficiary of more than three decades of government-funded cancer drug development, had invested nowhere near "hundreds of millions of dollars" in bringing Taxol to market. Only after it received FDA approval did the company begin to invest substantial sums in Taxol—mostly on clinical trials aimed at expanding its use. In 2002, shortly after being sued by twenty-nine state attorneys general for delaying access to generic versions of the drug, chief executive officer Peter R. Dolan wrote a public letter to his employees claiming that Bristol-Myers had invested more than $1 billion since beginning its work on the drug's development eleven years before. Most of that money had been spent in six hundred postmarketing trials involving more than forty thousand patients, which were aimed at refining and expanding its potential uses.[51]

None of that investment represented risk capital. It represented a small portion of the ongoing sales of the new product. In its first full year on the market, Taxol generated nearly $600 million in sales. By 2001, Bristol-Myers was selling more than $1 billion of Taxol a year and had reaped more than $8 billion in total sales since the drug's approval. It was the first billion-dollar blockbuster in the history of cancer chemotherapy. Taxol had done more than extend lives. Bristol-Myers's price on the government's discovery turned cancer into a lucrative market.

In the wake of the Taxol discovery, numerous new players jumped into the hunt for anticancer drugs. By the mid-1990s, years of basic biological research into the molecular mechanics of cancer had turned up a range of potential therapeutic targets. The biotechnology revolution on Wall Street had simultaneously turned up hundreds of new companies, flush with venture capital funding, who were willing to explore the possibilities. Sometimes their lead compound—it could be a traditional small molecule drug, a monoclonal antibody that used the body's immune system to hit its target, or a recombinant protein—was developed in academic labs with government funding. Sometimes the targeted therapy was rooted in a private firm's own discoveries. But most often the potential therapy was the product of a collaboration between the two, facilitated by the technology transfer process established under the Bayh-Dole Act.

The shifting landscape forced NCI to reevaluate its own drug-hunting strategy. Richard Klausner, who became director of NCI in 1996, began placing bets on academic researchers who had developed potential targeted therapies but had failed for one reason or another to hook up with a drug company. "We were looking for the strength of the science. It could be anything: a peptide, a small molecule, a biological entity, a vector. We wanted to evaluate it through peer review that said it made sense as a cancer drug, based not on market consideration but only on the idea it was aimed at a target and there was data suggesting it might have an effect on cancer cells," he said. Using its virtual drug company skills, the agency backed a drug candidate through the various development stages, knowing that some company would pick it up if it ever became viable. In the first five years of the new program, the agency backed over fifty compounds with several reaching clinical trials.[52]

Despite those efforts, the Pharmaceutical Research and Manufacturers Association 2001 survey of cancer medicines in development revealed how much the landscape had been transformed over the previous decade. The trade group counted 402 cancer drugs and vaccines under development at 170 pharmaceutical and biotechnology companies. NCI, either alone or in partnership with a private firm, accounted for just ninety-three of those potential therapies. Most of the major pharmaceutical companies had a few entries on the roster. But the vast majority of candidates were being developed by companies with names like ImmunoGen, Intracel, SuperGen, and NeoPharm—small biotechnology firms whose financial prospects hinged on hitting a home run with the one or two drug candidates in their portfolios.[53]

To some longtime participants in the cancer wars, the locus of innovation had permanently shifted. "Initiative and creativity have moved to the private sector," Sam Broder, the former head of NCI, said. "There is just no way of getting around it, and anyone who tells you otherwise is on a different planet. What was done in the early seventies was necessary, even in retrospect, but that doesn't mean we should do it that way now."[54] After leaving NCI in 1995, Broder worked for a time with a company seeking to bring a generic version of Taxol to market before joining Celera Genomics' drug discovery team as its chief medical officer.

But Klausner, who left NCI in 2002 to lead the Bill and Melinda Gates Foundation's program for developing drugs for the less developed world, believes the government still has a major role to play in the hunt for new drugs. "We could support the only laboratory big enough for the entire drug industry, which is everyone," he said during 2001, the war on cancer's thirtieth anniversary year. "That's the right-size laboratory for discovering pharmaceuticals. That doesn't mean there isn't a role for a drug discovery in a drug company. But there's no way for one company to keep track of all the biology that's out there."[55]

Recent experience suggests the financial incentives that drive private firms won't be sufficient to overcome the hurdles that inevitably stand in the way of researchers seeking to bring new cancer drugs to market. The first targeted molecules that made it through the regulatory process required something as old as science itself—the passion of dedicated researchers who wouldn't take no for an answer.

Dennis Slamon is one such researcher. Son of a disabled West Virginia truck driver, he attended the unheralded Washington and Jefferson College in Washington, Pennsylvania, before his good grades earned him a full scholarship to the University of Chicago Pritzker School of Medicine, where he simultaneously earned a doctorate in cell biology. After completing his residency, he gravitated to a junior faculty position at the University of California at Los Angeles, at the time considered a backwater in cancer research. Slamon, who preferred lab work to treating patients, began collecting tumor specimens and dreamed of finding oncogenes, which by the time he arrived in the late 1970s had become the hottest topic in cancer research.

In the mid-1980s, Slamon hooked up with Axel Ullrich of Genentech, an experienced gene cloner who had isolated several oncogenes believed to be associated with cancer. Ullrich visited UCLA to present his work in isolating and cloning epidermal growth factor (EGF), which regulates cell growth and overpopulates the surfaces of some cancers. The gene had been discovered by Massachusetts Institute of Technology scientists and cloned by three different labs. But Genentech, which in those days was not far removed from its entrepreneurial roots, gave Ullrich a free hand to pursue the target. He began sending his gene samples to Slamon to test against the DNA extracted from his collection of tumor cultures to see if they could find a match.

In 1986, Slamon hit pay dirt. Actually, it was an undergraduate research assistant in his lab named Wendy Levin who made the discovery since Slamon couldn't afford his own graduate students or postdocs. Ullrich's gene for the human-epidermal-growth-factor receptor-2 (Her-2) matched a protein on the surface of some breast and ovarian cancer cells. A normal breast cell has about sixty thousand Her-2 receptors on its surface. But on a cell with a Her-2 mutation, there were more than a million, each telling it to divide. The result was a particularly virulent form of the disease that hits about one in four breast cancer patients.[56]

While other cancer researchers were dismissing his results as nonreproducible, Slamon began a full-court press to develop monoclonal antibodies aimed at the receptor that might jam up its machinery. The immune system produces antibodies when an invader like a virus or bacteria enters the body. They latch onto a receptor on the invader and stop it from functioning. After isolating the antibody, scientists can use recombinant technology to manufacture it in bulk (the multiple expression of a single antibody is called a monoclonal antibody) so they can give it as a drug. Georges J. F. Köhler and César Milstein—joint winners of the Nobel Prize—developed that critical technology at Cambridge University in the mid-1970s with the support of the British government's Medical Research Council. Within a decade it found widespread use in university and industry labs around the world. Slamon asked at least three different industrial labs and a similar number of academic labs to make a monoclonal antibody aimed at the Her-2 receptor. "We wouldn't restrict ourselves to any one person or lab," Slamon recalled in an interview more than a decade later, "including ones we developed ourselves." Ullrich's Genentech lab won the race.[57]

Slamon ran into his first roadblock. Genentech had been down the cancer road before. It had invested heavily in interferon in the early 1980s based on the media-inflated hype that it was the ultimate cure for cancer. But its alpha-interferon turned out to be effective only against hairy cell leukemia, an extremely rare form of the disease. It licensed the product to Roche, which soon showed it was effective against hepatitis B and Kaposi's sarcoma (the skin lesions that were the first manifestations of full-blown AIDS) and reaped the rewards from the drug. Genentech's other anticancer drugs—recombinant versions of gamma-interferon and tumor necrosis factor—failed to show results.

By the late 1980s, Genentech was also a company rapidly shedding its feisty start-up status. Kirk Raab, a former Abbott marketing executive, had taken over the company's reins in the mid-1980s. The company finally had two FDA-approved drugs in its portfolio—human growth hormone and an anticlotting medicine—and the science-driven agenda of its early years was giving way to the Wall Street imperative for sales and profits. It farmed out most of its clinical trials to contractors, leaving it ill-suited to bringing a brand new drug to market.

A few years later the government began investigating the company for the unethical and possibly illegal promotion of its two FDA-approved products. A congressional subcommittee investigation found the company had granted stock options to outside scientists testing its anti-blood-clotting medicine. Genentech's overly aggressive sales force used those tests to push sales of the wildly expensive biotech drug even though subsequent trials by nonaffiliated scientists showed it was no better than a much cheaper and older drug. To push human growth hormone, its other product, the company set up a program to measure millions of school children, hoping to convince parents with short kids to put them on the drug.[58]

It wasn't until 1995, when Genentech's board ousted Raab and installed Arthur Levinson, a first-rate scientist who had done his post-doctoral work under oncogene pioneer Michael Bishop at UCSF, that the company put Herceptin on its front burner. Commenting on the scandals surrounding the firm at the time of his takeover, Levinson said, "We haven't always been proud to work here."[59]

Slamon's relationship with the company bridged that troubled history. Ullrich quit Genentech in 1988, in part because he was frustrated by the company's refusal to dedicate resources to investigating the Her-2 cancer connection. Over the next several years, Slamon repeatedly traveled to the Bay Area to haunt the corridors of the biotechnology firm, looking for anyone interested in the drug. It limped along with support from Michael Shepard, who had joined Genentech right out of graduate school in 1980 and replaced Ullrich. Shepard complained bitterly about his lack of support inside the firm. "They were really very allergic to cancer," he said.[60] The program also had support from Levinson, who was moving up the ranks of Genentech's research department, and a vice president of manufacturing, whose mother was dying of breast cancer. Frustrated by the company's slow pace, Slamon looked to NCI for assistance. Still skeptical about targeted therapies, the agency's drug development program said no. "Antibodies had been tried in the past and weren't successful. They said [my proposal] was derivative, not very innovative, and not very new. It got the usual knocks," he recalled.[61]

Slamon would not have made it through those rocky years without support from Hollywood, a story that in itself speaks volumes about the serendipitous road to therapeutic innovation.[62] In the early 1980s, Brandon Tartikoff, the creator of *Cheers* and *Hill Street Blues* and a cancer survivor, felt a swollen gland in his neck. Fearing a recurrence of Hodgkin's disease, he went to a top physician at UCLA who told him everything was fine. Unconvinced, Tartikoff called his former roommate at Yale, a physician who had been Slamon's roommate in medical school. The referral got made, and after Slamon reviewed the slides, he correctly diagnosed the cancer's recurrence. He put Tartikoff on a drug regimen that kept the disease in remission for well over a decade.

Over those years, the Tartikoff and Slamon families grew close. Their kids attended the same schools. Brandon's wife, Lilly, an accomplished ballet dancer whose career was cut short by injury, decided to devote her life to raising money for Slamon's lab. She worked her connections in

Hollywood and eventually convinced Revlon chairman Ronald Perelman, who made billions peddling cosmetics, to do more for women beyond donating money for a dermatology clinic. "You give millions for zits but nothing for breast cancer," she told him.[63] Perelman's foundation held its first Fire and Ice Ball in 1990, a black-tie five-hundred-dollars-a-plate affair that attracted more than a thousand of Hollywood's glitterati. Between 1989 and the drug's approval in 1998, Revlon would raise more than $13 million to support Slamon, who would later say that it would have taken another decade to bring the drug to market without the foundation's help.[64]

The clinical-trials collaboration between a reluctant Genentech and an eager Slamon that took place over the 1990s was a fitful one. The earliest trials for determining a safe dose of a drug now called trastuzumab (trade name Herceptin) justified one of the more important claims for the superiority of targeted therapies. Other than a mild allergic reaction treatable with antihistamines, the drug had almost no side effects. As soon as word of the nontoxic therapy got out, the company found itself besieged by volunteers for its clinical trials and in a nasty confrontation with breast cancer treatment activists. Modeling themselves after the AIDS activists, groups like the National Breast Cancer Coalition, led by breast cancer survivor Frances Visco, demanded that Genentech make the drug available to desperately ill women on a compassionate use basis. The company at first refused. Genentech also resisted Slamon's recommendations that they combine Herceptin with several different chemotherapy agents in critical third-stage trials in the hopes of finding the best regimen.

The bitterness spilled out when the results of the third-stage trial were announced at the annual meeting of the American Society for Clinical Oncology in Los Angeles in May 1998. Four hundred sixty-nine women whose metastatic breast cancer tumors overexpressed the Her-2 gene had received either traditional chemotherapy or chemotherapy combined with Herceptin. The response rate (the tumors shrank by at least half) increased from 29 percent of patients on chemotherapy alone to 45 percent in the Herceptin group. The disease did not resume progressing for 7.2 months on average in the Herceptin group compared to 4.5 months in the group on chemotherapy alone. The median survival time for patients in both groups was indistinguishable—about two years.[65]

The drug wasn't a slam dunk, but it was better than existing therapies and bound to gain FDA approval. Slamon made only a brief presentation at the press conference and refused to attend the party given that night by Genentech to celebrate the trial's results. "This drug could have come to market anywhere from four to six years earlier if people had believed in the data early on," he said. "I thank my lucky stars for some people in Genentech like Shepard. But there were others who didn't believe in it."[66] Subsequent trials using Herceptin alone showed the poisonous chemotherapy could be eliminated from the regimen entirely without increasing a patient's risk. Moreover, using the drug in one of the regimens that Slamon initially proposed (but was rejected by Genentech) decreased the death rate by 30 percent.[67]

Herceptin, one of the first targeted therapies that had been derived from three decades of basic science, was no magic bullet. It was only useful for a fourth of breast and ovarian cancer patients, with no clear indication of how long its benefits last. But it was an improvement over previous therapies, and for that, tens of thousands of women every year could be thankful. Genentech later claimed it spent from $150 million to $200 million on developing Herceptin. Within three years of its approval in September 1998, it was generating twice that in annual sales.[68]

Dennis Slamon's experience was far from unique. Many FDA-approved cancer therapies have had to overcome scientific skepticism and commercial reluctance, and in nearly every case a dedicated academic researcher made it happen. Tamoxifen, the earliest approved targeted therapy and the most widely prescribed medicine for women with breast cancer, would not exist were it not for Northwestern University's V. Craig Jordan, whose indefatigable work with the antiestrogenic compound began in the mid-1960s.

Jordan first encountered tamoxifen as a student intern for England's ICI Pharmaceuticals (now part of AstraZeneca). It was the swinging 1960s, and the estrogen blocker had been developed as a potential birth-control pill. It flopped when ICI clinicians discovered to their chagrin that tamoxifen actually enhanced the chances of pregnancy among subfertile women. However, one of its developers, Arthur Walpole, who was Jordan's doctoral adviser, believed the drug might have anticancer properties. Cancer surgeons had discovered in the 1930s that removing the ovaries—the primary source of estrogen—induced tumor regression in about a third of advanced breast cancer patients. In the mid-1950s, Elwood V. Jensen of the University of Chicago helped identify the estrogen receptor on breast and uterine cells and subsequently theorized that breast cancer patients who responded to ovary removal had developed mutant cells with an overabundance of estrogen receptors.

Drawing on that theory a decade later, Walpole encouraged his prized pupil to pursue using estrogen-blocking tamoxifen as a cancer therapy. "Charged with producing birth-control agents, he could not pursue the notion himself," Jordan recalled. "They weren't a cancer company. They had no history in this area. It was not seen to be a big market, maybe a few hundred thousand dollars at the most."[69]

Early clinical trials showed tamoxifen reduced tumors temporarily in about a third of patients with late-stage breast cancer. Since the drug had very few side effects, the British government allowed its use in 1973, with the U.S. government following suit five years later. NCI funded the U.S. trials; ICI provided the drug. Lois Trench, an NCI researcher who later went to work for ICI, was the main advocate for the drug within the agency.

Jordan, meanwhile, moved to the United States, first to the Worcester Foundation for Experimental Biology in Massachusetts and eventually to Northwestern University, where he continued working with the drug. Early on, he and his coworkers discovered that it was actually a by-product of digested tamoxifen that blocked estrogen from latching onto the cancer cells (one variation of the metabolite would become ralox-ifene, sold by Eli Lilly under the trade name Evista, for treatment of osteoporosis).

Jordan next turned to using tamoxifen for adjuvant, or additional, therapy after breast cancer surgery. "The drug, we hoped, would destroy micrometastases—undetectable tumor cells that had already spread around a woman's body and that, left unopposed, could evolve into fatal masses," he said. But for how long? A year of adjuvant therapy wasn't enough, he quickly discovered. It took years of clinical trials, many of them funded by NCI, to determine that five years of postoperative therapy worked best, reducing the recurrence of cancer by nearly 50 percent.

In 1993, NCI launched a massive Breast Cancer Prevention Trial among 13,388 postmenopausal women to assess tamoxifen's impact among women who had never had breast cancer. Six years later, the FDA approved its prophylactic use based on the results of that trial, which showed tamoxifen cut the risk nearly in half.[70] Once Eli Lilly's raloxifene was approved for osteoporosis prevention, NCI launched a major comparison trial to see if it worked better than tamoxifen at breast cancer prevention, which as of this writing is still underway. "This is the strength of America," said Jordan in a thick British accent that has survived his three decades in the United States. "It has made the commitment to find solutions to this problem. The government and taxpayers' money has been well served in this case."[71]

The poster child for targeted therapies is Gleevec, a small-molecule drug that originated in the Swiss labs of Ciba-Geigy, which is now part of Novartis Pharma AG. When the drug was first approved for chronic myeloid leukemia (CML) in May 2001, the press proclaimed a new era in cancer therapy, "the first fruits of some three decades of investment in research into the basic biology of cancer."[72] Yet once again, after stripping away the hyperbole, one finds that it took a dedicated independent researcher, aided by desperate patients, before a reluctant drug company delivered on the promise of its proprietary product.

CML, marked by an explosion of white blood cells up to fifty times greater than normal, strikes about eight thousand people in the United States a year, most of them in their fifties and sixties. People live on average about six years after developing the disease. In the late 1960s and early 1970s, researchers at the University of Pennsylvania discovered that the white blood cells in CML patients were marked by a chromosomal mutation—named the Philadelphia chromosome after the place of its discovery—where a small fragment of one chromosome had shifted onto its neighbor. It took another decade before researchers identified the gene disrupted by the transfer. It turned out to be a gene that triggered cell division. The mutated gene produced a cell surface receptor, one of the hundreds of tyrosine kinase signaling proteins produced in the body, whose switch was permanently turned on or at least was hyperactive. "We knew then that we had our molecular target for CML," said Owen Witte of UCLA, one of the researchers credited with the discovery.[73]

Witte spent most of the 1980s trying to interest drug companies in developing inhibitors without success. Most firms weren't interested in diseases with small patient populations. Companies like Novartis that were developing tyrosine kinase inhibitors focused their attention on receptors implicated in many cancers or those involved in heart disease. But in 1993, Brian Druker, newly recruited to Oregon Health Sciences University in Portland from Harvard Medical School, where he had studied CML, heard that one of the Novartis inhibitors that had been developed to block another receptor was active against the mutant kinase.

He called the company and convinced Nicholas Lyden, the drug's synthesizer, to send him samples of STI-571, which would become known as Gleevec. It proved extraordinarily potent in the test tube against CML cultures. Over the next five years, Druker became a transcontinental lob-byist demanding that Novartis conduct the preclinical work needed to get the drug ready for human testing. Lyden was on his side, but the small patient population meant he had little clout inside the firm. Testing the drug for animal toxicity; determining how fast it cleared the body; developing a soluble derivative—at every stage of its early development, Druker and Lydon had to push the company to move the drug along.[74]

Four years into the process, Lydon left the company to start his own firm, leaving no one inside Novartis eager to champion STI-571's cause. Though the drug was ready to test for safety and proper dosing in hu-mans, Druker had to fight with Novartis to make enough drug to conduct the trial. Voices inside Novartis resisted, arguing the company would be better off focusing on diseases that affected larger patient populations. "I forced them to call the question," Druker recalled. "I couched it in terms of 'make a decision': either get it into clinical trials or license it to me." Druker, whose research throughout the 1990s was supported by NCI and the Leukemia and Lymphoma Society, convinced the company to produce enough drug to conduct at least one trial. "It was entirely my own lob-bying that got the trial going," he said.[75]

In December 1999, he reported the startling preliminary results to the nearly ten thousand physicians attending the American Society of Hematology meeting in New Orleans. Every one of thirty-one patients given the drug had their blood counts return to normal, and nine of twenty patients treated for five months or longer had cleared the cancer-ous white blood cells from their systems entirely.

Even before that meeting, word of the experimental drug's remarkable success had begun rocketing through the CML patient community, largely via the Internet. The patients mounted a massive letter-writing campaign to Novartis headquarters demanding the company begin pro-ducing more drug. One patient submitted a petition to chief executive officer Daniel Vasella with more than four thousand signatures. NCI director Klausner, meanwhile, called Vasella to suggest Novartis collab-orate with the government on trials testing STI-571 against gastrointesti-nal stromal tumors (GIST), a rare stomach cancer, since it also overex-pressed the rogue receptor targeted by the molecule.

Stunned by the response, Vasella overrode his go-slow managers and ordered production of commercial quantities of the drug. It would be used for the next round of clinical trials and given free to desperately ill patients in a compassionate use program. "I told people not to worry about excess supplies of STI-571 that might never be sold," Vasella told the *Wall Street Journal.* "People had been trying to manage the testing program in a controlled way. We want to get this drug available to patients quickly, and to do that you simply can't stick to bureaucratic rules." He also approved clinical trials to test the drug against GIST, but rejected NCI's offer of help in its initial trials.[76]

A few months after the New Orleans meeting, STI-571, now known as Gleevec, became the best-known cancer drug in the world in the wake of publication of the completed studies in the *New England Journal of Medicine.* They showed fifty-three of fifty-four patients with CML responding to the drug. A companion study, had it received the same coverage in the press, might have dampened some of the enthusiasm. It showed that while the drug worked for about two-thirds of patients who had reached the crisis phase of the disease, virtually all of them within a year's time saw their white blood cell counts begin to mount—a sure sign of resistance by cells with the Philadelphia chromosome. Still, the FDA granted its approval for the drug in near record time and a year later also approved it for GIST.[77]

The drug was clearly better than interferon, the previously approved first-line therapy against the disease. But would the fast-growing cancer cells figure out a way around it, even in the patients diagnosed early in the disease who responded well to the drug? "The relapse rate after ten years could be 25 percent or 85 percent. The problem is you can't predict," Druker said. "If you draw a straight line from our early experience, you'd get 15 to 25 percent after ten years. But the rate could accelerate."[78] He has turned his attention to understanding and characterizing the mutations that survive in those patients, so chemists can one day design a drug that when used in combination with Gleevec might halt the cancer entirely.

The hope that numerous targeted cancer therapies would soon come cascading out of industry's labs suffered a series of setbacks shortly after Gleevec's approval. Two companies developing drugs aimed at EGF receptors, which proliferate in a number of major cancers, failed spectacularly during 2002. The FDA rejected AstraZeneca's Iressa, which had shown early promise in patients with lung cancer, when longer clinical trials showed no effect on survival. An advisory committee would later recommend approval based on a single study that showed it shrank tumors in fourteen of 139 patients who had already failed two other therapies.

One skeptic on the committee who voted against approval, Thomas Fleming, chairman of the biostatistics department at the University of

Washington, complained that the committee had been unduly influenced by a well-orchestrated parade of patient testimonials at the meeting. "When you have conducted an expanded access program involving more than twelve thousand patients, as the sponsor for Iressa had done, wouldn't you expect you could run out such a show, even when an intervention has at best very trivial effects?" he told *The Cancer Letter*, a newsletter that closely monitors developments in the cancer therapeutics industry. "I remember hearing many such testimonials for laetrile after tens of thousands of U.S. patients had traveled to Mexico to receive this agent in the late 1970s, until scientific trials were conducted that established laetrile provided no benefit."[79]

The second fiasco involved ImClone System Inc.'s Erbitux, which also targeted EGF. The company became a household word when insiders dumped its stock after receiving an FDA letter warning that its new drug application was inadequate. ImClone chairman Samuel Waksal downplayed the agency's concerns when he finally made the FDA letter public. The previous fall, he had negotiated a $2-billion deal with Bristol-Myers that made the medical entrepreneur and Manhattan socialite a millionaire many times over.

For a few days after the FDA's letter, Waksal's public reassurances stabilized the company's stock. But after *The Cancer Letter* published the details of the FDA letter, which showed the company's clinical trials would have to be repeated, the resulting publicity and stock price collapse led both Congress and federal prosecutors to launch investigations. Waksal eventually resigned from ImClone and pleaded guilty to securities fraud and bank fraud, while Bristol-Myers took control of its troubled Erbitux project.[80]

The inventor of Erbitux was John Mendelsohn, director of the M. D. Anderson Cancer Center. His story paralleled the remarkable tales of Slamon, Jordan, and Druker—but only up to a point. It began in the 1970s at the University of California at San Diego, where he went to teach and conduct research after earning his undergraduate and medical degrees from Harvard. The oncogene revolution set off by the Bishop-Varmus discovery put him on the path of searching for uncontrolled growth signals in cancer cells. He focused on EGF since it proliferated wildly in many cancers. He eventually developed a monoclonal antibody that could latch onto the EGF receptor and stop it from functioning.

Though he started the NCI-funded cancer center at San Diego and did his most creative work there, the agency turned down his requests for further funding. Targeted therapies simply weren't on the agency's radar screen in those days. So, like Slamon, he turned to private foundations, and by the mid-1980s had used their money to develop a potential drug that worked well in cancerous mice. Once he published his mouse studies, NCI began supporting his work. By the late 1980s Mendelsohn had a version of the large protein molecule that wouldn't provoke severe immune reactions when injected into humans.[81]

UCSD, which owned the patent, initially licensed the drug to a small biotechnology start-up called Hybritech. Eli Lilly bought the company in 1992, but rejected working on the promising drug. The license reverted to UCSD. Mendelsohn, meanwhile, moved on to become the chairman of the department of medicine at Memorial Sloan-Kettering in New York. In an effort to rejuvenate work in his potential therapy, he hooked up with Samuel and Harlan Waksal, ambitious brothers who had started ImClone Systems Inc. in 1985 with a goal, as Harlan later told *Business Week*, to "focus on infectious diseases, cancer, and diagnostics, make some products, get rich, and retire early."[82]

Samuel Waksal had worked at NCI and held research posts at Stanford, Tufts, and Mt. Sinai Medical Center before starting ImClone. But he was, according to some of his contemporaries, nothing more than a slick scientific salesman, a fast talker who could dazzle his colleagues with his knowledge of the latest advances without actually conducting his own research. Mendelsohn didn't learn until later that his partner was forced from each of those positions after being accused of falsifying data, and that his brother Harlan in the early 1980s was convicted of possessing cocaine with intent to distribute, although the conviction was overturned on appeal.[83]

What was apparent from the beginning was that the Waksal brothers had virtually no experience developing drugs.[84] Yet just when the experimental cancer therapy was about to go into clinical trials, Mendelsohn essentially withdrew from day-to-day involvement. While he wanted to push his experimental cancer therapy, he also wanted to pursue his career within the cancer establishment. In 1996, he accepted the top job at M. D. Anderson Cancer Center in Houston. Erbitux became a drug whose scientific champion couldn't play a hands-on role in its development. Physicians at the institution would eventually take part in the clinical trials of Erbitux. But as a member of ImClone's board of directors, with a financial stake in the firm and a potential recipient of royalties, Mendelsohn could play no role in either designing or implementing the studies. To do so would have violated conflict-of-interest guidelines he put in place shortly after joining the world famous center.[85]

The Waksals announced the findings of their original studies at the annual meeting of ASCO, which met in San Francisco in June 2001. Nearly a quarter of patients with colon cancer who had failed chemotherapy saw their tumors shrink by at least half when treated with Erbitux and chemotherapy, the company's clinicians reported. The ebullient sponsors hired the Doobie Brothers to entertain the more than fifteen thousand practicing oncologists at the meeting. The buzz generated a cover story in *Business Week* and a glowing profile on CBS's *60 Minutes*.

Six months later, the FDA weighed in with its evaluation. The data was inadequate and uncontrolled. The evaluators couldn't tell if the benefits came from the traditional chemotherapy agent used in the trial or Erbitux. Even the choice of patients was suspect. Not only did the agency refuse to consider the new drug application, they noted in their nine-page letter that the company had been repeatedly told in the months leading up to the application that the trials would probably have to be repeated.[86]

"We screwed up," Waksal told an investors' conference a few days later. Within a few months, Bristol-Myers would bounce him from the floundering firm. Mendelsohn, who gave a keynote lecture to the ASCO meeting in Orlando a few months later and was called before Congress several times to explain his actions during the drug's development, was more upbeat. Erbitux was still a good drug, he insisted. At ASCO, he cited one study showing that all six patients with head and neck cancer responded to a combination of Erbitux and cisplatin. Yet when the full study was released a few days later, it showed just one patient out of forty-four achieving a complete response and just five (11.4 percent of patients) had a partial response that lasted long enough to reach clinical significance.[87] In the fall of 2002, Mendelsohn defended the Waksals and ImClone's actions before an oversight subcommittee of the House Energy and Commerce Committee. "The protocol was developed with the advice of medical oncologists from some of the world's greatest institutions, twenty-seven of which participated in carrying it out," he testified. Praising ImClone and Bristol-Myers for launching a new round of trials, he said his greatest regret was that "Erbitux will not be available for patients who need it as soon as we had originally hoped."[88]

Are targeted therapies just one more failure on the cancer crusade's long and winding road? Or are they another incremental step toward more beneficial and more benign treatments that might one day turn many cancers into manageable chronic illnesses? And why is Gleevec so successful, while Erbitux or Iressa seem to have so little impact? To Brian Druker, Gleevec's champion, the answers can be found in the science that preceded the drugs. More than thirty years of research went into understanding the Philadelphia chromosome and its impact on CML. "Just because you know what targets your drug hits, doesn't mean you've got a good drug," he said. "You've got to have a good target and I don't think we have that many good targets. We have a huge amount of work to do to validate good targets. I think there will be good targets in each cancer. But the current list is extremely short in my book."

Druker questions weather the EGF receptor will turn out to be a good target for cancer drugs. It may take years, perhaps decades of additional investigation before the process of angiogenesis in tumors is well understood. "We have pseudo-empiricism in most cancers," he said. "It's like taking your car to a mechanic. He looks under the hood and says, 'I see you have this part here. If I replace it, your car will run better.' You say, 'Is that part broken?' The mechanic says, 'I don't know, but it might be.'" Many of the new cancer drugs are targeting things in cancer cells that may or may not be driving that cancer. "I think the paradigm will work," he said, "but we're not ready in most cancers with the right targets."[89]

Jordan, whose career is synonymous with tamoxifen, believes a successful recipe for developing drugs must include investigator passion. During our long discussion, I asked him how he has stayed motivated to work on the same drug for more than thirty years. "If you had five hundred people with this kind of passion, this is how you make progress. Just by throwing money at various things and buying mercenaries to work on that problem doesn't solve the problem. The following week, they'll work on something else if there is more money over there," he said. "You have to want to do it without the money."[90]

Ellen Vitetta has brought that kind of passion to her study of non-Hodgkin's lymphoma, which strikes about forty thousand Americans annually. Over the past two decades, she has studied the cancer, worked on developing a monoclonal antibody that would seek it out, and developed a poison derived from castor beans to attach to the antibody that, hopefully, will kill the cancer. She calls it immunotoxin therapy. A graduate of the New York University School of Medicine, she worked briefly with Kohler and Milstein at Cambridge before moving on to the University of Texas Southwestern Medical Center in Dallas.

What sets her lab apart is that it does all the work of translating her basic science into potential therapies in-house. "We develop the antibodies, we test them, we take them in preclinical trials in primates, we manufacture them in the academic institutions, we do all the FDA testing in-house. We are an entire drug company within an academic institution, and we do it all on federal grants [of about $2 million a year]," she said. Her lab has about a half dozen drugs in its pipeline. "When they begin to emerge, the drug companies begin sniffing around. Some of them want a license; some want to share in the trials; some want to sponsor the research and let us do the work; some want the rights if it ever reaches the finish line. My own view is I don't want them telling me what to do. I want to do this in a scientifically driven way."[91]

The story thus far has focused on documenting the government's role in fostering basic science and the early steps of the drug innovation process. It has shown how taxpayer-funded directed research played the leading role in the battle against some of the nation's most pressing health care problems like AIDS and cancer. In almost every case, pharmaceutical and biotechnology companies also played critical roles in bringing new drugs to market. Sometimes the role began early in the process, in chemically synthesizing a new drug. Sometimes it began late in the process, when the new drug was well along in clinical trials. Sometimes the private firms invested large sums in the process. Sometimes participation cost the drug company next to nothing.

So a central question remains: Do the steps drug companies play in bringing an innovative drug to market demand the extraordinary sums industry pours (over $30 billion in 2001) into research and development? Does the cost of these steps justify the high cost the industry charges the public for drugs?

The next two chapters seek to answer those questions. But first we must go back to the earliest days of the modern pharmaceutical industry to trace the history of an industry practice that has nothing to do with bringing innovative medicines to market, a practice that at the dawn of the new century accounted for more than half of all industry research and development.

PART THREE

BIG PHARMA

8

Me Too!

President Franklin Delano Roosevelt had every reason for optimism in the winter of 1936. He had just won reelection in a landslide, and the prospects for the more far-reaching of his New Deal reforms never looked brighter. But just before Christmas, close aides brought word that his only son, Franklin Delano Jr., had a bad case of tonsillitis. With her son's fever soaring, Eleanor Roosevelt called in White House physician George Tobey Jr. He feared the worst. The infection had seeped into the blood, which in those days was a potentially fatal condition.

More out of desperation than any sense that it might help the young man, Tobey gave the president's son a new German drug called Prontosil. When news of the drug first appeared in the medical literature a year earlier, most American doctors scoffed. How could a derivative of a chemical dye cure a bacterial infection? But to Tobey's surprise, young Roosevelt's fever quickly subsided. A few days later the press heralded both the medicine and the miraculous recovery in the first family. "New control for infections," the *New York Times* headlined its front-page story. The era of wonder drugs was underway.

Prontosil not only heralded the modern era of drug therapy, it ushered in the modern era of drug marketing. It helped transform the Depression-era pharmaceutical industry from a sprinkling of small firms peddling a handful of cures (an early 1930s symposium listed only seven diseases amenable to drug treatment) to the modern corporations that we know today: vertically integrated giants that can develop, produce, and, most important to their bottom lines, market drugs.

Prontosil was discovered by Gerhard Domagk, a young physician on the staff of Bayer Laboratories in Elberfeld, Germany. Inspired by the pioneering work of fellow countryman Paul Ehrlich, who had discovered the first drug treatment for syphilis, Domagk spent five years screening hundreds of Bayer's industrial dyes and their derivatives for their antibacterial properties. Five days before Christmas 1932, he discovered that one of his red dyes cured a handful of mice that he had infected with deadly streptococcus. Over the next two years, while ignoring the social upheavals around him that brought Adolf Hitler to power, Domagk and physicians on the staff of the local hospital injected dozens of patients with the new drug. It not only killed streptococci but had powerful effects on patients suffering from a host of life-threatening infections like rheumatic and scarlet fever, which had been the scourge of children for centuries.

Domagk published the first report about his miraculous cures in February 1935 in an obscure academic journal. Researchers around the world immediately began trying to replicate his results. A husband-and-wife team in France soon discovered that it wasn't the dye that killed the streptococci, but one of its constituent chemicals, which only became active after the patient metabolized the original drug. The active ingredient in Prontosil, they discovered, was sulphanilamide, a common industrial chemical that was no longer patented and that no one had ever thought to test against bacteria.

Within months, every drug company in the world began synthesizing their own versions of sulfanilamide. Bayer was left without any financial remuneration for the pioneering research of Domagk and his colleagues. German dictator Adolf Hitler's health ministers, meanwhile, heaped scorn on his extraordinary achievement. They called the medicine quackery and in late 1939 forced Domagk to write a letter to the Caroline Institute in Stockholm turning down his Nobel Prize.[1]

As war clouds gathered over Europe, dozens of companies in England, France, Germany, and the United States began peddling their own versions of the miracle sulfa drugs. These first copycat drugs, usually called me-too drugs by industry insiders, created a problem that has bedeviled the industry thereafter—the propensity for some of the newer versions of the drug to be less safe than the ones that already existed. In 1937, a small Tennessee firm named Massengill and Company started making a liquid form of the medicine because it believed southerners and children preferred it that way. Since sulfanilamide did not dissolve in water or alcohol, company chemists opted to suspend the drug in diethylene glycol, an industrial solvent used to make antifreeze. No one at the company thought to test the product for safety before it began selling the concoction. Later testimony showed that no one at the company even bothered to look up diethylene glycol in a textbook. Within weeks of the medicine's initial marketing, more than one hundred people were dead, most of them children. When questioned by the dozens of reporters who poured into Tennessee to cover the tragedy, the company's president refused to take responsibility. His chief chemist committed suicide.[2]

The incident led an outraged Congress to alter the 1906 Pure Food and Drug Act. The original Progressive Era legislation, which had been created in response to public outrage over contaminated food, had drugs in its title but did little to regulate the industry. The Massengill tragedy put an end to that. For the first time, companies were required to prove to an expanded Food and Drug Administration (FDA) that their drugs were safe for human consumption before they could put them on the market.

The advent of FDA drug regulation radically transformed the pharmaceutical marketplace. Companies began marketing their wares directly to doctors—either through advertising in medical journals or through office visits (called detailing in the trade because the salesmen provided physicians with the latest details on new medicines) instead of through the traditional channels, which to that point had been largely newspaper and magazine advertising.

The result was intense competition among many companies in the still limited marketplace for scientifically proven medicines. Detailers would crowd physicians' offices, leaving behind free samples and various trinkets. But it was very difficult to differentiate their products. Every version of the new sulfa drugs, for instance, had basically the same medical outcome. Textbook economics took over. The price of the new sulfa drugs plunged.

The pattern was repeated when the first miracle antibiotics came along in the years immediately after World War II. The government, which had developed the mass production techniques for penicillin as a wartime measure, licensed the drug to five firms. Those firms engaged in a fierce competition for sales. Between 1945 and 1950, the price of penicillin plunged from $3,955 to $282 a pound.

The pattern happened yet again with the next generation of antibiotics. In the late 1940s Selman Waksman and his colleagues at Rutgers University in New Brunswick, New Jersey, developed streptomycin, a derivative of bacteria-killing microbes that he had found in soil. Waksman, a soil botanist, made his discovery by pursuing the reasonable assumption that soil must contain something that killed bacteria since they didn't survive burial. His drug proved to be the first effective treatment for tuberculosis, earning Waksman the Nobel Prize and making him America's most celebrated research scientist until Jonas Salk and the first polio vaccine came along in the mid-1950s. But unlike Salk, who would refuse to patent the polio vaccine ("Could you patent the sun?" Salk answered Edward R. Murrow when he was asked who owned the vaccine on *See It Now*), Waksman patented streptomycin and licensed it to Merck Research Laboratories in nearby Rahway, whose engineers and scientists had done much of the production work.

Waksman's decision to seek a patent on his discovery represented a second watershed event in the evolution of the modern drug industry. For the first time, the Patent and Trademark Office (PTO) gave seventeen-year exclusivity to the chemical modifications and the processes that created a product—streptomycin—that in its raw state had been part of nature. Merck wouldn't benefit from that decision, however. Worried about a public backlash against a private company generating massive profits from scientific research conducted at a public university, Waksman convinced Merck to return the license for streptomycin to the nonprofit Rutgers Research Foundation. The drug was then licensed broadly and sold generically. The price of the miracle drug soon fell to rock-bottom levels, a repeat of the penicillin story.[3]

The industry recognized it had to deal with its disastrous experience with the first three antibiotics. A number of firms had already deployed chemists to develop new microbe killers using Waksman's techniques. Three firms quickly came up with new medicines comparable to streptomycin. They patented the results despite the fact the uses of the new drugs were virtually indistinguishable from their predecessors. However, without the government or Waksman to prod them, they refused to license the new medicines to other firms. Given the similarity in medical outcomes from the various antibiotics now on the market, an intense competition for market share should have broken out. But this time, just the opposite occurred. The price of the new drugs, marketed as improved versions of the generic antibiotics penicillin and streptomycin, soared.

A decade later, the Federal Trade Commission launched a massive investigation into the antibiotic cartel. It turned up overwhelming evidence showing the industry refused to compete against one another on price even though every company was charging far more than the cost of production and a reasonable return on its investment. Yet the agency refused to crack down. In essence, it accepted industry's argument that it was sufficient that competition took place in arenas other than price, such as the frequency of dosage or the method of getting the drug into the body. "The producers regained this market power by differentiating their products along the lines that any other consumer good is differentiated," economic historian Peter Temin wrote. "Since the therapeutic effects of the drugs appeared to be identical, other—more familiar—quality dimensions had to be employed. So the firms intensified their advertising, their detailing, and their reliance on company identities. The postwar pattern of integrated drug companies competing by introducing and marketing new drugs was beginning to take shape."[4]

Throughout the 1950s, drug companies, often drawing on the latest research emerging from academic labs but sometimes relying on their own resources, discovered class after class of new medicines. Antidepressants, antacids, anti-inflammatory medicines, antihistamines, and new chemicals for controlling blood pressure became mainstays of the modern medicine chest. Whenever one company broke new ground, other firms in the industry would introduce copycat versions of the original molecule within a very short time. The me-too drugs almost always entered the market at the same or within a few percentage points of the innovator's price.

By the early 1960s, popular anger over the high price of drugs led Senator Estes Kefauver of Tennessee to hold a series of hearings on the drug industry's behavior. A Yale-trained lawyer who had arrived in Washington in the late 1930s as an idealistic New Dealer, Kefauver by the early 1950s had became one of Washington's most powerful and closely watched senators, largely because of his well-publicized attacks on organized crime. But after his support for civil rights and principled opposition to the demagogy of Senator Joseph R. McCarthy cost him a shot at the presidency, he turned his attention to abusive corporate practices, using his chairmanship of the Senate Subcommittee on Antitrust as a platform. "I keep feeling that mergers, consolidations, and cooperation between large blocs of economic power are on the increase, and that this is bound to lead to total abuse of our free-enterprise system, and inevitably, to total state control—in short, statism," he told *New Yorker* writer Richard Harris in 1961. "That is something none of us want."[5]

In a series of hearings between 1960 and 1962, Kefauver focused public attention on the drug industry's penchant for spending much of its time and resources developing copycat drugs, which, in defiance of every economics textbook, rarely resulted in competition on price. He called numerous medical professionals and former industry executives to testify. At one point, Kefauver pressed the former head of research at E. J. Squibb to estimate how much corporate drug research was driven by the desire to come up with me-too drugs. The retired executive replied that "more than half is in that category. And I should point out that with many of these products it is clear while they are on the drawing board that they promise no utility. They promise sales."[6]

Ironically, the 1962 amendments to the Food and Drug Act that resulted from the hearings did little to curb the industry's penchant for pursuing me-too drugs. They required drug companies for the first time to prove their drugs were not only safe but effective. That change was put into effect largely because of the thalidomide tragedy, which came to light as the hearings were drawing to a close and was only prevented in the United States by the stalling tactics of an eagle-eyed FDA physician.

The first great era of drug discovery, then, which stretched roughly from 1935 to the mid-1960s, could also be called the era of molecular modification. Once a researcher—often in the public sector—identified a new chemical class that was effective against a disease state, every major drug company put chemists to work coming up with their own versions that could do roughly the same thing. "The great drug therapy era was marked not only by the introduction of new drugs in great profusion and by the launching of large promotional campaigns but also by the introduction of what are known as 'duplicative' or 'me-too' products," noted pharmacologist Milton Silverman and physician Philip R. Lee of the University of California at San Francisco. Surveying the drug scene in the early 1970s, they counted more than 200 sulfa drugs, more than 270 antibiotics, 130 antihistamines, and nearly 100 major and minor tranquilizers. Most of the new drugs "offer the physician and his patient no significant clinical advantages but are different enough to win a patent and then be marketed, usually at the identical price of the parent product, or even at a higher price."[7]

The biotechnology revolution of the late 1970s and 1980s and the NIH-funded explosion of knowledge about cellular interactions set off a second wave of drug innovation. Drawing from the government's vast investment in biomedical research since the end of World War II, medical researchers promised unique cures for the chronic diseases that had become the leading causes of death: heart disease, cancer, diabetes, and dementia. Cover stories in the nation's popular magazines and newspapers heralded the exploits of scientific medicine, often focusing on the drug companies that were bringing the new products to market. No longer would the drug industry focus on developing and marketing me-too drugs that did little more than cloud physicians' judgments and crowd pharmacists' shelves. A new era of miracle drugs was at hand, the companies' press releases suggested.

Progress on delivering on those promises was slow, however. A handful of the new biotechnology products, such as erythropoietin, human growth, and blood clotting factors, which hit the market in the first decade after biotechnology's emergence, certainly were unique. Physicians for the first time were able to replace or enhance patients' supplies of naturally occurring proteins by injecting artificial versions.

The handful of genetically engineered medicines that emerged in the first two decades of the biotechnology revolution were also unique in an economic sense. In 1980 the Supreme Court in *Diamond v. Chakrabarty* liberalized the nation's intellectual property laws by allowing the patenting of living things. (The case involved a patent on an oil-eating bacteria.) The young start-up companies that manufactured the proteins were now able to protect themselves against me-too competition by surrounding their inventions with gene and gene-process patents. For this new class of medicines, companies no longer had to rely on marketing and cartel-like behavior to ensure against a sharp decline in prices due to competition from me-too drugs. They could rely on the exclusivity granted by patent law. There would be only one genetically engineered version of a therapeutic protein.

By the mid-1970s, traditional pharmaceutical companies were also beginning to take advantage of the burst of knowledge generated by the government's generous funding of academic research during the postwar years. Firms introduced a number of new drugs and new classes of drugs, which they advertised as clearly superior to the older drugs on pharmacists' shelves. A 2001 survey of 225 physicians ranked the top innovations in medicine over the previous thirty years, putting several new medicines near the top of the list. A majority of doctors ranked angiotensin converting enzyme (ACE) inhibitors for controlling blood pressure and statins for lowering arterial plaque-forming cholesterol levels among the top six medical inventions. About 40 percent of the doctors thought the new antidepressants and new antacids were clearly superior to older medications aimed at the same symptoms. However, the physicians weren't convinced that every new class of medicine represented a significant medical advance. The same survey showed fewer than 2 percent of doctors considered nonsedating antihistamines, calcium channel blockers, and erectile dysfunction drugs as major innovations.[8]

As each new class hit the market, however, whether or not it represented a therapeutic improvement over older medicines, the leading pharmaceutical companies reverted to their now familiar pattern of introducing roughly comparable products. Their sometimes vicious marketing competition resulted in a divvying up of the market but rarely competition on price. By the early 1990s, drug prices, like health care costs generally, were soaring at double-digit rates. When the Clinton administration put health care reform at the top of its political agenda, drug prices came under increasing public scrutiny. For the first time since Kefauver, the industry's me-too research practices were being called into question.

But this time industry officials used a new set of arguments in their response to the charge that they wasted research dollars on copycat drugs. Many of the new me-too drugs had fewer side effects than their predecessors, industry officials claimed. They also suggested that individual patients responded differently to drugs, so me-too drugs offered an alternative for people who did not respond to other drugs in that class. "There's no such thing as a 'one-size-fits-all' drug," a typical handout from the Pharmaceutical Research and Manufacturers of America (PhRMA), the industry's main trade association, said. "Each patient is unique and may respond to the same drug differently. What works for one person does not necessarily work for another. Physicians and patients benefit from a variety of medicines available to treat each ailment."

The Clinton administration's top drug officials were unimpressed by those arguments. Amid the 1993–94 health care debate, David Kessler, the activist head of the FDA, and a team of FDA drug reviewers published a scathing response to the industry's claims for the latest generation of me-too drugs. "In today's prescription-drug marketplace a host of similar products compete for essentially the same population of patients," they wrote in the *New England Journal of Medicine*. Reviewing the 127 new drugs approved between 1989 and 1993, Kessler and his team found that "only a minority offered a clear clinical advantage over existing therapies. Many of the others are considered me-too drugs because they are so similar to brand-name drugs already on the market."

"Pharmaceutical companies are waging aggressive campaigns to change prescribers' habits and to distinguish their products from competing ones, even when the products are virtually indistinguishable," the article continued. "This is occurring in many therapeutic classes—antiulcer products, angiotensin-converting-enzyme inhibitors, calcium-channel blockers, selective serotonin-reuptake-inhibitor antidepressants, and nonsteroidal anti-inflammatory drugs, to name a few. Victory in these therapeutic-class wars can mean millions of dollars for a drug company. But for patients and providers it can mean misleading promotions, conflicts of interest, increased costs for health care, and ultimately, inappropriate prescribing."[9]

No drug class illustrated Kessler's concerns better than the great stomach acid wars of the 1990s. The problems of heartburn, sour stomach, and acid indigestion are as all-American as ordering takeout pizza and beer after a long day at an aggravating job. The usual cure is a nonprescription acid neutralizer that can be purchased anywhere and in almost every form imaginable, from crunchy tablets to chalky liquids. But for some patients, the condition is chronic, often leading to stomach ulcers, gastroesophageal reflux disease (the backflow of stomach acid into the esophagus), and eventually erosive esophagitis. In those cases, doctors often prescribe one of the more powerful new medicines that arrived on the scene in the late 1970s through early 1990s, which attack the problem at its source—the production of acid—rather than relying on a neutralizer once it is already in the stomach. In recent decades, these prescription antacids have been among the pharmaceutical industry's most broadly prescribed and lucrative medicines.

The first class of prescription antacids to come along targeted histamines, whose production in the stomach is triggered by the presence of food. European scientists discovered histamines in the 1930s, and over the next several decades academic scientists on both sides of the Atlantic linked various histamines with complex body processes including the regulation of blood pressure, bronchial reactions, and the production of stomach acid. In 1937, a French academic discovered the first inhibitor of histamine, and over the next decade scientists came up with a number of comparable drugs. The most famous member of the class was diphenhydramine, sold over the counter today as Benadryl. It was developed by a U.S. academic scientist and later provided the chemical basis for the wildly popular antidepressant fluoxetine, more commonly known by its trade name, Prozac.

The first industry scientist to conduct systematic studies on histamine blockers was James Black, who worked at Smith, Kline, and French in the 1960s and 1970s. Black began his career as an academic pharmacologist in Glasgow, but during the 1950s he moved to Great Britain's ICI Pharmaceuticals (the drug wing of the mammoth Imperial Chemical Industries), where he helped develop the first drugs that could block adrenaline's effect on the heart. While still an academic, he had shown that there were at least two cell receptors that bound to adrenaline, but only one—the beta-receptor—was present on the heart muscle. His ICI team developed the first beta-blocker, propranolol. When it was introduced in 1962, it was considered a major breakthrough in the treatment of high blood pressure and heart disease.

After moving on to Smith, Kline, and French, Black applied the same dual-receptor concept to the histamines that were unleashed by the presence of food and sent signals for the production of stomach acid. European academic researchers had shown that the first generation of antihistamines, while useful for allergic reactions, did not block the secretion of stomach acid. Positing there must be at least two receptors, Black began synthesizing analogues of a histamine blocker that might block only the histamine receptor that triggered action in the stomach. Eight years and seven hundred chemicals later, Black came up with his first drug for blocking the stomach histamine (H_2) receptor. He spent several more years of fiddling before coming up with one that was useful as a drug. He called it cimetidine, which is sold under the trade name Tagamet. Other companies soon jumped on the bandwagon. In 1984, scientists at Glaxo won FDA approval for ranitidine (Zantac), which was similar chemically to cimetidine but had fewer side effects. It soon became the best-selling drug in the world, surpassing SmithKline's Tagamet and generating billions of dollars in sales for Glaxo.[10]

While Black and his imitators were pursuing H_2 antagonists, academic scientists began looking for the engines in the stomach cells that actually produced the acid. In 1977, George Sachs, a Scottish physician who taught at the University of Alabama at Birmingham, attended a symposium in Sweden, where he presented his work on the ion-exchange mechanism in stomach cells that produced acid. He called it the proton pump. After his talk, a young scientist from Astra Pharmaceuticals approached the podium. "This Swedish person asked me a question that was intriguing," Sachs recalled. "He had found a compound that inhibited the gastric pump in rats. They sent me a couple of compounds. My lab discovered the acid pump was the target. We also discovered that the drugs were converted into active form by the acid. In 1978, we went there, told them the mechanism, and started a tight collaboration that resulted in the synthesis of omeprazole (trade name Prilosec) as a candidate drug."[11]

The drug's development was delayed when some early safety experiments with omeprazole generated tumors in mice. Company officials feared the new drug might be a carcinogen. But low-dose experiments in monkeys and later humans dispelled those fears, and widespread clinical trials resumed. The FDA approved it for sale in 1989, with Merck acting as Astra's marketing agent in the United States.

By the early 1990s, the companies that made competing versions of the new antacids were battling over a $7-billion-a-year market. The leading firms began pouring hundreds of millions of research dollars into clinical trials in an effort to prove that their product was better than the competition. There is little interest among elite scientists in conducting these types of studies, although many medical professionals at the nation's academic medical centers take part in order to raise money for their labs. Many times the results aren't even published in the literature, or when they are, they appear in second-tier journals that receive little notice from the mainstream of the profession.[12]

By the end of 1994, Astra, Glaxo, and SmithKline had sponsored hundreds of studies on the relative merits of Prilosec, Zantac, and Tagamet. One reviewer counted 293 clinical trials comparing the drugs. He concluded that proton-pump inhibitors were marginally more effective at healing ulcers, with cure rates at 94 percent after four weeks for Prilosec compared to 70 to 80 percent for the H2 antagonists. The cure rate for Prilosec fell to 84 percent after eight weeks, and for some types of ulcers and conditions, the cure rates were statistically indistinguishable.[13] Despite the similarities between the drugs, Astra and Merck used the results to launch a massive marketing push for its proton-pump inhibitor, which soon turned Prilosec into the best-selling medicine in the world. By 2000, it was racking up nearly $5 billion a year in sales in the United States alone. TAP Pharmaceuticals' me-too proton-pump inhibitor Prevacid, launched in 1995, was the third-best-selling medicine in the United States with more than $3 billion in sales.[14]

Astra's research team wasn't through with heartburn yet. With the company's patent on Prilosec set to expire in 2001, company officials knew that generic manufacturers would line up to manufacture the lucrative pill. As early as 1995, Astra officials launched a massive research project to come up with a successor to their wildly popular purple pill (the color became a mainstay of its advertising campaigns). It would be best if they came up with a better drug, company scientists knew. But with an 80-percent cure rate for the existing antacids, a better mousetrap would be hard to find.

The company never considered one possible approach, which had been percolating in the world of academic medicine for more than a decade. In the years since the discovery of H2 antagonists and proton-pump inhibitors, scientifically inclined academics had moved away from interfering with the mechanisms for generating stomach acid. In 1983, Barry Marshall, then working at the Royal Perth Hospital in Australia, had isolated the *Helicobacter pylori* bacteria that flourished in the excess stomach acids of gastritis and ulcer patients. He believed it was the root cause of ulcers. After returning to the United States to a post at the University of Virginia, he used NIH funding to establish the Center for the Study of Diseases Caused by *Helicobacter pylori*. Over the course of the next decade, Marshall and other scientists showed that the bacteria, which infects about half the world's population, was the leading cause of stomach and intestinal ulcers, gastritis, and stomach cancer. The center even developed regimens of common antibiotics that could eliminate the minor infection.

Unfortunately, no pharmaceutical company championed the cure. They had no interest in eliminating the cause of ulcers with a short, cheap course of generic antibiotics when they could make billions of dollars treating their chronic recurrence with expensive prescription antacids. As one NIH analyst put it: "A one-time antibiotic treatment regimen to eliminate *H. pylori*, as opposed to long-term maintenance with H2-antagonist drugs, recurrence, and sometimes surgery as a last resort, is an obvious benefit both to the patient and to the health care insurers. However, [promoting this approach would lead to] the possible decline in sales."[15]

Instead of pursuing this potential cure for ulcers, Astra scientists launched Operation Shark Fin, an effort to find a drug to replace Prilosec after it came off patent and became generically available. At first they tried drug combinations and oral suspensions, but they didn't work any better and were less convenient. Finally, Astra scientists created a molecule that was, in essence, half of Prilosec. They dubbed it Nexium. In doing so, they used a process that by the late 1990s had become one of the drug industry's chief strategies for extending patents, a strategy that was garnering an increasing share of industry research-and-development budgets.

The process is based on a quirk in the chemistry of organic molecules. Scientists have long known that most organic molecules come in two shapes because their carbon atoms arrange themselves in six-sided rings. The side chains of atoms that make the molecule unique can attach themselves to either side of the symmetrical rings. The result is a mixture of two versions of the molecule, each with the same chemical formula, but different in that they are mirror images of each other, much like a person's left and right hands. Each version is called an enantiomer (science literature occasionally refers to them as isomers). Sometimes only one enantiomer is active against the disease. The other causes unwanted side effects or is inactive. Drug companies could not do much about it until the early 1990s when chemists developed a way of separating the two sides. That deft piece of chemistry was pioneered by K. Barry Sharpless of the Scripps Research Institute in La Jolla, California, Ryoji Noyori of Nagoya University, and William S. Knowles of Monsanto Company, who jointly shared the 2001 Nobel Prize for chemistry.

The new process succeeded in rescuing some drugs that had been sidelined for their unwanted side effects. In 1992, for instance, the FDA ordered Merrell Dow, which later became part of Aventis, to put a warning label on its allergy drug terfenadine (Seldane) after adverse reaction reports began pouring into the agency. Doctors who prescribed the nonsedating antihistamine for their allergy patients reported many terfenadine users had suffered severe heart palpitations after taking the drug. Six years and at least eight deaths later, it was withdrawn from the market. But the drug was resuscitated when a specialty chemical company called Sepracor separated the two enantiomers of terfenadine for Aventis, which was then able to continue marketing the safe but active half. They called it Allegra. Sepracor later performed the same trick for Johnson and Johnson after its allergy drug astimezole (Hismanal) suffered a similar fate.

Operation Shark Fin's Nexium, marketed as the new purple pill, was nothing more than one of Prilosec's enantiomers. But unlike the antihistamines that had to be withdrawn from the market, Prilosec had no major side effects. It was even possible that both of Prilosec's enantiomers became active in the stomach. Getting rid of half of the drug would provide no significant clinical benefits for patients. All it provided was a new chemical entity—in reality half the old entity—that could be patented separately and submitted to the FDA for approval.

Recognizing the inadequacy of their solution, Astra scientists launched a desperate search for some way to differentiate the Nexium and Prilosec. They authorized four wildly expensive studies comparing the two drugs against erosive esophagitis. If Nexium proved to be a better drug for that one indication, they would at least earn a unique label from the FDA and give company detailers some talking points when they were out visiting physicians. It wasn't a foolproof strategy, however, since a worse outcome would have to be reported on the label. "You spend $120 million studying the thing, and it could have come out worse," one Astra official told the *Wall Street Journal.* "You're scared as hell." The company won its bet, but by the thinnest of margins. By comparing the two drugs at equal doses, Astra discovered the more slowly metabolizing Nexium healed 90 percent of patients after eight weeks compared to 87 percent for Prilosec. Two of the studies did not show Nexium to be a better drug and were never released to the public.[16]

Sachs, the codiscoverer of the proton-pump mechanism, who had worked closely with Astra to develop Prilosec, provided a final epitaph for the hundreds of millions of dollars that the company, now called AstraZeneca, had poured into Nexium research. "Both enantiomers in the end would appear to be equally active at the pump," he told me in an interview. "Once they are activated, they are no longer enantiomers anyway. They are the identical molecule."[17] Though medically irrelevant, the costly research paid off for AstraZeneca. While the company deployed its patent attorneys to delay generic firms from selling Prilosec, it sought FDA approval for Nexium, which arrived in 2001. Once on the market, the company's detailers, backed by a massive television advertising blitz, convinced thousands of physicians to switch their patients to the new purple pill, which like Prilosec, sold for about four dollars a dose.[18] The company then convinced the FDA to allow Prilosec onto the over-the-counter market, thus frustrating the generic manufacturers and giving Nexium free rein as the prescription—and presumed stronger—antacid.

The Prilosec-to-Nexium transition exemplified a common industry practice. Throughout the 1990s, the drug industry poured billions of research dollars into developing alternatives to drugs that were approaching the end of their patent terms. In most cases, the alternatives were little changed from the originals. The better the original sold, the more likely it was that the company would devote considerable research resources to generating a copycat version with renewed patent life.

Another example that garnered considerable public attention was Schering-Plough's Claritin, one of the antiallergy medicines developed in the early 1980s as a nonsedating alternative to an earlier generation of antihistamines. By the late 1990s, the drug was generating over $2 billion a year in sales for Schering-Plough, a figure that was growing rapidly because of the 1997 legalization of direct-to-consumer advertising. To reach the estimated thirty-five million allergy sufferers in the United States, Schering-Plough poured hundreds of millions of dollars a year into ads for the drug. Consumers were encouraged to ask their doctors for a pricey prescription—it cost eighty dollars for a month's supply— that, according to the original studies submitted to the FDA, worked only marginally better than a placebo.

Though you would never know it from the television advertisements featuring handsome women frolicking through flowering fields oblivious to the pollen-laden air, the FDA's reviewer was openly skeptical about the drug's efficacy at the low dose offered by Schering-Plough. The company, which tested the drug on thousands of patients, needed a low dose to ensure that it would be nonsedating, which was the only way the new drug would be able to gain a toehold in the already crowded antihistamine market. But at the low, nonsedating dose, clinical trials showed that only 43 to 46 percent of Claritin users gained relief of allergy symptoms compared to a third of patients on a sugar pill. A separate study that asked doctors to assess the patients on the placebo found that 37 to 47 percent of them had a "good to excellent response to treatment," which as a practical matter was no different than those who took the real pill.[19]

In addition to questioning its marginal medical significance, other reviewers at that late 1980s FDA hearing worried that Claritin, whose generic name is loratadine, might be a carcinogen. It took the company several more years of studies before it could dispel those fears. Finally, in 1993, the drug was approved. The delays actually proved to be an auspicious event for Schering-Plough. In the early 1990s, patients on Seldane and Hismanal, the first nonsedating antihistamines to hit the market, began turning up in hospital emergency rooms because of the drugs' violent interactions with other drugs and the development of life-threatening heart irregularities. By the time Claritin hit pharmacists' shelves, there was pent-up demand for a safe alternative, and the new drug immediately jumped to number one in sales in its class.

Yet in the late 1990s, as Claritin neared the end of its patent term, Schering-Plough launched a massive lobbying campaign in Washington to get an extension on its patent. The company claimed the long delays at the FDA had robbed it of years of market exclusivity. Aware of the history, Congress rebuffed Schering-Plough's frequent requests.

Forced to fall back on research and development, Schering-Plough scientists took apart loratadine to see what made it tick. They discovered the active part of the drug was actually a metabolite of the whole molecule, which became active in the stomach after patients began digesting the pill. They patented this metabolite, called it desloratadine, and filed a new drug application with the FDA. It was approved in late 2001, just months before the expiration of loratadine's patent. The company launched a massive advertising campaign that convinced millions of their customers to switch to the new, equally expensive but no more effective drug. Then, to frustrate the generic companies getting ready to sell loratadine, Schering-Plough announced it would begin selling Claritin as an over-the-counter allergy remedy.[20]

Public-sector science has sometimes pushed industry researchers down the road to better medicine, only to discover as they neared the end of their labors that they developed yet another me-too drug. During the late 1990s, few drug classes received more media attention than a new pain reliever known within the medical community as Cox-2 inhibitors. The original members of this new drug class were Celebrex, made by G. D. Searle (later bought by Pharmacia), and Vioxx, made by Merck. In 2001, Pharmacia came out with a follow-up drug to Celebrex called Bextra.

One of the discovers of the mechanism behind the new drugs was Philip Needleman, a professor of pharmacology at the Washington University School of Medicine in St. Louis who went on to become chief science officer of Pharmacia. While still an academic, Needleman, whose NIH support began in 1977 and lasted for nearly twenty years, surmised there must be a specific enzyme that caused inflammation and pain around arthritic joints and traumatic injuries. Scientists had already discovered an enzyme called cyclo-oxygenase—or Cox for short—that triggered the production of prostaglandins, which in turn caused swelling. Existing painkillers like aspirin and ibuprofen (known in the medical literature as non-steroidal anti-inflammatory drugs, or NSAIDs) reduced the pain by blocking the action of Cox and limiting the production of prostaglandins. But scientists like Needleman hypothesized there had to be at least two versions of Cox, including one that produced enzymes for protecting the digestive tract from stomach acid. A tiny proportion of patients who took NSAIDs, which blocked the Coxes indiscriminately, suffered from gastrointestinal bleeding and, in the worst cases, ulcers.

By the late 1980s, scientists working in industry and government labs around the United States had identified the Cox specific to swelling, which they dubbed Cox-2. They then turned to finding the gene that expressed Cox-2. If they could produce the protein through genetic engineering, they would be able to give medicinal chemists at pharmaceutical houses a powerful tool for producing large volumes of a juicy drug target. In 1992, three teams of NIH-funded scientists at the University of Rochester, Brigham Young University, and the University of California at Los Angeles, each working independently, discovered the gene. But only Donald Young at the University of Rochester thought to file for a patent on it, which was granted by the PTO in April 2000.[21]

Needleman, meanwhile, had moved across town to Monsanto (though he continued receiving NIH grants until 1995 as an adjunct professor at Washington University, according to NIH records). He eventually became president of G. D. Searle after it was acquired by the bigger chemical company. His main focus at Searle became developing a Cox-2 inhibitor, which later became Celebrex.

Merck's road to a Cox-2 inhibitor also began in 1992 when Peppi Prasit, a Thai-born medicinal chemist who was working in the company's Montreal office, saw a scientific poster at a small medical conference. The poster reported the latest research from a Japanese company that was trying to come up with a painkiller that targeted the newly discovered Cox-2 enzyme. That summer, Prasit replicated its work in his own lab. His work excited Edward Scolnick, the director of Merck's research division, who authorized a major search for its own version of the molecule. By 1994, it had discovered Vioxx. A dosing glitch in clinical trials slowed its race to market, which it lost to Searle by a few months.[22]

Though billed as super-aspirins, the Cox-2 inhibitors provided no more pain relief than over-the-counter aspirin, ibuprofen, or prescription naproxen, which were the most popular NSAIDs on the market. This inconvenient fact was overlooked by the new drugs' marketers. In the spring of 2002, Pfizer Inc. chief executive Henry McKinnell, whose company comarketed Celebrex, awarded PhRMA's highest research award to the four scientists who developed the drug. "Thanks to their pioneering work, millions of people throughout the world who were once crippled with arthritis can now work, walk, garden, and do all the little things that make life worthwhile," he said, even though they were no more able to perform those tasks than if they had popped a couple of over-the-counter ibuprofen.[23]

The only medically legitimate selling point for the Cox-2 inhibitors was the premise that the newer drugs would eliminate the ulcers and even deaths that on rare occasions resulted from the prolonged use of generic painkillers. Yet the FDA didn't allow them to claim that in their advertising or literature since the clinical trials failed to turn up evidence that the new drugs were safer than NSAIDs. The package insert, which goes out with every prescription, contained the same warning label as all the other NSAIDs.

Yet FDA oversight didn't stop the companies from launching a surreptitious marketing campaign claiming otherwise. Articles, often written by scientists who had conducted the companies' clinical trials, flooded the medical literature about the major public health hazard posed by the traditional NSAIDs.[24] Relying on extrapolations from small group studies, one physician claimed that NSAID use resulted in forty-one thousand hospitalizations and thirty-three hundred deaths a year among the elderly. Another put the death rate at five times that level. Meanwhile, other articles reported the results from small clinical trials for Cox-2 inhibitors that hinted the new drugs might prevent the side effects.

The higher number of deaths from NSAIDs rapidly found its way into the popular press as the drugs neared FDA approval and the companies began gearing up their marketing campaigns for their "super-aspirins." Reporters, anxious to jump on the bandwagon of the next medical miracle, never read the fine print. "Pain-Killers Promise to Be Tummy-Friendly," read the headline on a typical story heralding a medicine that promised "new arthritis relief."[25] A more circumspect *Business Week* article pointed out that "Celebrex is no more effective at relieving pain that the commonly prescribed NSAIDs" but went on to state that "it's less likely to cause the stomach bleeding and ulcers experienced by about 30 percent of patients on the older treatments."[26] By the time Vioxx got its FDA approval, the *Washington Post* was reporting that NSAIDs were responsible "for 107,000 hospitalizations and the death of 16,500 people every year."[27]

Sales exploded the instant the FDA gave the okay for the drugs' makers to rev up their marketing machines. Commercials featuring frisky seniors flooded the airwaves. Detailers inundated doctors with free samples. Millions of people pestered their physicians to give them prescriptions for the new drugs, requests that fell on receptive ears. Wall Street's stock analysts considered the rollouts of Celebrex and Vioxx the most successful drug launches in pharmaceutical industry history. Within a year of its launch, Celebrex was generating more than $2 billion a year in sales for Pharmacia and its comarketer Pfizer. Merck's Vioxx was right behind with about $1.5 billion. Arthritis pain relief medicine that had once cost pennies a day was now costing millions of patients and their insurers nearly three dollars a pill.

Amid all the hype, two questions remained unexplored: Were the traditional NSAIDs really as dangerous as a growing volume of medical reports claimed? And did the Cox-2 inhibitors solve the problem?

Reviewers of medical studies for peer-reviewed journals sometimes apply what is called a face test to check the validity of extrapolation studies that draw broad conclusions based on the sampling of small groups. Are there any statistics out there that call into question the validity of the extrapolation study? In 1999—the year the two Cox-2 inhibitors were approved for sale to the general public—the Centers for Disease Control reported in its annual survey that fewer than six thousand Americans died the previous year from all forms of gastrointestinal bleeding disorders, including ulcers. That's ten thousand fewer than the claims in some of the NSAID studies. It is possible that at least a few of those six thousand bleeding-ulcer deaths were from something other than NSAID use. After all, contemporary accounts of Alexander the Great's untimely passing—he died at age thirty-two from acute abdominal pain—suggest he suffered a perforated peptic ulcer after several days of binge drinking.

Moreover, the assertion that many NSAID users suffer gastrointestinal distress from the painkillers was never proven to the FDA's satisfaction. The government-mandated package insert for one popular prescription NSAID warns users that 1 percent of users will experience some gastrointestinal problems anywhere from mild to severe within three to six months, and 2 to 4 percent will have such problems after one year. But even that may overstate the case. A recent study in Scotland that followed more than fifty thousand people over fifty years of age for three years found that 2 percent of NSAID users were hospitalized for gastrointestinal problems after using the drugs for a prolonged period of time, compared to 1.4 percent of people who took no drugs at all.[28]

In a final attempt to manufacture proof that Cox-2 inhibitors were safer than traditional NSAIDS, Pharmacia and Merck launched postapproval clinical trials that compared Celebrex and Vioxx against several older prescription and over-the-counter NSAIDS. Since so few NSAID users suffered from gastrointestinal tract problems, the trials had to be enormous—more than eight thousand patients each—in order to get statistically valid results. The first published accounts of the trials seemed to justify their enormous cost. The Vioxx trial, which compared the new drug to naproxen over a period of about nine months, cut the incidence of gastrointestinal bleeding and ulcers from 4.5 incidents per 100 patient years (100 patients taking the drugs for a year) to 2.1 incidents. The Celebrex trial, which allowed patients to continue taking aspirin, published only six months of data (although the trial lasted for thirteen months) and found the incidence rate fell from 1.5 to 0.9 incidents per 100 patient years. When the latter study appeared in the *Journal of the American Medical Association* in September 2000, an accompanying editorial called the new Cox-2 inhibitors "a welcome addition to the therapeutic armamentarium" that might benefit an "enormous number of individuals . . . who do not take aspirin."[29]

Reviewers soon began poking holes in the industry-funded studies. Many of the patients enrolled in the trials had other risk factors for developing ulcers. They, like Alexander the Great, were drinkers, for instance. Patients without those risk factors had less than a half of 1 percent chance of developing gastrointestinal tract problems on NSAIDS. Even in the higher-risk group, the Vioxx study suggested "that forty-one patients needed to be treated for one year to prevent one such event." The Celebrex study, meanwhile, because of its short duration, had "no statistically significant difference between the groups."[30]

When the regulators got their hands on the data in the studies, things took a turn for the worse from the drugmakers' perspective. It turned out the patients on Vioxx developed serious heart problems at three times the rate of those on naproxen, the traditional NSAID that it had been compared to in the study. Merck quickly pointed out that the overall rate of heart problems remained small and probably meant that the new "super-aspirins" did not provide the same cardiovascular benefits as taking older NSAIDs like naproxen, aspirin, and ibuprofen, which reduce the blood-clotting factor in the blood while fighting pain and inflammation.[31]

The FDA was not impressed by that logic. To the regulators, the new data suggested that for every patient saved from gastrointestinal complications by taking Vioxx, two patients would develop a potentially life-threatening heart condition. In April 2002, the FDA ordered Merck to revise its Vioxx label to contain the new warning. The FDA also said the new study didn't warrant removing the gastrointestinal complications warning that had been slapped on Vioxx's label when it was initially approved—and whose removal was the whole purpose of the giant study.[32]

The Celebrex study, meanwhile, received the most damning evaluation possible. Its organizers were accused of junk science in the influential *British Medical Journal.* A year after the study appeared, it reported that Celebrex's allegedly superior safety profile over the two NSAIDs in the company-funded study had been based on just six months of data, even though many patients had remained in the study for more than a year. If the entire data set was evaluated, the Celebrex patients developed just as many ulcers as the generic and over-the-counter competition. "I am furious. . . . I looked like a fool," M. Michael Wolfe, a noted gastroenterologist at Boston University, told the *Washington Post.* Wolfe had written the glowing editorial in the *Journal of the American Medical Association* that accompanied the report on the original study.[33]

After a Swiss scientific team reviewed the entire study, it concluded in the *British Medical Journal* that the original protocols of the study "showed similar numbers of ulcer-related complications in the comparison groups and that almost all the ulcer complications that occurred in the second half of the trials were in users of celecoxib (Celebrex)." Pointing out that all the authors of the original study were industry-funded and more than thirty thousand copies of the erroneous study had been distributed to physicians around the world, the editorial charged that "publishing and distributing overoptimistic short-term data using post hoc changes to the protocol . . . is misleading. The wide dissemination of the misleading results of the trial has to be counterbalanced by the equally wide dissemination of the findings of the reanalysis according to the original protocol. If this is not done, the pharmaceutical industry will feel no need to put the record straight in this or any future instances."[34]

As the twenty-first century dawned, the drug industry's search for new drugs to replace old ones coming off patent became frenzied. There were fifty-two drugs with more than $1 billion in sales in 2000, but forty-two were slated to lose their patent protection by 2007. The drugs that account for fully half the industry's sales were on the cusp of low-cost, generic competition. But instead of looking for truly innovative medicines, which are dependent on the maturation of biological understanding and even then are difficult to find, an increasing share of the industry's research and development budgets turned to the search for replacement drugs—drugs that would provide fairly similar medical benefits to patients as the drugs losing their patent protection, drugs that could be positioned in the marketplace as "new and improved" medicines. This chapter anecdotally documented some of the more broadly prescribed and financially significant examples. But as we'll see in the next chapter, the effort was pervasive.

Before turning to the economics of me-too research and the extent to which it dominated industry's budgets for research and development, it is worth noting that the aggressive search for me-too medicines also drove the rapid rise in marketing expenses at drug companies. If one only looks at what the industry refers to as marketing expenses—the free samples, detailing, direct-to-consumer and professional journal advertising—totals rose 71.4 percent to $15.7 billion between 1996 and 2000, with direct-to-consumer ads representing the fastest growing expense. If one expands the definition of marketing to include continuing medical education, physician support meetings, and the postmarketing research (sometimes called fourth-phase clinical trials), which are aimed almost exclusively at expanding sales of the drugs by getting them into the hands of more doctors, then the total marketing budgets among drug industry firms may have exceeded $40 billion. Meanwhile, research-and-development budgets rose at a slower pace—52.7 percent—to $25.7 billion.[35]

By decade's end, with drug costs soaring at double-digit rates, these skewed priorities—which were a major component in the rising cost of drugs— were again drawing fire from the guardians of scientific integrity. "The industry depicts these huge expenditures as serving an educational function," the *New England Journal of Medicine* editorialized.

> It contends that doctors and the public learn about new and useful drugs in this way. Unfortunately, many doctors do indeed rely on drug-company representatives and promotional materials to learn about new drugs, and much of the public learns from direct-to-consumer advertising. But to rely on the drug companies for unbiased evaluations of their products makes about as much sense as relying on beer companies to teach us about alcoholism. The conflict of interest is obvious. The fact is that marketing is meant to sell drugs, and the less important the drug, the more marketing it takes to sell it. Important new drugs do not need much promotion. Me-too drugs do.[36]

9

The $800 Million Pill

B y the late 1990s, the pharmaceutical industry's penchant for pursuing drugs of limited incremental value had reached a tipping point.

The Food and Drug Administration (FDA) approved anywhere from twenty-five to fifty new drugs (new molecular entities in FDA parlance) per year throughout the 1990s. In 2001 and 2002 the pace fell off sharply to fewer than twenty new drugs a year. While there was a handful of legitimate medical advances in any given year, the FDA designated the majority of new drugs as having "limited or no clinical improvement" over existing drugs. In 2002, for instance, just seven of seventeen new drugs were rated a priority by the FDA, which indicated they represented a legitimate medical advance. To a growing number of critics, me-too drug development had become what the drug industry was all about.

According to textbook economics, the new competition from me-too drugs should have triggered intense price competition. But that is not how it worked most of the time. The companies offering the me-too drugs usually priced their products relatively close to the price of existing drugs and relied on the power of their marketing departments to determine how they would fare, especially if they were the second or third entry in a relatively new market. Indeed, not much had changed from the days when the Federal Trade Commission investigated the antibiotic cartel. While one survey of twenty me-too drugs introduced between 1995 and 1999 argued their arrival did in fact herald price competition, a close examination of the data revealed that prices on a dozen of the latest entrants were within 10 percent of the median price of existing drugs in the class, and in eight cases there was no price break at all.[1]

As drug sales soared, criticism of me-too drug development mounted. The critics fell into two camps that had one thing in common: They both had to pick up the tab for the rising cost of pharmaceuticals. The noisiest protests came from angry senior citizens. Stoked by consumer groups and an issue-hungry Democratic Party, elderly Americans staged well-publicized buying trips to Canada and Mexico, where they could purchase cheaper medicine from price-controlled systems. But as drug expenditures rose, they were joined by a quieter but potentially more effective group: the nation's employers, medical insurance companies, and pharmacy benefit managers. They were seeing their own bottom lines, which had been eroded by the skyrocketing price of drugs for their workers, retirees, and enrollees, and they wanted something done about it.

How bad was it? Retail spending on prescription drugs doubled in just five years, reaching $154.5 billion in 2001. At the beginning of the new century, pharmaceuticals accounted for nearly one in every ten dollars spent on health care, nearly twice what it had been two decades earlier. The government agency that pays the nation's Medicare and Medicaid bills projected drug spending would soar to 14 percent of all health care costs by 2010 unless something was done to check the upward spiral.

What was behind runaway drug spending? Prices rose only modestly, so that wasn't the major problem. Utilization soared. Physicians prescribed medicines at a breakneck pace to an aging, overweight, and out-of-shape American people suffering (to judge from prescription patterns) in near epidemic proportions from high cholesterol, high blood pressure, allergies, depression, arthritis, and diabetes.

Neither party to the transaction—the doctors nor the patients—had the time, knowledge, or inclination to pay close attention to the scientific sophistry behind many of the new drugs coming on the market to treat these conditions, which were often little different from the drugs they were replacing or may not have been needed at all. They just wanted the best. "The industry introduces improved versions of existing drugs, and new often means more expensive," *Newsweek* opined in a cover story that sought to explain the rising cost of medicine to its readers. "When it comes to their own health, people want Starbucks, not Maxwell

House, and medical decisions aren't like other economic choices: Americans like to have the best, and will pay for it if they possibly can."[2]

An unprecedented rise in drug industry promotional spending stoked the grassroots demand for the pricier drugs. The legalization of direct-to-consumer advertising in 1997 allowed firms to peddle their wares on television, radio, and in newspapers and magazines. Ad spending tripled from $788 million in 1996 to $2.5 billion in 2000.[3]

As drug entrepreneurs have known since the days when traveling salesmen pushed unregulated patent medicines at circus sideshows, advertising works. Consumption of the latest antacids, anticholesterol agents, antidepressants, antihistamines, and painkillers reached unprecedented levels. The average American consumed eleven prescriptions in 2000, up from seven just a decade earlier. And for every one hundred office visits, doctors prescribed 146 drugs in 1999, up from 109 prescriptions in 1985. The fifty most heavily advertised drugs accounted for nearly half the increase in spending in the final year of the decade.[4]

A few doctors rebelled against the trend, especially those worried about the frail elderly who consumed the most drugs. Study after study appeared in the medical literature documenting widespread misuse of medicine by seniors, whether they got their drugs in hospitals, nursing homes, or physician offices. Anywhere from 12 to 40 percent of prescriptions were deemed "inappropriate," according to the studies. Physicians either prescribed the drugs incorrectly (sometimes the wrong drug, sometimes the wrong dose, sometimes no prescription was needed at all) or the drugs caused violent side effects because of their interaction with other drugs the seniors were already taking. One survey of eleven drugs whose labels specifically cautioned against their use in seniors found that more than one million elderly individuals took at least one of those inappropriate medicines.[5]

But the industry's marketing blitz drowned out the skeptics. Sales soared, and as they did, the industry's profits surged to unprecedented levels. Indeed, year after year *Fortune* magazine ranked the pharmaceutical industry number one in its annual survey as the most profitable businesses in the nation (belying the notion that there was inordinate risk in investing in pharmaceuticals). Like clockwork, the industry returned somewhere between 23 and 25 percent of its total revenue in profits.[6]

As a first step in trying to halt the cost spiral, insurance companies and employers began raising copayments and forced tiered payment plans onto their beneficiaries. In a tiered payment plan, consumers pay a low copayment if they purchase off-patent generic drugs, a moderate copayment if they purchase brand-name drugs included on the insurance company's formulary (a list of approved drugs), and the highest copayment if their doctors prescribe one of the high-priced, heavily advertised drugs that the insurance company has determined isn't worth the money. The strategy borrowed a page from the managed care revolution of the early and mid-1990s, which had succeeded in holding down overall health care costs for a few years.

But like the managed care industry's ability to hold down costs—which collapsed after an angry backlash from consumers in the form of a Patient Bill of Rights movement—the tiered-payment plans were doomed to failure. The theory behind such tiered payment plans is that they will reduce consumption by making average citizens feel the pain of rising costs. If consumers knew the real price of the prescriptions, they would begin demanding lower-cost alternatives or eliminating purchases of medicines of borderline necessity, so the theory went. While incentive schemes work in some marketplaces, they have little to no effect on drug consumption patterns. The schemes' fatal flaw lies in the fact that patients don't make the ultimate buying decision in the medical marketplace (although they can influence it by demanding their doctors prescribe the drug they heard about last night on television). Kefauver recognized the problem as early as 1959 during his first hearings on monopolistic drug prices. "The drug industry is unusual in that he who buys does not order, and he who orders does not buy," he had complained.[7] The ultimate choice of drugs was made by doctors, and they were increasingly being influenced by the industry's army of seventy thousand detailers who plied them with free samples, free dinners, and education seminars in exotic locales.[8]

The industry, meanwhile, didn't turn the other cheek to the insurance companies' assault on its profitability. To defend the massive cash flow generated by the new and largely redundant drugs, it replied to its critics in the same way that it had for decades. "If one were to awaken any one of a thousand drug executives in the dead of night and ask him where all those profits went, the answer would undoubtedly be 'Research,'" Richard Harris wrote in his 1964 account of the Kefauver drug company investigations. "For most of the witnesses at the hearings who used it tirelessly—and, as far as that goes, for many who heard it—the word seemed to have the force of an incantation."[9]

Alan F. Holmer, president of the Pharmaceutical Research and Manufacturers Association (PhRMA), trumpeted the modern variant of the incantation in congressional testimony and in numerous interviews with the press as the new battle over drug pricing heated up. "The industry is spending more than $30 billion annually on research and development [the 2002 projection], with about 80 percent of this investment dedicated to the advancement of scientific knowledge and the development of products, compared to about 20 percent that is devoted to improving and/or modifying existing products," he asserted in a *USA Today* article. "This research and development builds on the steady introduction over the years of innovative medicines that have enabled patients all over the world to lead longer, healthier, and more productive lives. Life expectancy is increasing; infant mortality is decreasing; disability rates among the elderly are falling; and progress is continuing against many diseases. A leading reason: major pharmaceutical breakthroughs in the 1990s."[10]

Most public health experts, whose voices were rarely heard in the debate, dismiss those claims as a gross exaggeration. Life expectancy rose more slowly in the 1990s than in any other decade of the twentieth century, and no studies have concluded recent gains were the result of better drugs. The average person at birth could expect to live just 49.2 years in 1900. That rose ten years to 59.3 by 1930, largely due to improvements in living conditions, especially improved sanitation. It rose another ten to 69.9 by 1960, and while antibiotics played a role in improving health in the middle years of the century, many of the major victories over infectious disease were recorded before the first wonder drugs came along, again as a result of improved living conditions.

Between 1960 and 1990—an era bracketed by the end of the first great era of drug discovery and the arrival of the biotechnology and molecular biology revolutions—the rate of increase in life expectancy gradually tapered off. Life expectancy stood at 75.4 in 1990, which meant that in the thirty years leading up to that point the average lifespan had increased at half the rate of earlier epochs. And between 1990 and 2000, the average person's lifespan rose only to 76.9 years, making the last decade—a time when American spending on pharmaceuticals rose at its fastest pace ever—the slowest in terms of improving life expectancy. Indeed, at the current rate of increase, the average American won't live to be eighty until 2020, which will undoubtedly leave the world's richest country significantly behind a number of European and Asian nations. "The rise in life expectancy over the last quarter-century is associated with declining death rates at middle and older ages—a product of improved lifestyles and better treatments for major fatal diseases," said Jay Olshansky, a professor of public health at the University of Illinois at Chicago and coauthor of *The Quest for Immortality*. "Some pharmaceuticals contributed to this, such as treatments for cancer and stroke, but evidence for [drugs'] impact on the life expectancy in the United States is lacking." A far more compelling argument to explain recent gains can be made for the public health campaign against smoking.[11]

However, the American public has not exhibited much interest in pursuing public health methods of disease control in recent years. Public health officials have long recognized that obesity is a major contributor to heart disease (the nation's number-one killer) and diabetes (number six). But the government has done little to promote a national campaign to combat the dietary and sedentary habits behind the epidemics. While President George W. Bush appeared on the cover of *Runner's World* magazine to promote fitness, a survey of educators showed mandatory physical education continues its downward descent in the nation's schools. A majority of students take physical education for just one year during their high school years. In half the states, children can substitute electives like bowling and band.[12]

The crusade to cut back on carcinogens in the environment, which had begun in earnest in 1962 with publication of Rachel Carson's *Silent Spring*, by the early twenty-first century had become a rear-guard action by a government unwilling or uninterested in confronting powerful corporate interests. Government regulators, caught between corporate lobbyists, who claimed only 2 percent of cancers came from man-made chemicals dumped into the environment, and environmentalists, who insisted it was at least half, all but halted their efforts to root out potential carcinogens from the environment.[13]

Meanwhile, the identification of therapeutically valid targets for combating cancer, Alzheimer's, and arthritis—the major scourges of old age—continued to baffle scientists. Most Americans, fed a steady diet of news extolling the latest advances in the nation's medical laboratories, took it on faith that treatments for the diseases that threatened the well-being of their golden years would ultimately be found in a bottle. The drug industry appealed directly to those hopes when it argued that its prices and profit margins had to be maintained if promising therapies for those conditions were ever going to be brought to market. In defending their huge research-and-development budgets, the industry trade group's officials pointed out its member firms in 2001 had more than a thousand drugs and vaccines in development, including 780 for senior citizens, 400 for cancer, and 120 for heart disease and stroke.[14] Bringing any one of those projects to a successful conclusion would require vast expenditures of funds—by the latest count, more than $800 million per successful therapy.

This breathtaking statistic, invoked by industry officials—as in Kefauver's day—with the force of an incantation, rested on studies of the cost of new drug development that had been conducted over two decades by the Tufts University Center for the Study of Drug Development. The center was started in the mid-1980s by a group of economists who were largely funded by the drug industry. They surveyed industry research-and-development officials to come up with their estimate for drug development costs. In the initial study, released in 1991, they randomly picked ninety-three new chemical entities under development at a dozen big drug companies and asked the firms to report their research-and-development expenditures on each stage of development for each molecule. They then divided the total expenditures by the number of drugs in the group that eventually gained approval from the FDA—thus factoring in the price of failure—to come up with an average cost per new drug. Their first study pegged the total cost per new drug at $114 million (measured in 1987 dollars).

They then adjusted that cost for the time needed to secure approval. Economists call this adjustment the opportunity cost of capital. It assumes that the money invested in research and development today, which won't have a payoff for many years down the road, could have been spent on other things or turned back to shareholders as additional profit. The opportunity cost of research-and-development spending increased the final estimate to $231 million per new drug (or $318 million in 2000 after adjusting the price for inflation).[15]

Tufts's most recent estimate was released in November 2001. The average new drug now cost $802 million. The clinical-trial phase of drug development was largely responsible for the rapid increase, the study's authors asserted. The cost of testing drugs in humans rose at an annual rate of nearly 12 percent in the 1990s, five times faster than the preclinical stages where companies identified drug targets and tested them for toxicity and bioavailability in animals. "The increased focus on developing drugs to treat chronic and degenerative diseases has added significantly to clinical costs," said Joseph E. DiMasi, the Tufts economist who was the lead author of the study.[16]

The rapid increase in the drug industry's clinical trials expenditures merits a closer look, especially since publicly funded clinical trials had a very different experience. The Division of AIDS within the National Institute for Allergies and Infectious Diseases ran more than seventeen hundred clinical trials between 1992 and 2001, spending nearly $1.5 billion on the treatment, care, and testing of nearly one hundred thousand AIDS patients in the trials. Yet the average cost per enrollee did not keep pace with the rate of inflation, rising just 11 percent over the entire decade.[17]

The National Cancer Institute (NCI) also proved to be a more efficient provider of clinical trials services than the private sector. Throughout the 1990s, clinicians working with NCI frequently complained about insurers' unwillingness to pay for the additional cost of treating terminally ill cancer patients willing to take experimental medicines. Senator James Jeffords, chairman of the Committee on Health, Education, Labor, and Pensions, demanded the Government Accounting Office look into how much it really cost. The government watchdog agency surveyed the medical directors at eleven of NCI's forty-eight designated comprehensive cancer centers and concluded "the additional costs of clinical trial protocols may not be great." Average costs per patient were $24,645 for the first year for trial enrollees, compared to $23,964 for patients receiving standard care. The report went on to cite a 1999 survey by the American Society of Clinical Oncology that showed the additional costs per patient in an NCI-backed trial was just $750 compared to $2,500 for standard care costs for a patient who enrolled in a cancer trial sponsored by private industry.[18]

Why were expenses for industry-run clinical trials rising at such a rapid rate? One reason was an explosion in the number of trials whose sole purpose was to help companies market their drugs. CenterWatch, a newsletter that monitors clinical trials, estimated drug manufacturers spent $1.5 billion in 2000 to test medicines already approved by the FDA—the fastest growing component of clinical trials spending. Some trials were undertaken to provide company salespersons the veneer of science when countering rival claims in the marketplace. Bristol-Myers Squibb, for instance, spent tens of millions of dollars to prove its cholesterol-lowering statin was no different than Merck's statin in protecting against heart disease even though it didn't lower cholesterol quite as much. Other trials— dubbed seeding trials—were designed to get more physicians using an approved drug or to encourage them to use it for other indications.[19]

Most of these postmarketing trials were never submitted to the FDA because they did not have placebo controls or were not rigorously designed. But in conducting the trials the companies did get to ply participating physicians with the drug, share the results with other physicians through detailing, and employ public relations and advertising firms to herald the results at major conferences. The trend drew a sharp rebuke from the editors of thirteen of the nation's leading medical journals. "Patients participate in clinical trials largely for altruistic reasons— that is, to advance the standard of care," the joint editorial said. "In the light of that truth, the use of clinical trials primarily for marketing, in our view, makes a mockery of clinical investigation and is a misuse of a powerful tool."[20]

As the debate heated up in Congress over a prescription drug benefit for Medicare, Public Citizen/Congress Watch, which was started by Ralph Nader, published a detailed critique of the Tufts assumptions. Complaining that the drug industry had never opened its books to congressional or outside investigators, the Public Citizen researchers argued that research and development ought to be considered an expense, not an investment, as per accounting purposes (accountants deduct expenses as they occur; investments are depreciated over time since it is assumed their useful life extends beyond the year of purchase). The Naderites suggested an alternative method for calculating the cost of drug development. They divided the total number of new drugs approved between 1994 and 2000 into total industry spending on research and development. They came up with pretax research expenses of $108 million per new drug. Adjusting for the tax deductibility of research-and-development expenses, they pegged the actual cost per new drug at $71 million. The industry's oft-repeated claim that lower prices would slow new drug development was nothing more than "a misleading campaign to scare policy makers and the public," the report said.[21]

Though the industry's main trade group wasn't the author of the original Tufts study, it rose to the Tufts researchers' defense. PhRMA hired the accounting firm of Ernst and Young to debunk Public Citizen's methodology. Citing an introductory textbook on corporate finance, the accountant-consultants at Ernst and Young pronounced "the cost of capital a valid cost that must be accounted for when evaluating any investment. . . . When a pharmaceutical firm's management decides on behalf of its investors whether to pursue a research-and-development project, it evaluates whether the project is a better use of capital than alternative investments. The justification for the Public Citizen's omission of this cost is not clear," their report concluded. They also rejected the tax argument since "the value of the associated tax deduction will vary depending on the particular financial profile of the business incurring the expense, which may be limited in its ability to take deductions."[22]

Should companies evaluate research-and-development investment the same way they do capital projects like new factories, office buildings, and computers? The arguments are not as clear-cut as the Ernst and Young consultants would suggest. According to generally accepted accounting principles (which are used for filings to the Securities and Exchange Commission and Internal Revenue Service), research costs must be deducted from income in the year in which they are incurred. For income tax purposes, therefore, they are a deduction, not an investment. "These companies don't want to capitalize it because there is a huge subsidy when the government allows developers to write off immediately all their research and development expenses," said Baruch Lev, a professor of finance at the Stern School of Business at New York University and a leading expert on accounting for intangible property like patents and research and development. "If you spend more, you get to write it off immediately. No one questions it because people regard greater research-and-development costs as a good thing."[23]

Unfortunately, the evidence suggested the drug industry was not doing better with the additional sums being poured into research and development. In the late 1990s, the health insurance industry, which was paying much of the tab for the rising cost of drugs, formed a new research center to evaluate the new products rolling off the pharmaceutical industry's production lines. In May 2002, the National Institute for Health Care Management issued a report called "The Changing Patterns of Pharmaceutical Innovation." It was the first time that any outside group had systematically evaluated the usefulness of the drug industry's latest "new and improved" offerings.

The group's consultants used the FDA's classification system for ranking new drugs to sort out the usefulness of the latest medicines. Under the 1992 Prescription Drug User Fee Act (PDUFA), the government had imposed fees on drug makers when they submitted their new drug applications. Industry had pushed the plan as a way to speed up the review process at the chronically underfunded agency. Before PDUFA, the agency had a three-tier system for allocating its reviewers. They classified new drugs as a significant medical advance, a modest medical advance, or no medical advance at all. Under the new system, the FDA divided the new drug applications in two classes—priority and normal—and gave the applications of higher-rated drugs a faster review.

While the new ratings could be subjective, the agency appears to have bent over backwards to grant priority status to new drugs in order to please industry lobbyists. Company press releases routinely stated they were pursuing priority designation for a new drug and trumpeted the success when they gained it. For instance, Celebrex and Vioxx, which provided a potentially minor improvement in side effects but no painkilling benefits over previous drugs in their class, received priority status, as did the erectile dysfunction drug Viagra. The diabetes drug Rezulin gained fast-track approval status in 1997 even though an FDA examiner warned that it might cause heart and liver damage. A Pulitzer Prize–winning series in the *Los Angeles Times* later revealed that Rezulin caused at least thirty-three deaths and was kept on the market by Warner-Lambert despite there being at least nine other drugs for the condition.[24] (The Rezulin case highlighted one of the enduring truths about me-too drugs: Users of the new molecule were exposed to greater safety risks than consumers using tried-and-true drugs already on the market. Every one of the thirteen drugs withdrawn from the market for safety reasons during the 1990s failed to meet a medical need that wasn't already served by a number of drugs already on the market. In some cases, there were already more than a dozen drugs in the class.)[25]

But even with a number of companies lobbying their me-too drugs into fast-track designations, the study from the National Institute for Health Care Management found that just 24 percent of the 1,035 drug applications approved by the FDA between 1989 and 2000 earned priority review. If one looked at just the new chemical entities in the group— new drugs that had the greatest likelihood of providing physicians with a meaningful alternative—the industry's overall output still couldn't be deemed innovative. The FDA gave priority status to just 42 percent of the 361 new chemical entities introduced over the twelve-year period.

Moreover, the pattern of FDA designations over the course of the decade suggested the industry's vast increase in research-and-development expenditures in the late 1990s had increasingly gone to pursuing me-too drugs. While seventy-three of the 149 (or nearly half) new drugs introduced by the industry between 1989 and 1994 were considered high priorities for agency reviewers, only eighty, or just 38 percent, of the 212 new molecular entities put in the nation's medicine chest over the next six years received the priority designation. The pace of new drug introduction had picked up, but the pace of innovation was slowing down. There was indeed something coming out of all that new money being poured into research and development. But from a medical point of view, the output was no more significant than when research-and-development budgets had been half of their fin de siècle level. "The plain fact is that many new drugs are altered or slightly changed versions of existing drugs, and they may or may not be all that much better than what's already available," Nancy Chockley, president of the National Institute for Health Care Management, told the press conference where she released the report. "Consumers should be more aware of that."[26]

The industry's main trade group immediately attacked the study as nothing more than an effort by the insurance industry to deny people new and innovative medicine, claiming the priority ranking system was only a management tool for the FDA to allocate its scarce resources. "If priority were routinely granted, the concept would lose its meaning," the PhRMA report said. "Just because an application is subjected to a standard review does not mean it is not an important innovation or valuable addition to physician's treatment options."[27] Having multiple drugs in a therapeutic class offers choice, the group said. Patients respond differently to similar drugs, which may have different side effects. And with response rates to drugs below 50 percent in many categories (painkillers, antidepressants, and antiallergy drugs are especially notable in this regard), patient trial and error can provide important clinical benefits.

Finally, PhRMA accused the insurance industry–funded group of deliberately skewing its results by failing to include the 130 vaccines and biotechnology-derived drugs approved by the FDA over the twelve years in the study. Since they were reviewed by a separate division of the federal agency, biotech drugs were not part of the priority review system. By failing to count them, "the study incompletely and inaccurately portrays pharmaceutical innovation."[28]

It was a curious assertion. Only a few of the larger and more successful biotechnology companies belonged to PhRMA, and the trade group's annual compilation of industry research-and-development efforts did not include biotech. The surveys from the Biotechnology Industry Organization, on the other hand, counted nearly fifteen hundred firms in the sector, most of them quite small and unprofitable. Yet the entire biotech industry generated just $20.7 billion in sales in 2001, less than one-seventh the sales of brand name and generic drugs combined. Funded largely by venture capital and initial public stock offerings, biotech firms spent an estimated $15.7 billion on research and development—nearly 60 percent of the total spent by big drug companies.[29] Furthermore, an increasing share of the research budgets at big pharmaceutical firms—some observers estimate the total may be as high as 30 percent—was being invested in collaborations with biotechnology companies. Even in-house research efforts at traditional drug companies were increasingly concentrated on using genomics to identify new targets for traditional medicinal chemistry.[30] Clearly, biotechnology will play a much bigger role in pharmaceutical innovation in the years to come.

But as documented in chapter 1, successful biotechnology companies like Amgen, which alone accounted for a quarter of biotechnology drug sales, were just as prone to developing marginally significant drugs (longer-lasting versions of its two big sellers, Epogen to stimulate for red blood cell production and Neupogen to stimulate white blood cell production, for instance) as their big pharmaceutical cousins. Even unsuccessful biotech companies have begun looking to develop me-too drugs to generate sales when their primary research efforts fail to pay off.

Human Genome Sciences, the high-profile biotechnology firm run by former NIH-funded AIDS researcher William Haseltine, failed in its first four efforts at turning its portfolio of gene patents into marketable proteins because it poorly understood how those proteins impacted the underlying diseases. The company then turned to developing longer-lasting versions of biotech products already on the market, such as human growth hormone and interferon alpha for hepatitis C. Dismissing concerns that the strategy might embroil the company in endless patent litigation, Haseltine said in 2002 that "the way we look at it, we are a protein and antibody company, and we pick the best drug. If the best drug is an improved version of an existing drug, that's O.K."[31]

Human Genome Sciences' experience with its gene patent portfolio was hardly unique. As the giddiness over the Human Genome Project's successful completion began to wear off, medical researchers in both the public and private sectors confronted a sobering reality. Medical progress from biotechnology, genomics, and ongoing research into cellular processes would be slow in arriving and incremental in nature. "We're well past the low-hanging fruit," lamented Fred Hassan, chairman of Pharmacia Corporation, just one month after the genome announcement. "It's getting very difficult to get easy wins." Two years later, his tune was even sadder. "People got way too excited about the genome being unlocked. Five to ten years from now, it might help our product flow. In the meantime, the industry is going to go through rough times."[32]

The bottom line was that despite record levels of research-and-development spending, the industry's vaunted pipelines were running dry. The industry received just seventeen new drugs approvals in 2002. And, increasingly, the new drugs were not much changed from their blockbusters, the drugs that earned more than $1 billion a year and were on the verge of losing their patent protection.[33]

The insurance companies and Naderites weren't the only ones questioning the pharmaceutical industry's assertion that it cost $800 million to develop a new drug. Public health activists concerned about developing new drugs for the most prevalent infectious diseases in poor countries also wanted a true picture of the cost of pharmaceutical innovation.

In the years immediately after the development of the AIDS cocktail, health advocates around the world turned their attention to gaining access to these expensive drugs for the more than forty million people in developing countries who have the disease. Since they have no money and their governments cannot afford developed world prices, organizations like UNAIDS, the World Health Organization, and some governments turned to generic manufacturers and drug company philanthropy for their antiretrovirals.

But HIV/AIDS represented only one of the major infectious disease killers ravaging the less developed countries of Africa, Asia, and Latin America. Almost as many people have died each year from tuberculosis and malaria—diseases that have been largely eliminated in advanced industrial countries. Yet unlike AIDS, which represents a large market in the developed world, these diseases were largely ignored by the global pharmaceutical industry—not because there were no patients, but because the millions of sick people had no money. Where there's no money, there's no market, and where there's no market, there's no private investment in drug development.

Yet the need for new drugs to combat the world's most deadly infectious diseases is acute. Tuberculosis today infects eight million people a year, 77 percent of whom do not have access to medicine. The result is two million deaths a year, many of which could be avoided with antibiotics that cost less than one hundred dollars per course of treatment. However, the course of treatment is long, and resistance to the drugs is growing. Despite the pressing need, there have been no new medicines to address this age-old scourge in decades.

Malaria, the third-leading cause of death in developing countries, infects more than three hundred million people every year and kills an estimated one million to two million people. Chloroquine, the standard treatment since the 1940s, is increasingly ineffective because of resistance. Again, no new drugs for malaria are in the private sector's pipeline. Leishmaniasis, an immune-system disease that is transmitted by sand flies, has infected more than twelve million people in eighty-eight developing countries. Leishmaniasis-related conditions, including diarrhea and pneumonia, kill more than five hundred thousand people a year. The standard course of treatment—a derivative of the heavy metal antimony—costs $150 and has brutal side effects. As with malaria, no new drugs have been developed to combat this disease since the 1930s.

Unlike AIDS, which knows no borders, these killers have largely been confined to the developing world (although the occasional immigrant shows up on U.S. shores carrying the bugs, which invariably sends government health officials into a deep panic). As a result, major pharmaceutical companies have largely ignored them. The international humanitarian group Doctors without Borders surveyed the world's eleven largest pharmaceutical firms and found that of the 1,393 new drugs introduced in the last quarter-century, only thirteen treated tropical diseases that are the biggest killers in the developing world. The humanitarians had found a way to shame drug companies into providing HIV drugs at cost to the developing world. But how could they get them to invest $800 million to develop drugs that didn't already exist for people who didn't have much money?

The Global Alliance for TB Drug Development, launched at a meeting of global tuberculosis (TB) activists in Cape Town in February 2000, decided to make its own estimate of the cost of drug development. The group brought together academic researchers, government agencies, nongovernmental organizations, well-heeled philanthropists (the Bill and Melinda Gates and Rockefeller Foundations are championing alternative approaches to finding drugs to solve developing world health problems) and a handful of industry representatives. The nonprofit's goal was the development of new and more effective TB regimens by 2010.

The Global Alliance's strategy called for scouring the world's academic and industry labs for promising TB drug candidates and bringing the most promising ones through the drug development process. The TB bacteria's genome has been sequenced. Researchers (primarily academics funded by NIH) have identified targets. The group's managers figured they could contract with research organizations in both the public and private sectors to do the rest of the work. Finding them wouldn't be hard. In recent years, big pharmaceutical companies had increasingly farmed out their research to smaller players. They looked to biotechnology start-ups to find their drug targets. They contracted with firms like Quintiles International and Parexel to conduct clinical trials.

The Global Alliance proposed to do the same thing with one major difference. They would control the intellectual property to ensure that the new TB drugs could be made broadly available at low prices to those who needed them most. "The Alliance's goal is to come up with a new, faster-acting anti-TB medicine by the year 2010 that is affordable to people in endemic countries," said Maria Freire, the former head of NIH technology transfer who was hired to run the group. "We are a not-for-profit, international public-private partnership utilizing the best practices of industry to develop the drugs, but with a different ultimate bottom line."[34]

But would Bill Gates's foundation have to invest $800 million to develop a new TB drug? The Global Alliance commissioned a team of former drug company executives to build their own model of what it costs to develop new drugs. Their October 2001 report, "The Economics of TB Drug Development," directly challenged the Tufts studies, which had dominated the field of pharmaceutical economics in the prior decade. They surveyed contract research organizations that specialize in microbiology, toxicology, and drug metabolism. They used the Tufts estimate for drug discovery and extrapolations from the cost of government-run clinical trials. They allowed for failures at every stage of development and inflated the final figure to account for the time value of money.

Though Global Alliance's methodology was very similar to the Tufts study, their bottom line was very different. "The total costs to discover and develop a new anti-TB drug is roughly estimated to range from $115 million to $240 million. However, it is generally accepted that discovery and development of a new drug to treat TB will require an international, collaborative effort that allows costs to be shared by multiple organizations, lowering ultimately the investment burden borne by a single agency or company," the report said.[35]

On closer inspection, the Global Alliance's numbers actually jibed with the Tufts studies. The industry-funded academics never factored out research on me-too drugs. They didn't take into account the cost of developing the enantiomer version of raceimate drugs whose only purpose is to extend the patent life of a medicine. They never considered the waste of resources when an industry research budget pays for clinical trials whose only purpose is to get doctors to prescribe their medicine instead of someone else's. In short, if the industry-funded academic economists at Tufts had factored out the half of industry research that is more properly categorized as corporate waste, their number would have been similar to that of the Global Alliance.

10

The Future of Drug Innovation

On December 17, 2002, some of the nation's leading heart physicians gathered at the National Press Club in downtown Washington, D.C., to unveil the latest news from the frontlines of antihypertensive research. Heading the panel of thought leaders were physicians from the federal government's National Heart, Lung, and Blood Institute, which had just completed an eight-year-long test of four different blood-pressure control medications. Each drug in the trial represented a major class of antihypertensives. The trial enrolled more than forty thousand older Americans, making it by far the largest and best-controlled study of antihypertensive drugs in medical history.

The results made all the evening newscasts and the next day's front pages. Generic diuretics (so-called water pills), which had been introduced in the 1950s and cost less than ten cents a day, had proved slightly superior to still-on-patent calcium channel blockers and angiotensin converting enzyme (ACE) inhibitors, which cost consumers anywhere from 75 cents to $1.75 per day. The fourth drug, a patented andrenergic blocker, was dropped from the trial when it became clear that patients on the drug fared substantially worse than people on the other drugs. The elderly and near-elderly people who took diuretics suffered slightly fewer heart attacks and strokes than comparable groups on the costlier medicines. While a majority of elderly Americans needing blood control medication eventually take two or more drugs, the doctors on the dais reported that the test results indicated people with high blood pressure should start off with the tried and true—and cheaper—diuretics. If physicians followed that advice, drug consumers across the United States would save billions of dollars annually since most doctors started patients on the patented drugs hawked by drug companies.

Despite the widespread media coverage, medical practice did not change dramatically over the ensuing months. With a $10-billion market at stake, the drug industry's sales force fanned out across the country to continue pushing the pricier pills (there are more than one hundred blood-pressure control medicines on the market). The government had spent $80 million on the study (dubbed ALLHAT for the Antihypertensive and Lipid-Lowering Treatment to Prevent Heart Attack Trial), but it had no detailers ready to hand out copies of the report, not to mention the coffee mugs, pens, and mouse pads that pharmaceutical marketers routinely leave behind in physicians' offices. "It will take quite a while for dissemination of the results to take place," said Curt Furberg, a professor of public health at Wake Forest University and chairman of the ALLHAT panel. "But we're going to go full press with what we call academic detailing and, hopefully, we'll have a major impact."[1]

With so much money at stake, it was inevitable that the ALLHAT study would not be the last word on antihypertensive medicines. Two months later, physicians in Australia released the results of a smaller comparative study, which was also government funded. Their results showed ACE inhibitors were slightly better than diuretics. The 6,083 Australian patients were almost all white (the U.S. study mirrored the U.S. population that takes blood control medicines—35 percent were black) and contained fewer smokers or patients with diabetes or coronary heart disease, conditions that made it more likely high blood pressure would lead to heart attacks and strokes. Still, the study's results gave the industry's detailers the ammunition they needed. An editorial written by Edward D. Frohlich, a leading hypertension specialist, who was also an industry consultant, appeared in the prestigious *New England Journal of Medicine*. It cautioned against "allowing newscasts to declare immediately which class of drugs is best. . . . Physicians must focus on the individual patient's clinical responses."[2]

For the vast majority of people needing blood pressure control, however, the most important lesson offered by the dueling studies was not whether one drug was marginally better than the other. The medical bottom line was that several classes of medicines worked just about the same. The major difference was that using the generic drug as initial therapy for high blood pressure could save the American health care system and patients billions of dollars a year without a reduction in the quality of health care.

For the new Medicare prescription drug benefit to become both financially meaningful and affordable to taxpayers, the government must hold down the spiraling cost of drugs by reforming the pharmaceutical innovation system. One way to do that is for the government to conduct more trials like ALLHAT. If the industry knew that its "new and improved" medicines might one day face exposure as no better or not much different than cheap generics, its research managers might be less inclined to spend billions of dollars every year pursuing me-too drugs. Instead of wasting time, money, and scientific talent on such fruitless pursuits, the industry could focus on real innovation.

For decades leaders of the industry have argued that the high cost of medicine reflects the huge risks it takes to innovate. But as I have sought to demonstrate in the previous chapters of this book, much of the risk in drug innovation has been borne by the public and nonprofit sectors, which conduct virtually all the long-term basic research and much of the applied research that generate the scientific insights needed to create genuinely innovative therapies.

The risk of failure in those arenas is extremely high. Significant breakthroughs, uncommon in any field, are especially rare in medicine. They depend on insights gained from the long, convoluted, and serendipitous process known as scientific discovery. Sometimes these insights can be hastened along by targeted programs of applied research, as happened with the successful campaign against AIDS. But as the war on cancer shows, even the weight of massive government spending and the mobilization of thousands of scientists and clinicians in the public and private sectors cannot will a pharmaceutical breakthrough into existence. The humbling results of decades of cancer research reveal the absurdity of the drug industry's claim that new drug therapies for the diseases of great concern to the American public—heart disease, cancer, Alzheimer's, diabetes—inevitably depend on the public's willingness to continue pouring huge sums into industry's coffers.

The stories recounted in this book further suggest the most significant breakthroughs of recent times have another common element that can never be purchased. Look behind any major medical advance and you will almost always find a committed scientist or group of scientists, people who have dedicated their careers to understanding a disease or biochemical pathway. It is lonely work, and the bench scientists and clinicians who do it successfully often find themselves swimming against the tide of conventional wisdom. It is that kind of intellectual bravery that ultimately provides the insights needed to create a new drug or therapy.

Eugene Goldwasser was haunted by doubts over the many years he spent nights and weekends sifting through sheep's blood in his search for erythropoietin. But at the end of his career, he had the satisfaction of knowing his work had led to one of the best-selling drugs in the world. But for every Goldwasser, there are a dozens of researchers like cancer specialist Ellen Vitetta, who after twenty years still doesn't know when she might find success for her antibody-based drug delivery system.

It is scientists like her who will eventually unlock the mysteries of America's most pressing medical problems. What are the biochemical processes that trigger most of the more than one hundred forms of cancer, and which ones can be interrupted without causing unacceptable harm to the patient? Nearly thirty years after discovery of the first oncogene, basic scientists are still searching for answers to those questions. They must be answered before drug developers can come up with highly effective therapeutic agents. The same is true for dementia, the slow deterioration of mind that has robbed more than four million seniors of their dignity and placed tragic burdens on their families and caregivers. New drugs based on only a partial understanding of the natural history of the disease have been approved by the Food and Drug Administration (FDA) despite offering only the most marginal improvements in the underlying condition of patients.[3] It may take decades of basic research to truly understand the mysteries of the brain. The same can be said for dozens of rare medical conditions, many of them with genetic origins. Scientists are no closer to a treatment for cystic fibrosis today than they were in 1991, when the gene responsible for the condition was first identified.

The stories recounted here also show that the fifty thousand scientists and support staff in the research-and-development laboratories of the pharmaceutical and biotechnology industries play a crucial role in the development of new drugs. Once the public sector has identified and validated a cellular target suitable for pharmaceutical intervention, industry's skilled biochemists and protein synthesizers often develop the complex molecules that go into clinical trials. Its physicians often shepherd the drug candidates through the difficult process of proving efficacy to regulators' satisfaction. But even in these applied research arenas, as the stories in this survey have shown again and again, public and nonprofit-funded bench scientists and clinicians wind up playing critical roles. Would Genentech or Novartis have pursued their latest cancer drugs in the absence of the dogged determination of Dennis Slamon or Brian Druker? It is doubtful.

Getting the drug industry to focus more of its resources on significant research will require major changes in the current system for funding clinical trials and approving new drugs. The existing incentives encourage companies to pursue alternative versions of existing drugs without regard to how the new drugs compare to those already on the market. The result is an overcrowded medicine chest, where the primary source of information for physicians comes from studies commissioned by the companies peddling the drugs. Oftentimes the studies are published in obscure journals with scant or poor peer review, leading at least one longtime observer of industry-supported academic clinical trials to conclude many are "secondary science."[4]

Doctors need good science driving their medical decisions, not secondary science. Congress should create an independent institute on clinical practice within the National Institutes of Health (NIH) whose major purpose is to conduct clinical trials that compare existing medicines. The new institute's major goal would be to generate best-practice guidelines for physicians. When in the course of disease progression should drug therapy begin? What drugs among the many out there work best? Which ones should be tried when frontline therapies fail? What are the most successful combinations of drugs? ALLHAT was just the tip of the iceberg. These questions arise in virtually every area of medicine, from cancer chemotherapy to arthritis pain relief. With NIH budgets above $27 billion a year, the agency can afford to redirect a modest 5 percent of those funds (more than $1 billion a year) to the vital task of generating and disseminating information about the best clinical use of modern medicines. An alternative funding mechanism would be to levy a 1 percent surtax on prescriptions, which would generate a similar amount but provide a return in cost savings many times over.

The new institute would also become the primary sponsor of clinical trials designed to look for new uses for old drugs. Hundreds of drugs that are now off patent and manufactured by generic pharmaceutical companies are sold at prices only slightly higher than their manufacturing cost, leaving the generic manufacturers with no incentive (and no money) to conduct trials that might validate new uses of the medicines. Yet physician-researchers who routinely use generics in their practices often see potential new uses, some of which are revolutionary in their implications. Unfortunately, they have few places to turn for funding to test the validity of their observations.

A case in point is the potential use of steroids for septic shock or sepsis, the systemic blood infection that kills more than two hundred thousand patients in hospitals every year. In 1987, G. Umberto Meduri, a physician on the staff of the University of Tennessee hospital in Memphis, discovered one of his patients with sepsis responded to an accidental dose of a generic steroid. For the next fifteen years, he fruitlessly sought funds from drug companies and NIH to conduct a major study. The small studies he was able to cobble together were snidely attacked by physicians associated with Eli Lilly and Company, which had spent years developing a biotechnology product to fight the disease. Eli Lilly's drug Xigris, which costs nearly seven thousand dollars per patient, was eventually approved in 2001 after tests showed it reduced mortality by about 20 percent. Only after a small French test indicated steroids were just as effective did NIH finally show interest in sponsoring Meduri's trial.[5] An institute whose mission included sponsorship of such trials would not be so reluctant.

The new institute would also apply one of the main lessons learned from decades of clinical trials for cancer and AIDS drugs. Diseases of complex origin often require combinations of drugs to produce improved patient outcomes. The rapidly advancing fields of genomics and proteomics have enabled scientists to begin identifying the multiple inter- and intracellular pathways that constitute the cascade of events in many diseases. A targeted drug or antibody that intervenes at just one link in that chain may not be sufficient to have an impact. Yet drug companies, whose research departments have their eyes firmly fixed on the regulatory goal line of drug approval, have little incentive to test their new drug in combination with other firms' products. The dream of a magic bullet—and the financial rewards its discovery might bring—lives on. The new government institute would be the perfect vehicle for overcoming these institutional barriers to testing combinations of drugs produced in different laboratories.

Finally, the new institute could become an objective source of information about the true economic value of new medicines. If taxpayers are to provide a universal yet affordable Medicare drug benefit, managers of the system—whether it is the government, pharmacy benefit managers, or the insurance industry—will need some way of saying no to drugs that deliver too few benefits at too high a price or saying no to high-priced drugs whose benefits can be obtained elsewhere at lower cost. That will entail establishing a formulary, a list of preferred drugs that limits physicians' prescription choices. One stream of science to inform decisions about what drugs go onto a formulary can come from comparative clinical trials like ALLHAT.

But independent medical economists should also begin asking whether the high prices of some of the latest medicines are worth the benefits. Studies have shown that ubiquitous drug advertising and hyperactive industry marketing practices have led physicians to overprescribe many medicines, especially to senior citizens. The emerging field of pharmacoeconomics, which evaluates the worth of new medicines by comparing their cost to a dollar figure placed on their health and social benefits, has so far been dominated by economists who either work for or are funded by the drug industry. Studies funded by a neutral source may come up with different answers. "It is important for physicians to have better information about the relative cost effectiveness of prescription drugs, especially those that are new to the market," wrote Stuart Altman, a professor at Brandeis University and a member of the National Bipartisan Commission on the Future of Medicare. "This requires sustained government funding of appropriate research and successful methods of communicating the findings to physicians."[6]

The FDA is another important arena for reform of the drug innovation process. Its guidelines should be amended so that the regulatory approval process contributes to physicians' understanding of the best way to use new drugs.

The basic guidelines for drug approval have not changed much since 1962, when proof of efficacy was added to the 1937 stricture that drugs must be proven safe before they can be prescribed. Subsequent changes have shortened the time it takes to get new drugs to market. User fees have allowed the FDA to increase the number of examiners on the job and substantially reduced the amount of time between the filing of a new drug application and the agency's eventual decision. Responding to the demands of AIDS activists, the FDA now approves many drugs based on surrogate markers of clinical improvement. But the government has not expanded the basic requirements of safety and efficacy.

The government should add a third component to the testing regime for experimental medicines. The current gold standard of double-blind, placebo-controlled trials should be amended to require that new drugs be measured against other therapies where they exist, which is in most drug classes. For most life-threatening conditions like cancer, something similar is already in place for ethical reasons. No researcher can deny a dying patient an existing drug or combination of drugs that is known to extend life, even if only for a few months, in the name of testing a new drug whose efficacy is still unknown. But drug companies routinely test new drugs for chronic conditions without giving the patients existing therapies. Adding an extra cohort of patients to those trials—one that compares the new drug to the best drug on the market—will provide regulators and physicians with crucial information about the best uses for the new drug.

These reforms of the government-driven research agenda would help focus the drug industry's research and development budget—which grew to more than $30 billion in 2002—on truly innovative medicines. Providing physicians, consumers, and payers with better information will force drug companies to pare back meaningless and therefore wasteful projects. Consumers could ultimately save billions of dollars through lower drug costs.

Some industry critics have concluded that the only way to hold down the rising cost of drugs is to impose price controls on the industry.[7] Such proposals are not likely to find a receptive audience on Capitol Hill and in any case would provoke the industry to mobilize its massive public relations and lobbying army in opposition. Better information is one way to avoid the contentious debate that would inevitably accompany and probably doom any price control proposals.

Many of these reforms will sound punitive to an industry that has become accustomed to the current regulations governing the drug approval process. The existing regime gives drug and biotechnology companies maximum flexibility in the marketplace while—outside an adverse events-reporting system—paying almost no attention to how drugs actually get used by physicians and patients. As the government intervenes to create better-informed consumers, it will inevitably reduce spending on drugs (or at least hold down the rate of increase in spending). One can only hope the industry will offset those lost revenues by reducing wasteful marketing and advertising expenses and paring back research projects designed with markets and not medicine in mind. The goal is to get industry focused on real innovation. Improved regulations are one way to do that.

At the same time, the government can take steps to lower industry's cost of developing new medicines. One way to do that is through reform of the nation's patent laws. Since the Supreme Court legalized life-form patents in 1980, the Patent and Trademark Office (PTO) and the courts have liberalized life-science patent claims to the point where they may now be hindering innovation and frustrating competition. A case in point is the widespread patenting of single nucleotide polymophisms (SNPs), the minor variations in genes that account for hair or eye color but may also prove useful in diagnosing some genetic diseases or in predicting individual responses to drugs. Drug companies have recognized the costs these patent holders may one day impose on real innovators should their SNPs get incorporated into the application of a successful therapy. The SNP patent holders are nothing more than toll collectors on the highway to innovation.

To avoid such costly roadblocks, the biggest players in the drug industry have set up the nonprofit SNP Consortium. Its goal is to catalogue all known SNPs and put them in the public domain "without intellectual property restrictions." By the end of 2001, it had found more than 1.5 million, five times more than initially anticipated.[8]

What is true for SNPs is equally true for genes. The standard argument in favor of broad patenting of genes is that they give small biotechnology firms the intellectual property portfolios needed to attract investment for research. However, more than two decades after the start of the biotechnology revolution, the low-hanging fruit of one gene/one protein/one recombinant drug are long gone. Identifying the gene behind a protein that is involved in a disease's progression is only one step in the long-term basic research that may ultimately reveal how to intervene with a chemical, protein, or gene therapy. Allowing one firm (whether it makes the discovery itself or licenses it from NIH or a university on an exclusive basis) to lock up one step in the process could preclude other researchers from pursuing research in that field. It certainly will deter other companies, thereby delaying innovation by limiting scientific competition. At the very least, it will set up gene patent holders as parasitic rent collectors on the products of any subsequent developments that make use of the patented genetic information, needlessly increasing the future cost of drugs.[9]

Things have gotten so far out of hand at the PTO that it is now issuing patents on metabolic processes. In 2000, University of Rochester scientists won a patent for research conducted years earlier on the receptor that is blocked by Cox-2 inhibitors, the heavily advertised painkillers sold by Pfizer Inc. and Merck. The university then sued the drug giants, hoping to skim some of the enormous profits generated by the drugs, which are no better than off-patent ibuprofen in relieving pain. Two years later, Pfizer won a patent on the enzyme inhibited by its erectile dysfunction drug, which would effectively preclude other companies from developing similar drugs for decades. Pfizer immediately sued the two companies developing alternatives to Viagra for patent infringement. These claims may not stand up in court. A federal judge in Rochester in March 2003 dismissed the university's patent claim. The patent "identifies some compounds that *might* [emphasis in the original]) work," but it "amounted to little more than a starting point, a direction for further research," wrote U.S. District Judge David Larimer. How many such patents are out there? It is hard to know. But it is clear that rather than tightening patent requirements as it promised around the time the Human Genome Project's completion was announced, the PTO has continued widening the scope of life-science claims.[10]

It is simple common sense to state categorically that genes, proteins, and metabolic pathways are products of nature, just like the law of gravity. Understanding their role in the biochemical events behind human functions and malfunctions (disease) is the stuff of basic science, no more patentable than Isaac Newton's observations about why the apple fell from the tree. Yet by using the latest technologies like advanced gene sequencing machines, companies or university-based scientists have filed patent claims on thousands of genes with only the vaguest knowledge of their roles in a particular disease. Basic research scientists are claiming ownership of the biological processes that make up life itself, pushing back the frontiers of patentability to the point where it can only impede research and increase its cost.

Congress should redress these loopholes in the patent laws by reinvigorating the requirement that the hand of man and usefulness be present in any invention. If a research entity (public or private) comes up with a drug, a monoclonal antibody, or an artificial protein that can affect a disease, it should be patentable. But in an era when there are multiple methods of making the same protein, and multiple methods, both through recombinant proteins and traditional drugs, of affecting a metabolic pathway, allowing patents on either the genes or the pathways will only serve to impede competition and further research.

Industry officials will allege that these reforms will dry up pharmaceutical innovation. For more than half a century, the drug industry has successfully argued that the high cost of medicine is a price the public must pay if it wants to see the next generation of wonder drugs emerge from its labs. But in recent years, scientists have emerged to challenge that notion in the only places where it matters—in the laboratory and in the clinic.

The problem they are seeking to solve is the dearth of new drugs aimed at diseases of the developing world. Few drug companies are interested in coming up with new drugs for tuberculosis. Nor is there significant private sector research into malaria or leishmaniasis, sometimes known as black fever. No new drugs have been developed for these and a number of other diseases in decades, even though they are the world's most prevalent maladies. Why? The people who contract them have almost no money. And without the financial incentive of a potentially lucrative market, the private sector has not invested in research.[11]

Yet there are plenty of potential new drugs. Some are sitting in academic labs awaiting a commercial developer. Some are gathering cobwebs on industry shelves. Paromomycin, for instance, was the first new antibiotic effective against black fever to come along in years. The disease strikes millions of people in the developing world every year, with a particularly virulent strain called kala azar endemic in parts of India. An Italian firm had invented the drug in the 1980s but never developed it. Pharmacia Corp. also rejected further research after it gained rights to the drug through a merger. Eventually Pharmacia gave the rights to paromomycin to the World Health Organization, which conducted a few early-stage clinical trials. But the United Nations agency ran out of money, and once again a promising cure got shelved.[12]

But in 2001, the Institute for OneWorld Health picked up where private companies and government agencies had left off. The nonprofit drug development company was launched in 2000 by Victoria Hale, then a forty-year-old pharmacologist and former FDA official who had gone to work for Genentech after her stint in government. Her personal and professional experiences drove her to the nonprofit world. A friend's thirteen-year-old daughter had died of a rare cancer when experimental therapies went unexplored because no company was interested. She knew there are drugs, including some in her own firm, with the potential to affect millions of people around the world. But they couldn't draw a nickel in private investment. "I was increasingly frustrated by the fact I had enormous success in drug development, but companies were deciding to walk away from drugs that could save lives. It was time to give it a shot. There was so much to be gained and so many opportunities that existed," she told me. "It was time for me to try."[13]

Paromomycin became her institute's first major drug development program. Promising to turn over manufacturing rights to a generic manufacturer in the developing world should it gain regulatory approval, the institute raised more than $6 million from the Bill and Melinda Gates

Foundation and the federal government to pursue a third-stage clinical trial. The institute, whose staff has expertise in the full range of drug development tasks, has since licensed other drugs that were languishing in private-sector labs.

One such drug is a protease inhibitor aimed at Chagas disease, a blood-borne parasite that infects more than sixteen million Latin Americans a year and can lead to fatal heart problems. The drug had initially been developed as a potential anti-HIV drug by Axys Pharmaceuticals, a small biotech firm. After scientists at the University of California at San Francisco discovered its potential by screening it against the Chagas organism, they began searching for someone to develop it. The rights to the drug eventually landed in the hands of Celera Genomics, which bought Axys. But that firm, rich with cash from its human genome–based stock offering, had no interest in pursuing it. Hale negotiated a nonexclusive license on behalf of OneWorld Health, which will turn over manufacturing rights to generic firms in the developing world if the drug makes it through clinical trials. "We're a team of pharmaceutical scientists who've come together to move drugs forward that would never otherwise reach the market," Hale said. "And we have no stockholders."[14]

Hale and her colleagues at the Institute for OneWorld Health are not alone. The Global Alliance for TB Drug Development, which commissioned the drug development cost study outlined in the previous chapter, is pursuing similar strategies to develop new drugs for that age-old killer. The Sequella Foundation was founded in 1997 by Carol Nacy to develop new vaccines against tuberculosis. Nacy, who honed her immunology skills at Walter Reed Army Institute of Research before becoming chief scientific officer at Entremed, echoed Hale's belief in the ability of nonprofits to carry the ball through the entire drug and vaccine development process. "If I don't look and smell like the Amgen of the future, I can't get the venture capitalists to even look at me," she said.[15] John Erickson, who developed one of the first protease inhibitors against HIV for Abbott Laboratories on an NIH grant, recently set up the Institute for Global Therapeutics. He wants to use his skills in structure-based drug design to develop drugs for resistant strains of HIV, which have emerged as a major problem wherever large-scale use of the AIDS triple cocktail has been deployed.

Can these nonprofit drug developers, funded by governments and wealthy foundations, get the job done? In recent years, the pharmaceutical industry has begun farming out the many tasks of drug development. An entire industry of contract research organizations has sprung up to cater to the various steps of the drug development process. There are companies that specialize in drug design and medicinal chemistry, genomics and proteomics, animal toxicity testing, and human clinical trials. These firms can just as easily be employed by nonprofit drug developers as by big pharmaceutical firms. And if the Global Alliance's estimates for the cost of drug development are accurate—and the anecdotal evidence in this book suggests they are—then it can be done at a far lower cost than the public has been led to believe.

Unless the government helps the pharmaceutical industry by reforming its drug approval process in a manner that fosters innovation, the prognosis for the industry is grim. The pace of new drug development slowed appreciably in the early years of the twenty-first century, and many knowledgeable observers were pessimistic about the industry's ability to turn the situation around. For the foreseeable future, pharmaceutical innovation will reside in universities, independent research institutes, and some biotechnology companies, according to Jürgen Drews, the former president of global research at Hoffmann–La Roche. In his recent book, he pointed out that almost all the large pharmaceutical firms were going through mergers and buying small firms for their expertise and were using both processes as a way of centralizing their research staffs. "Such a path represents the subordination of research to particular strategies determined by market forces and the enterprise as a whole," he warned.

> What, then, will it mean to subordinate research to the requirements of the market? It means that long-range problems have been subordinated to short-term needs, that the innovative must take a back seat to the tried and true; but above all, this subordination of research signals a reversal of the classical roles played by research and marketing. The contributor of ideas— research—will become a receiver of instructions, while the implementer of new concepts in the marketplace—marketing—will become the contributor of ideas. But these ideas won't go very far, since they reflect the marketplace, which is to say that they reflect today, if not yesterday, and never the truly novel.[16]

The nonprofit drug developers searching for cures for the diseases of the developing world understand that dynamic well. At her blackboard in Rockville, Maryland, just a few miles up the road from NIH, Carol Nacy of the Sequella Foundation drew a time line on which she placed the various stages of drug research. She then drew a circle around the earliest and longest part of her time line. "The technologies that have fifteen to twenty years of basic science behind them are the ones that end up making a product," she said. "Our success rate in moving ideas forward depends on those fifteen to twenty years of biology."[17]

What is true for diseases of the developing world is equally true for the diseases that plague the industrialized world. If the pharmaceutical industry continues to insist on double-digit revenue and profit growth year after year in the name of going after the 150th blood pressure control drug or the twentieth pain medication, then the public can assert with some confidence through the legislative process that that kind of innovation is not worth the cost.

There are other paths to new drugs. The AIDS cocktail, the few successes of the war on cancer, the enzyme replacement therapies developed at NIH, and the burgeoning movement to develop low-cost drugs for the developing world are the proof. When the scientific knowledge about a cancer or Alzheimer's disease or a rare genetic disorder matures to the point where a therapeutic intervention becomes possible, there will always be somebody ready and willing to develop it.

Notes

INTRODUCTION

1. Amgen Inc., 10-K (2002) filing with the Securities and Exchange Commission, Mar. 10, 2003. Amgen's profits were calculated by subtracting the $2.99-billion in-process research-and-development write-off for its acquisition of Immunex Inc. from its 2002 aftertax net operating loss of $1.39 billion.

2. Interview with Mark Brand, Sept. 10, 2001.

3. Amgen press release, "FDA Approves Amgen's Aranesp for Anemia Associated with Chronic Renal Failure," Sept. 18, 2001, http://www.amgen.com/news/news01/pressrelease010918.html (accessed Oct. 15, 2003).

4. Georgetown University Center on an Aging Society, "Prescription Drugs, a Vital Component of Health Care," Data Profile no. 5, Sept. 2002; Henry J. Kaiser Family Foundation, "The Medicare Program, Medicare and Prescription Drugs," Oct. 2002. Dozens of news accounts featured the impact on the elderly of rising drug costs; see, for instance, Peter Jennings, "Bitter Medicine," *ABC-World News Tonight*, May 29, 2002.

5. The latest data from the Center for Responsive Politics Web site. See http://www.opensecrets.org (accessed Oct. 10, 2003).

6. Alan F. Holmer, prepared testimony, Senate Finance Committee, Mar. 22, 2000.

7. Alfonso Gambardella, *Science and Innovation: The U.S. Pharmaceutical Industry During the 1980s*, p. 14.

8. *Merck Annual Report*, chairman's message, 2002, http://www.merck.com/finance/annualreport/ar2002/chairmans_message.html (accessed Oct. 15, 2003).

9. Jürgen Drews, *In Quest of Tomorrow's Medicines: An Eminent Scientist Talks about the Pharmaceutical Industry, Biotechnology, and the Future of Drug Research*, p. 20.

1. THE LONGEST SEARCH

1. This and subsequent comments are from various interviews with Eugene Goldwasser conducted between 1999 and 2002.

2. The updated version of *Goodman and Gilman's The Pharmacological Basis of Therapeutics* (McGraw Hill, 2001), edited by Gilman's grandson, is still in print and has been translated into nine languages.

3. James Le Fanu, *The Rise and Fall of Modern Medicine*, pp. 112–13. See also chapter 7.

4. T. Miyake, C. K. Kung, E. Goldwasser, "Purification of Human Erythropoietin," *Journal of Biological Chemistry*, Aug. 10, 1977 [252(15)], 5558–64.

5. Eugene Goldwasser, "Erythropoietin: A Somewhat Personal History," *Perspective in Biology and Medicine* 40 (fall 1996): 18–32 (quote on p. 25).

6. Martin Kenney, *Biotechnology: The University-Industrial Complex*, p. 23.

7. Oral history with Niels Reimers, Bancroft Library, University of California at Berkeley, May 8, 1997.

8. Sandra Panem, *The Interferon Crusade*, p. 72.

9. Interview with George Rathmann, May 27, 2000.

10. Interview with Fu-Kuen Lin, July 25, 2000.

11. A detailed chronology of both Amgen's and Genetics Institute's search for the Epo gene is contained in *Amgen Inc. v. Chugai Pharmaceutical Co., Ltd., and Genetics Institute, Inc.,* U.S. District Court for the District of Massachusetts, decided Dec. 11, 1989.

12. Ibid., p. 12.

13. Interview with Daniel Vapnek, Sept. 26, 2001.

14. *Biotechnology News*, July 21, 1995.

15. Lin interview. Victor Cohn, "Revolutionary Gene Transfer Is Achieved," *Washington Post*, Apr. 11, 1980.

16. *Amgen v. Chugai and Genetics Institute*, p. 12.

17. William Rob Carlson, "Erythropoietin: The Development of a Pharmaceutical Product" (Ph.D. diss., Princeton University, 1988), p. 18. See K. Jacobs et al., "Isolation and Characterization of Genomic and CDNA Clones of Human Erythropoietin," *Nature*, Feb. 28, 1985.

18. The Amgen–Genetics Institute case would drag out until mid-1995, when the Supreme Court finally decided not to hear an appeal of the Appeals Court decision in favor of Amgen.

19. J. W. Eschbach et al., "Correction of the Anemia of End-stage Renal Disease with Recombinant Human Erythropoietin. Results of a Combined Phase I and II Clinical Trial," *New England Journal of Medicine*, Jan. 8, 1987.

20. Laura Johannes, "Unsolved Mystery: Cystic Fibrosis Gave Up Its Gene Twelve Years Ago: Where's the Cure?" *Wall Street Journal*, June 11, 2001.

21. Le Fanu, *The Rise and Fall of Modern Medicine*, p. 259.

22. Andrew C. Revkin, "Firm May Have Found Key to Treating Anemia; Rare Hormone Holds Promise for Kidney Ills," *New York Times*, Jan. 22, 1987.

23. House Ways and Means Committee, *Hearing on Health Care Costs*, 102nd Cong., 1st sess., Oct. 10, 1991.

24. Interview with Howard Grossman, Dec. 18, 2001. I interviewed Grossman during his presentation at the forty-first Annual Interscience Conference on Antimicrobial Agents and Chemotherapy (ICAAC) meeting in Chicago.

25. Interview with Daniel Vapnek, Sept. 21, 2001. By the end of the 1990s,

Amgen was repurchasing nearly $1 billion a year of its own stock, according to its 1999 10-K filing with the Securities and Exchange Commission.

26. Barry Stavro, "Amgen Faces Weighty Task with Fat-Reduction Drug," *Los Angeles Times*, Sept. 5, 1995.

27. *Biotechnology News*, Aug. 18, 1995.

28. Gina Kolata, "Hormone That Slimmed Fat Mice Disappoints as Panacea in People," *New York Times*, Oct. 27, 1999.

29. See John H. Klippel, "Biologic Therapy for Rheumatoid Arthritis," *New England Journal of Medicine*, Nov. 30, 2000. See also J. M. Bathon et al., "A Comparison of Etanercept and Methotrexate in Patients with Early Rheumatoid Arthritis," *New England Journal of Medicine*, Nov. 30, 2000; Larry Schuster, "Prescribing Pain Fighters Proving Big Headache for Joint Docs," *Biotechnology Newswatch*, Dec. 3, 2001; and Andrew Pollack, "Amgen Buys Biotech Rival Immunex for $16 Billion," *New York Times*, Dec. 17, 2001.

30. Klippel, "Biologic Therapy," Nov. 30, 2000.

31. Interview with Doyt Conn, May 23, 2002.

32. Garabed Eknoyan, professor of medicine at Baylor University and cochair of the National Kidney Foundation's Dialysis Outcomes Quality Initiative (DOQI), lists himself as a paid consultant to Amgen at continuing medical education seminars where he teaches; Allen Nissenson, a professor of medicine at UCLA and a member of DOQI, is on the company's advisory board. A full account of this issue can be found in Merrill Goozner, "The Making of a Star Drug," *Chicago Tribune*, May 24, 1999.

33. Interview with Allen Nissenson, Feb. 15, 1999.

34. Rhonda L. Rundle and Laura Johannes, "Ruling Against Transkaryotic Therapies Saves Amgen's Monopoly on Anemia Drug," *Wall Street Journal*, Jan. 22, 2001.

2. RARE PROFITS

1. Vannevar Bush, *Science, the Endless Frontier: A Report to the President* (Washington, D.C.: U.S. Government Printing Office, 1945).

2. A good example of that reasoning can be found in Jerome Groopman, "The Thirty Years' War: Have We Been Fighting Cancer the Wrong Way?" *New Yorker*, June 4, 2001. For more on the war on cancer, see chapter 7.

3. Daniel S. Greenberg, *Science, Money, and Politics: Political Triumph and Ethical Erosion*, p. 419.

4. Interview with John Barranger, Mar. 28, 2002.

5. This and subsequent comments from Roscoe Brady were gleaned from numerous interviews conducted during 2000, 2001, and 2002.

6. Office of Technology Assessment, *Federal and Private Roles in the Development and Provision of Alglucerase Therapy for Gaucher Disease*, Washington, D.C., 1992.

7. Brady interviews.

8. See Office of Technology Assessment, *Federal and Private Roles*, pp. 1-2.

9. Interview with Ernest Beutler, Mar. 15, 2002. Beutler is a thorn in Genzyme's side since he is the chief U.S. proponent of the idea that low doses of

enzyme are just as effective as Genzyme's recommended higher doses in treating Gaucher disease (see the discussion of price below).

10. Interview with John Barranger, Mar. 28, 2002. Of course, Amgen, where Fu-Kuen Lin was finishing his work at about the same time, did patent their gene's use for the expression of erythropoietin (see chapter 1).

11. Interview with Robin Ely Berman, June 13, 2002.

12. Brady interviews.

13. Carolyn H. Asbury, *Orphan Drugs, Medical versus Market Value*, p. 111.

14. Interview with Marlene Haffner, Apr. 12, 2002.

15. Office of Technology Assessment, *Federal and Private Roles*, p. 2.

16. Interview with Abby Meyers, Oct. 18, 2001.

17. *Congressional Record*, Apr. 1, 1993, vol. 138, no. 44, p. 1851.

18. Nancy Kassebaum and Howard Metzenbaum, "Wonder Drugs and Scare Talk," *Washington Post*, June 23, 1992.

19. Henri A. Termeer, "Pricing: The Cost of Miracles," *Wall Street Journal*, Nov. 16, 1993.

20. Patent and Trademark Office, Patent no. 5,236,838, granted Aug. 17, 1993. Office of Technology Assessment, "Federal and Private Roles," p. 13.

21. Interview with Roscoe Brady, June 6, 2002.

22. A list of orphan drugs, both those still under investigation and those approved, is available on the Web site of the Food and Drug Administration's Office of Orphan Products Development, http://www.fda.gov/orphan/designat/list.html (accessed Oct. 15, 2003).

23. Meyers interview.

24. Interview with David Calhoun, Mar. 16, 2002.

25. D. H. Calhoun et al., "Fabry Disease: Isolation of a CDNA Clone Encoding Human Alpha-Galactosidase A," *Proceedings of the National Academy of Science* (Nov. 1985): 7364–68.

26. Interview with Yiannis Ioannou, Mar. 25, 2002.

27. Patent and Trademark Office, Patent no. 5,356,804, granted Oct. 18, 1994.

28. FDA, Office of Orphan Products Development, Web site, http://www.fda.gov/orphan/designat/list.html (accessed Oct. 15, 2003).

29. Interview with Jack Johnson, president of the Fabry Information and Support Group, Feb. 27, 2002.

30. Interview with Frank Landsberger, June 4, 2002.

31. E-mail communication from Lowell Weiner, assistant vice president for public relations at Wyeth, which now owns Genetics Institute, June 4, 2002.

32. Interview with Richard Selden, Apr. 4, 2002.

33. Ioannou interview.

34. Selden interview.

35. Ibid.

36. Transkaryotic Therapies Inc. (TKT), initial registration statement with the Securities and Exchange Commission, Aug. 27, 1996.

37. Genzyme Corp., 10-K (1993–2001) filings with the Securities and Exchange Commission.

38. Raphael Schiffmann et al., "Enzyme Replacement Therapy in Fabry Dis-

ease," *Journal of the American Medical Association,* June 6, 2001; Christine M. Eng et al., "Safety and Efficacy of Recombinant Human a-Galactosidase: A Replacement Therapy in Fabry's Disease," *New England Journal of Medicine,* July 5, 2001.

39. Interview with Gregory Pastores, Mar. 27, 2002.

40. Genzyme Corp., 10-K (2001) filing with the Securities and Exchange Commission, Apr. 1, 2002.

41. Interview with Michael Russo, June 20, 2002.

42. Ibid.

43. Interview with Raphael Schiffmann, Jan. 14, 2003.

44. Otesa Middleton, "FDA Says Serono's Rebif Approval a Rare Case," *Dow Jones Newswires,* Mar. 8, 2002.

3. THE SOURCE OF THE NEW MACHINE

1. "Reading the Book of Life: White House Remarks on Decoding of Genome," *New York Times,* June 27, 2000.

2. Richard Preston, "The Genome Warrior," *New Yorker,* June 12, 2000, p. 66.

3. *New York Times* transcript of President Bill Clinton's press conference, June 27, 2000.

4. Kevin Davies, *Cracking the Genome,* p. 238.

5. Press conference, Capitol Hilton Hotel, Washington, D.C., June 26, 2000.

6. Thomas D. Kiley, "Patents on Random Complementary DNA Fragments?" *Science,* Aug. 14, 1992, p. 915.

7. Ibid.

8. Hearing of the House Judiciary Subcommittee on Courts and Intellectual Property, 106th Cong., 2nd. sess., July 13, 2000.

9. Press conference, June 26, 2000.

10. Davies, *Cracking the Genome,* p. 207.

11. Paul Jacobs and Aaron Zitner, "Genome Milestone: Cracking the Code," *Los Angeles Times,* June 27, 2000.

12. Cook-Deegan, *The Gene Wars,* p. 61. Cook-Deegan is quoting from F. Sanger, "Sequences, Sequences, and Sequences," *Annual Review of Biochemistry* 57 (1988): 1–28.

13. Ibid. (*The Gene Wars*), pp. 64–67.

14. Peter G. Gosselin and Paul Jacobs, "U.S. Officials Probe Cost of Genetic Decoder," *Los Angeles Times,* Feb. 16, 2000.

15. Cook-Deegan, *The Gene Wars,* p. 66.

16. David Fishlock, "How Applied Biosystems Produces Biotechnology Tools," *Financial Times* (London), Aug. 22, 1983, p. 5.

17. Huang was never included on the patent, which became a subject of litigation nineteen years later. MJ Research, which wanted to build a competitor machine using the technology, filed a *qui tam* suit against Applied Biosystems alleging it had overcharged the government for the machines. Michael Barbaro, "Patent Fight Erupts over Gene Machine," *Washington Post,* July 15, 2002.

18. Gosselin and Jacobs, "U.S. Officials Probe Cost of Genetic Decoder," *Los Angeles Times*, Feb. 16, 2000.

19. Cook-Deegan, *The Gene Wars,* p. 88.

20. Interview with Marvin Stodolsky, Aug. 24, 2000.

21. Interview with Lloyd Smith, Oct. 16, 2000.

22. Interview with Joseph Jaklevic, Jan. 26, 2002.

23. Ibid.

24. Interview with Richard Mathies, Sept. 15, 2000

25. Interview with Jingyue Ju, Oct. 15, 2000

26. Interview with Roy Whitfield, Oct. 16, 2000.

27. Interview with Mike Hunkapillar, July 9, 2002.

28. Nicholas Wade, "Scientist's Plan: Map All DNA within Three Years," *New York Times*, May 10, 1998.

29. Preston, "The Genome Warrior," p. 75.

30. Quoted in Davies, *Cracking the Genome*, pp. 91–92.

31. Interview with John Doll, July 3, 2002. My statistic of 1,300 patents comes from Doll's remarks.

32. Quoted in Tom Bethell, "A Map to Nowhere," *American Spectator*, Apr. 2001.

33. David P. Hamilton, "Myriad Genetics Unveils a Project to Catalog Every Protein in Humans," *Wall Street Journal*, Apr. 4, 2001.

34. Interview with Helen Berman, director of the Protein Data Bank, department of chemistry, Rutgers University, July 8, 2002.

35. Rebecca S. Eisenberg, "The Shifting Functional Balance of Patents and Drug Regulation," *Health Affairs*, Sept./Oct. 2001, p. 127.

36. Ibid.

37. Peg Brickley, "New Patent Worries Professors," *The Scientist*, July 22, 2002, p. 19.

38. Andrew Pollack, "Scientist Quits The Company He Led in Quest For Genome," *New York Times*, Jan. 23, 2002.

39. Patent and Trademark Office, U.S. Patent no. 6,410,294.

40. See, for instance, Lawrence K. Altman, "Cancer Doctors See New Era of Optimism," *New York Times*, May 22, 2001.

41. Interview with Susan Taylor, July 22, 2002.

4. A PUBLIC-PRIVATE PARTNERSHIP

1. National Institute for Allergies and Infectious Diseases, update, "Concorde Trial," Apr. 1, 1993, archived at http://www.aegis.com/news/niaid/1993/CDC93005.html (accessed Oct. 15, 2003).

2. John James, "Berlin Conference Overview," *AIDS Treatment News*, June 18, 1993.

3. I thank Jon Cohen, author of *Shots in the Dark: The Wayward Search for an AIDS Vaccine*, for what I consider to be the best of the many metaphors that have been used to describe the disease.

4. Stephen Fried, "Cocktail Hour," *Washington Post Magazine*, May 18, 1997.

5. The Vertex saga was documented in Barry Werth, *The Billion-Dollar Molecule: One Company's Quest for the Perfect Drug*. The molecule in the title was not the protease inhibitor but the drug aimed at curbing transplant rejections.

6. Interview with Robert Yarchoan, June 18, 2001.

7. Larry Kramer, "A Good News/Bad News AIDS Joke," *New York Times Magazine*, July 14, 1996; Andrew Sullivan, "When Plagues End," *New York Times Magazine*, Nov. 10, 1996; Christine Gorman, "The Disease Detective," *Time*, Dec. 30, 1996–Jan. 6, 1997.

8. Louis Galambos, "In the AIDS Fight, Big Is Beautiful: Only the Corporate Giants Can Afford the Cost of Innovation," *Washington Post*, Dec. 1, 1996.

9. Interview with John Erickson, June 21, 2001.

10. L. H. Pearl and W. R. Taylor, "A Structural Model for Retroviral Proteases," *Nature*, Sept. 24, 1987, pp. 351–54.

11. Interview with John McGowan, July 20, 2001.

12. Interview with Dale Kempf, Aug. 23, 2001.

13. Daniel J. Kevles, "The Changed Partnership," *Wilson Quarterly* 19 (summer 1995): 40–48.

14. *The Discovery and Development of Penicillin, 1928–1945*, Alexander Fleming Laboratory Museum (London), Nov. 19, 1999, p. 6.

15. Kenney, *Biotechnology*, p. 13.

16. Donald E. Stokes, *Pasteur's Quadrant: Basic Science and Technological Innovation*, p. 48; see also Kevles, "The Changed Partnership."

17. Stokes, *Pasteur's Quadrant*, p. 49.

18. See Kevles, "The Changed Partnership."

19. See Stokes, *Pasteur's Quadrant*, p. 135.

20. Cohen, *Shots in the Dark*, p. 179.

21. See, for instance, Groopman, "The Thirty Years' War" in *The New Yorker*, June 4, 2001, pp. 52–63; also, John C. Bailar and Heather L. Gornik, "Cancer Undefeated," *New England Journal of Medicine*, May 29, 1997, pp. 1569–74.

22. Cohen, *Shots in the Dark*, p. 6.

23. Peter S. Arno and Karyn L. Feiden, *Against the Odds: The Story of AIDS Drug Development, Politics and Profit*, pp. 37–46.

24. Letters to the Editor, *New York Times*, Sept. 28, 1989.

25. Arno and Feiden, *Against the Odds*, p. 54.

26. Interview with Lawrence Corey, Jan. 10, 2002.

27. John Thomas Mahoney, *The Merchants of Life: An Account of the American Pharmaceutical Industry*, p. 192. Frank Ryan, *The Forgotten Plague: How the Battle Against Tuberculosis Was Won and Lost*, p. 339.

28. Scolnick quoted in Louis Galambos and Jane Eliot Sewell, *Confronting AIDS*, The Business History Group and Johns Hopkins University, published by Merck Research Laboratories (undated), p. 8.

29. Galambos and Sewell, *Confronting AIDS*, pp. 16–17. Interview with Manuel Navia, June 15, 2001.

30. Michael Waldholz, "AIDS—The Race for a Cure—Tracking a Killer," *Wall Street Journal*, Feb. 16, 1989. See also Werth, *Billion-Dollar Molecule*, p. 32; and Navia interview.

31. Interview with Emilio Emini, Merck Research Labs, West Point, Pennsylvania, Nov. 8, 2001.

32. Werth, *Billion-Dollar Molecule*, p. 110.

33. Interview with Alexander Wlodawer, June 28, 2001.

34. Galambos and Sewell, *Confronting AIDS*, p. 20.

35. Mahoney, *Merchants of Life*, pp. 222–26.

36. Panem, *The Interferon Crusade*, p. 74.

37. Interview with Whaijen Soo, Aug. 14, 2001.

38. Ibid. Interview with Keith Bragman, July 6, 2001.

39. M. A. Navia et al., "Three-Dimensional Structure of Aspartyl Protease from Human Immunodeficiency Virus HIV-1," *Nature*, Feb. 16, 1989, pp. 615–20.

40. Interview with Noel Roberts, Aug. 8, 2001.

41. Ibid.

42. Ibid.

43. Interview with Miklos Salgo, Apr. 13, 2001.

44. Ibid., Aug. 8, 2001.

45. Drews, *In Quest of Tomorrow's Medicines*, pp. 15–16.

46. Ibid., p. 16.

47. Bragman interview.

48. Drews, *In Quest of Tomorrow's Medicines*, p. 16.

5. THE DIVORCE

1. Mahoney, *Merchants of Life*, pp. 129–42. See also *The Discovery and Development of Penicillin*, p. 6.

2. Julia Flynn Siler, "The Slipper Ladder at Abbott Labs," *Business Week*, Oct. 30, 1989.

3. See "Ferid Murad—Autobiography" on the Nobel Committee Web site: http://www.nobel.se/medicine/laureates/1998/murad-autobio.html (accessed Oct. 15, 2003).

4. Interview with Ferid Murad, Jan. 4, 2002.

5. Interview with Dale Kempf, Aug. 23, 2001.

6. Interview with John Erickson, July 13, 2001.

7. Interview with Dan Hoth, Sept. 6, 2001.

8. John Schwartz and John McCormick, "The CEO Who Won't Go," *Business Week,* May 7, 1990; Erickson and Murad interviews.

9. Susan Okie, "Scientists Return to NCI's Cutting Edge," *Washington Post*, July 27, 1990.

10. "AIDS Protesters Picket Pharmaceutical Firm," *San Francisco Chronicle*, Mar. 7, 1991. John James, "Clarithromycin: Accessible or Not?" *AIDS Treatment News*, Oct. 18, 1991; Kempf and John Leonard (Jul. 16, 2001) interviews.

11. Hoth interview.

12. Letter from Andre Pernet to Bruce Chabner, Dec. 19, 1991, obtained by Freedom of Information Act (FOIA) request. FOIA officials at the National Institute of Infectious Diseases said a similar correspondence between director Anthony Fauci and Pernet no longer exists.

13. For a comprehensive history of government policy toward intellectual property developed by the public sector, see Rebecca S. Eisenberg, "Public Research and Private Development: Patents and Technology Transfer in Government-Sponsored Research," *Virginia Law Review* 82 (Nov. 1996): 1663–1726.

14. For a complete discussion of the Bayh-Dole Act and its implications, see Peter S. Arno and Michael H. Davis, "Why Don't We Enforce Existing Drug Price Controls? The Unrecognized and Unenforced Reasonable Pricing Requirements Imposed upon Patents Deriving in Whole or in Part from Federally Funded Research," *Tulane Law Review* 75, no. 3 (2001): 631–93. See also Baruch Brody, "Public Goods and Fair Prices: Balancing Technological Innovation with Social Well-being," *The Hastings Center Report* 26 (Mar./Apr. 1996): 5–11.

15. Kenney, *Biotechnology*, p. 100.

16. Government Accounting Office, "Technology Transfer: Number and Characteristics of Inventions Licensed by Six Federal Agencies," June 1999.

17. Letter from Bruce Chabner to Andre Pernet, Jan. 7, 1992.

18. Interview with John Leonard, July 1, 2001.

19. Letter from Bruce Chabner to John Leonard, May 13, 1992.

20. Letter from John Leonard to Bruce Chabner, June 2, 1992 (the company nomenclature for the drug, A-77003, was redacted from the National Cancer Institute (NCI) response to my FOIA request). Also Hoth, Chabner, and Leonard interviews.

21. Hoth interview.

22. Hiroaki Mitsuya et al., "Targeted Therapy of Human Immunodeficiency Virus-Related Disease," *Journal of the Federation of American Societies for Experimental Biology* 10 (July 1991): 2369–81.

23. Interview with Emilio Emini, Nov. 8, 2001.

24. *AIDS Treatment News*, Nov. 22, 1991.

25. Emini interview.

26. See, for instance, Marilyn Chase, "Merck Setback Shows Problems with AIDS Drugs," *Wall Street Journal*, Nov. 26, 1991.

27. Erickson interview, Mar. 2, 2002.

28. Scolnick quoted in Galambos and Sewell, *Confronting AIDS*, p. 35.

29. Emini interview.

30. Yung-Kang Chow et al., "Use of Evolutionary Limitations of HIV-1 Multidrug Resistance to Optimize Therapy," *Nature*, Feb. 18, 1993, 650–54.

31. Jean-Pierre Aboulker and Ann Marie Swart, "Preliminary Analysis of the Concorde Trial" (letters to the editor), *Lancet*, Apr. 13, 1993, 889–90.

32. Steven Epstein, *Impure Science: AIDS, Activism, and the Politics of Knowledge*, p. 308.

33. Lawrence K. Altman, "Faith in Multiple-Drug AIDS Trial Shaken by Report of Error in Lab," *New York Times*, July 27, 1993.

34. Ibid.

6. BREAKTHROUGH!

1. These dates comes from NIH Grant Number 5U01AI027220-05 and U.S. Patent no. 5,343,866.

2. Interview with David Ho, Sept. 20, 2001.

3. D. D. Ho, et al., "Antibody to Lymphadenopathy-Associated Virus in AIDS," letter to *New England Journal of Medicine*, Mar. 7, 1985, pp. 649–50.

4. Ho interview.

5. Interview with Alan Perelson, Feb. 7, 2002.

6. Ho interview.

7. John S. James, "DDC/AZT Combination: Promising Early Results," *AIDS Treatment News*, Nov. 23, 1990.

8. A complete discussion of the AIDS surrogate marker issue is contained in Epstein, *Impure Science*, pp. 265–94.

9. Mark Harrington, *Ten Texts on Saquinavir: Its Rapid Rise and Fall*, June 16, 2001, Treatment Access Group, http://www.aidsinfonyc.org/tag/tx/saquinavirten.html (accessed Oct. 13, 2003).

10. Interview with Ann Collier, June 29, 2001.

11. Letter from Treatment Access Group, Gay Men's Health Crisis, AIDS Action Council, and AIDS Action Baltimore to David Kessler, June 16, 1994.

12. Warren E. Leary, "U.S. Gives Up Right to Control Drug Prices," *New York Times*, Apr. 12, 1995.

13. "Inside Roche: An Interview with Jürgen Drews and Whaijen Soo," Gay Men's Health Crisis' *Treatment Issues*, Dec. 1994.

14. Marlene Cimons and Thomas H. Maugh II, "New Drugs Offer Hope in Battle Against AIDS," *Los Angeles Times*, Feb. 1, 1995.

15. Henry E. Chang, "Conference Looks at HIV Drug Resistance," Gay Men's Health Crisis' *Treatment Issues*, Sept. 1995; Jules Levin, "Protease Inhibitors and Prevention of Cross Resistance," *AIDS Treatment News*, Oct. 6, 1995.

16. Interview with Keith Bragman, July 6, 2001.

17. Examiner's Report on Invirase (NDA 20-628), submitted to the Antiviral Drugs Advisory Committee, FDA, Nov. 7, 1995, p. 105. Transcript obtained through FOIA request, Apr. 5, 2002.

18. Pricing information obtained from the Cipla Web site: http://www.cipla.com (accessed Oct. 15, 2003).

19. Laurie McGinley, "First of New Class of AIDS Drugs Get FDA Approval," *Wall Street Journal*, Dec. 8, 1995.

20. Interview with John Leonard, July 17, 2001.

21. Theo Smart, "More Clinical Data on Protease Inhibitors," Gay Men's Health Crisis' *Treatment Issues*, Oct. 1995.

22. FDA, New Drug Application 20-659 (Norvir), p. 62. Obtained via FOIA request.

23. "Three Days that Shook the World," Gay Men's Health Crisis' *Treatment Issues*, Mar. 1996.

24. Galambos and Sewell, *Confronting AIDS*, p. 41.

25. Michael Waldholz, "Strong Medicine: New Drug 'Cocktails' Mark Exciting Turn in the War on AIDS," *Wall Street Journal*, June 14, 1996.

26. Galambos and Sewell, *Confronting AIDS*, p. 42.

27. Michael Waldholz, "Strong Medicine: New Drug Cocktails Mark Exciting Turn in the War on AIDS," *Wall Street Journal*, June 14, 1996.

28. Gabriel Torres and Dave Gilden, "Commentary: Studying Protease Inhibitors," Gay Men's Health Crisis' *Treatment Issues*, Aug. 1994.

29. "Roy Vagelos on AIDS Treatment and Drug Development," Gay Men's Health Crisis' *Treatment Issues*, Apr. 1994.

30. Galambos and Sewell, *Confronting AIDS*, p. 50.

31. Ibid., p. 51.

32. Ibid., p. 55n165.

33. Waldholz, "Strong Medicine."

34. Elyse Tanouye, "Short Supply: Success of AIDS Drug Has Merck Fighting To Keep Up the Pace," *Wall Street Journal*, Nov. 5, 1996.

35. Stephen Fried, "Cocktail Hour," *Washington Post Magazine*, May 18, 1997, p. 10.

36. The Global Alliance for TB Drug Development, "The Economics of TB Drug Development," Oct. 2001, p. 3.

37. See Fried, "Cocktail Hour."

38. Agouron Pharmaceuticals Inc., 10-K (1995, 1997, 1998) filings with the Securities and Exchange Commission.

39. Vertex Pharmaceuticals Inc., 10-K (1992–99) filings with the Securities and Exchange Commission.

40. David Brown, "Study Finds Drug-Resistant HIV in Half of Infected Patients," *Washington Post*, Dec. 29, 2001.

41. Thomas H. Maugh II, "AIDS Scientists Fight Rising Tide of Resistance, Risky Behavior," *Los Angeles Times*, Feb. 12, 2001.

42. Interviews with Erickson in Aug. 2001 and Mar. 2002 and various e-mail communications.

7. THE FAILED CRUSADE?

1. LeAnn D. Andersen et al., "Assessing a Decade of Progress in Cancer Control," *The Oncologist* 7 (2002): 200–204; see also Gina Kolata, "Study Sets Off Debate over Mammograms' Value," *New York Times*, Dec. 9, 2001.

2. All data drawn from NCI, *SEER Cancer Statistics Review, 1973–99*, http://www.seer.cancer.gov/; see also Robert N. Proctor, *Cancer Wars: How Politics Shapes What We Know and Don't Know About Cancer*, pp. 17–34.

3. Gina Kolata, "Hope in the Lab: A Special Report. A Cautious Awe Greets Drugs That Eradicate Tumors in Mice," *New York Times*, May 3, 1998. As of late 2002, one of EntreMed's anti-angiogenesis drugs was in Phase II clinical trials for a rare form of pancreatic cancer. The FDA provided financial support for the trial from a special fund set up to promote drugs for rare diseases.

4. Robert Bazell, *Her-2: The Making of Herceptin, a Revolutionary Treatment for Breast Cancer*, p. 25. He attributes the phrase to author Susan Love.

5. Unpublished briefing paper by Edward Sausville, director of the Developmental Therapeutics Program, Division of Cancer Treatment and Diagnosis, NCI.

6. Groopman, "The Thirty Years' War," p. 52.

7. Richard A. Rettig, *Cancer Crusade*, p. 98.

8. James T. Patterson, *The Dread Disease: Cancer and Modern American Culture*, pp. 88–90.

9. Ibid.

10. Ibid., p. 117.

11. Rettig, *Cancer Crusade*.

12. Ibid., p. 23; Patterson, *The Dread Disease*, pp. 130–31.

13. Rettig, *Cancer Crusade*.

14. Dudley's role is described in Patterson's book and in a short entry in the *Handbook of Texas Online*, Texas State Historical Association, http://www.tsha .utexas.edu/handbook/online/articles/view/JJ/fja44.html (accessed Oct. 15, 2003).

15. Norman Baker of Iowa, advertising that "cancer is curable," peddled his arsenic compounds through the mails. He eventually served four years in Leavenworth for mail fraud. Harry Hoxsey attracted thousands of dying patients to his Dallas clinic for a treatment that combined potassium iodide, red clover, poke root, prickly ash bark, and other herbal aids. It took the FDA more than two decades of litigation before it shut him down in 1960. The two were only the most famous of dozens of charlatans who "worked the cancer angle" in mid-twentieth-century America. See Patterson, *The Dread Disease*, pp. 106–8.

16. Bazell, *Her-2*, pp. 22–23.

17. Jordan Goodman and Vivien Walsh, *The Story of Taxol: Nature and Politics in the Pursuit of an Anti-Cancer Drug*, pp. 11–12.

18. Patterson, *The Dread Disease*, pp. 145–47, 195.

19. From a 1964 interview quoted in Patterson, *The Dread Disease*, p. 196.

20. Saul A. Schepartz, "The National Cancer Institute's Drug Development Program," Division of Cancer Treatment and Diagnosis, NCI; reprinted in *Cooperative Approaches to Research and Development of Orphan Drugs*, ed. Melvin H. Van Woert and Eunyong Chung (New York: Alan R. Liss Inc., 1985), p. 75.

21. Proctor, *Cancer Wars*, pp. 36–48.

22. Richard Kluger, *Ashes to Ashes: America's Hundred-Year Cigarette War, the Public Health, and the Unabashed Triumph of Philip Morris*, pp. 135–62.

23. Kluger, *Ashes to Ashes*, pp. 143–44.

24. See Kluger for a full history of the scientific battles over cigarette smoking and cancer. For a broader discussion of industry-funded science, see Proctor, *Cancer Wars*, esp. chapter 5, " 'Doubt Is Our Product': Trade Association Science."

25. Robert A. Weinberg, *Racing to the Beginning of the Road: The Search for the Origin of Cancer*, p. 31.

26. Weinberg, *Racing to the Beginning of the Road*, p. 57.

27. Panem, *The Interferon Crusade*, p. 12. At the outset of the biotechnology era, NCI funded numerous experiments with private companies seeking to use interferon against various cancers. It eventually found a use against hepatitis C and a few other minor indications, but it proved nowhere near as medically useful as initially expected. To an earlier generation of critics, the interferon experience was proof that government-led industrial policy in drug development was bound to fail.

28. Weinberg, *Racing to the Beginning of the Road*, p. 73.

29. Rettig, *Cancer Crusade,* pp. 156, 218.

30. Ibid., pp. 255–56.

31. Proctor, *Cancer Wars,* p. 137.

32. Ibid., pp. 57–61.

33. Ibid., p. 133.

34. Weinberg, *Racing to the Beginning of the Road,* pp. 83–84.

35. Interview with Vincent T. De Vita (director of NCI from 1980 to 1988), director of the Yale University Cancer Center, Aug. 12, 2002.

36. Michael Waldholz, *Curing Cancer,* p. 278.

37. Ibid., p. 43.

38. Ibid., p. 286.

39. Panem, *The Interferon Crusade,* pp. 35–74.

40. B. Rosenberg et al., "Inhibition of Cell Division in Escherichia Coli by Electrolysis Products from a Platinum Electrode," *Nature,* Feb. 13, 1965, pp. 698–99.

41. Arthur Allen, "Triumph of the Cure," *Salon.com,* July 29, 1999, http://www.salon.com/health/feature/1999/07/29/lance (Oct. 15, 2003); Lawrence H. Einhorn, "Update in Testicular Cancer" (unpublished paper, Indiana University Medical Center); and "NCI Role in the Discovery and Development of Marketed Anticancer Drugs" (unpublished paper, NCI).

42. Goodman and Walsh, *The Story of Taxol,* pp. 56–69.

43. P. B. Schiff, J. Fant, S. B. Horwitz, "Promotion of Microtubule Assembly In Vitro by Taxol," *Nature,* Feb. 22, 1979, pp. 665–67.

44. Goodman and Walsh, *The Story of Taxol,* pp. 115–19.

45. Marilyn Chase, "Clashing Priorities: A New Cancer Drug May Extend Lives," *Wall Street Journal,* Apr. 9, 1991.

46. Goodman and Walsh, *The Story of Taxol,* p. 158.

47. Interview with Joseph Rubinfeld, Dec. 3, 2002. Rubinfeld left Bristol-Myers Squibb to help start Amgen. In 2002 he was chief executive officer of SuperGen, which is seeking to commercialize anticancer drugs discovered at the Houston-based Stehlin Foundation, a nonprofit institute that has screened drug candidates for NCI for many years.

48. Hearing of the Regulation, Business Opportunity, and Energy Subcommittee of the House Small Business Committee, 103rd Cong., 1st sess., Jan. 25, 1993.

49. Ibid.

50. Ibid.

51. Peter R. Dolan, "Letter to Employees," Bristol-Myers Squibb, June 6, 2002, http://www.bms.com (accessed June 15, 2002).

52. Interview with Richard Klausner, July 16, 2002.

53. Pharmaceutical Research and Manufacturers Association, "2001 Survey: New Medicines in Development for Cancer," http://www.phrma.org/newmedicines/resources/cancer01.pdf (accessed Oct. 15, 2003).

54. Quoted in Groopman, "The Thirty Years' War," p. 63.

55. Klausner interview.

56. This account of the development of Herceptin is drawn largely from Bazell, *Her-2,* pp. 35–52. Also, interview with Dennis Slamon, Feb. 7, 2003.

57. Bazell, *Her-2;* Slamon interview.

58. See, for instance, Linda Marsa, *Prescription for Profits: How the Pharmaceutical Industry Bankrolled the Holy Marriage between Science and Business,* pp. 199–207.

59. Charles McCoy, "Genentech's New CEO Seeks Clean Slate—Levinson Takes Charge at Biotech Firm after Raab's Ouster," *Wall Street Journal,* July 12, 1995.

60. Bazell, *Her-2,* pp. 44–47

61. Slamon interview.

62. See, for instance, Craig Horowitz, "The Cancer Killer," *New York,* May 25, 1998, pp. 67–71.

63. Bazell, *Her-2,* p. 72.

64. Tara Parker-Pope, "Revlon Is a Cancer Drug's Unlikely Benefactor," *Wall Street Journal,* May 15, 1998.

65. For the trial's summary, see Herceptin's label, FDA, http://www.fda.gov/cder/biologics/products/trasgen020900.html (accessed Oct. 15, 2003).

66. Slamon interview.

67. C. L. Vogel et al., "First-Line Herceptin Monotherapy in Metastatic Breast Cancer," *Oncology* 61, supp. 2 (2001): 37–42; Slamon interview.

68. Herceptin generated $346.6 million in sales for Genentech in 2001. See Bernadette Tansey, "Judge Rules Against Genentech in Chiron Patent Suit," *San Francisco Chronicle,* June 28, 2002.

69. Interview with V. Craig Jordan, Sept. 11, 2002. See also V. Craig Jordan, "Designer Estrogens," *Scientific American,* Oct. 1998, pp. 60–67.

70. Gina Kolata and Lawrence M. Fisher, "Drugs to Fight Breast Cancer Near Approval," *New York Times,* Sept. 3, 1998.

71. Jordan interview.

72. Nicholas Wade, "Powerful Anti-Cancer Drug Emerges from Basic Biology," *New York Times,* May 8, 2001.

73. Jill Waalen, "Gleevec's Glory Days," *Howard Hughes Medical Institute Bulletin,* Dec. 2001, pp. 10–15.

74. Interview with Brian Druker, Jan. 17, 2003.

75. Druker interview. See also Wade, "Powerful Anti-Cancer Drug"; Waalen, "Gleevec's Glory Days"; and Stephen D. Moore, "Blood Test: News about Leukemia Unexpectedly Puts Novartis on the Spot," *Wall Street Journal,* June 6, 2000.

76. Moore, "Blood Test." See also G. D. Demetri et al., "Efficacy and Safety of Imatinib Mesylate in Advanced Gastrointestinal Stromal Tumors," *New England Journal of Medicine,* Aug. 15, 2002, pp. 472–80. The financial disclosure statements in the paper do not include NCI.

77. Brian J. Druker et al., "Efficacy and Safety of a Specific Inhibitor of the BCR-ABL Tyrosine Kinase in Chronic Myeloid Leukemia," *New England Journal of Medicine,* Apr. 5, 2001, pp. 1031–37. Also Brian J. Druker et al., "Activity of a Specific Inhibitor of the BCR-ABL Tyrosine Kinase in the Blast Crisis of Chronic Myeloid Leukemia and Acute Lymphoblastic Leukemia with the Philadelphia Chromosome," *New England Journal of Medicine,* Apr. 5, 2001, pp. 1038–42.

78. Druker interview.

79. "ODAC Advice Poses Challenge to FDA: Would Iressa Approval Erode Standards?" *The Cancer Letter*, Nov. 8, 2002.

80. "FDA Says Data Insufficient to Evaluate C225 Application," *The Cancer Letter*, Jan. 4, 2002.

81. For a detailed account of Erbitux's early development, see Catherine Arnst, "The Birth of a Cancer Drug," *Business Week*, July 9, 2001, pp. 95–102.

82. Ibid.

83. Geeta Anand, "History and Science: In Waksal's Past: Repeated Ousters," *Wall Street Journal*, Sept. 27, 2002.

84. Arnst, "The Birth of a Cancer Drug," p. 98.

85. Justin Gillis, "A Hospital's Conflict of Interest: Patients Weren't Told of Stake in Cancer Drug," *Washington Post*, June 30, 2002; "Mendelsohn Defends ImClone's Actions and His Role in Development of C225," *The Cancer Letter*, Oct. 18, 2002, p. 5.

86. *The Cancer Letter,* Jan. 4, 2002.

87. Ralph W. Moss, "Report from ASCO: Trials and Tribulations of a New Cancer Drug," *Cancer Decisions Newsletter*, July 29, 2002.

88. "Mendolsohn Defends ImClone's Actions," p. 3.

89. Druker interview.

90. Jordan interview.

91. Interview with Ellen Vitetta, Dec. 12, 2002.

8. ME TOO!

1. The best account I've found of the so-called Prontosil affair is contained in Frank Ryan, *Forgotten Plague*. See esp. pp. 98–120.

2. Milton Silverman and Philip R. Lee, *Pills, Profits, and Politics*, p. 86.

3. Peter Temin, "Technology, Regulation, and Market Structure in the Modern Pharmaceutical Industry," *Bell Journal of Economics* 10, no. 2 (1979): 429–46. See also Jane S. Smith, *Patenting the Sun: Polio and the Salk Vaccine*.

4. Temin, "Technology, Regulation, and Market Structure," p. 438.

5. Richard Harris, *The Real Voice*, p. 8.

6. Ibid., p. 79.

7. Silverman and Lee, *Pills, Profits, and Politics*, pp. 4–5.

8. Victor R. Fuchs and Harold C. Sox Jr., "Physicians' Views of the Relative Importance of Thirty Medical Innovations," *Health Affairs* 20 (Sept./Oct. 2001): 35.

9. David A. Kessler, Janet L. Rose, Robert J. Temple, Renie Schapiro, and Joseph P. Griffin, "Therapeutic-Class Wars: Drug Promotion in a Competitive Marketplace," *The New England Journal of Medicine*, Nov. 17, 1994, pp. 1350–53.

10. NIH, *NIH Contributions to Pharmaceutical Development, Case Study Analysis of the Top-Selling Drugs*, Office of Science Policy, Feb. 2000.

11. Interview with George Sachs, Mar. 29, 2001.

12. David Blumenthal et al., "Participation of Life-Science Faculty in Research Relationships with Industry," *New England Journal of Medicine*, Dec.

5, 1996, pp. 1934-39. Blumenthal and his colleagues asked more than two thousand teaching physicians about their relationships with industry and their publishing habits. Less than a third took money from industry. Scientists funded partially by industry published just as often as their publicly funded colleagues, except for the minority who took more than two-thirds of their money from industry. That minority published less often, were more likely to withhold information from colleagues, and were more likely to have generated trade secrets for their patrons.

13. Kevin Parent, *Postgraduate Medicine* 96 (Nov. 1, 1994): 53.

14. Henry J. Kaiser Family Foundation, "Prescription Drug Trends," Nov. 2001.

15. NIH, *NIH Contributions to Pharmaceutical Development,* pp. 12-13.

16. Gardiner Harris, "Prilosec's Maker Switches Users to Nexium, Thwarting Generics," *Wall Street Journal,* June 6, 2002.

17. Sachs interview.

18. Harris, "Prilosec's Maker."

19. Stephen Hall, "The Claritin Effect: Prescription for Profit," *New York Times Magazine,* Mar. 11, 2001.

20. Gardiner Harris, "As Blockbuster Claritin Goes Generic, Schering-Plough Pushes a Close Sibling," *Wall Street Journal,* Mar. 21, 2002. See also Scott Hensley, "More Than Ads, Drug Makers Rely on Sales Representatives," *Wall Street Journal,* Mar. 14, 2002.

21. Andrew Pollack, "Battling Searle, University Gets Broad Patent for New Painkiller," *New York Times,* Apr. 12, 2000.

22. Gardiner Harris, "When Its Patents Expired, Merck Didn't Merge—It Found New Drugs," *Wall Street Journal,* Jan. 10, 2001.

23. Pharmaceutical Research and Manufacturers Association, "Pharmaceutical Industry Honors Discoverers of Celebrex," press release, Mar. 25, 2002. Numerous studies in the academic literature have shown that Cox-2 inhibitors are no better than ibuprofen, diclofenac, and naproxen sodium for reducing aches and pains; see, for instance, A. J. Matheson and D. P. Figgitt, "Rofecoxib: A Review of Its Use in the Management of Osteoarthritis, Acute Pain and Rheumatoid Arthritis," *Drugs* 61, no. 6 (2001): 833-65; see also R. Hawel et al., "Comparison of the Efficacy and Tolerability of Dexibuprofen and Celecoxib in the Treatment of Osteoarthritis of the Hip," *International Journal of Clinical Pharmacology and Therapeutics* 4 (Apr. 2003): 153-64.

24. See for instance the special supplement to the *American Journal of Medicine,* Mar. 30, 1998.

25. Elizabeth Neus, "New Arthritis Relief: Pain-Killers Promise to Be Tummy-Friendly," *Chicago Sun-Times,* Oct. 28, 1998.

26. "Conquering Pain," *Business Week,* Mar. 1, 1999, p. 104.

27. "FDA Approves Pain Reliever with Fewer Side Effects," *Washington Post,* May 22, 1999.

28. Centers for Disease Control and Prevention, *National Vital Statistics Report* 47 (June 30, 1999); Susan Levenstein et al., "Stress and Peptic Ulcer Disease," *Journal of the American Medical Association,* Jan. 6, 1999; T. M. MacDonald et al., "Association of Upper Gastrointestinal Toxicity of Nonsteroidal

Anti-inflammatory Drugs with Continued Exposure: Cohort Study," *British Medical Journal*, Nov. 22, 1997.

29. David R. Lichtenstein and M. Michael Wolfe, "COX-2-selective NSAIDS: New and Improved?" *The Journal of the American Medical Association*, Sept. 13, 2000, pp. 1297–99.

30. Garret A. FitzGerald and Carlo Patrono, "The Coxibs, Selective Inhibitors of Cyclooxygenase-2," *The New England Journal of Medicine*, Aug. 9, 2001, pp. 433–42.

31. Melody Petersen, "Doubts Are Raised on the Safety of Two Popular Arthritis Drugs," *New York Times*, May 22, 2001.

32. FDA, "FDA Approves New Indication and Label Changes for the Arthritis Drug, Vioxx," press release, Apr. 11, 2002.

33. Susan Okie, "Missing Data on Celebrex: Full Study Altered Picture of Drug," *Washington Post*, Aug. 5, 2001.

34. Peter Jüni, Anne Rutjes, and Paul Dieppe, "Are Selective Cox-2 Inhibitors Superior to Traditional Nonsteroidal Anti-inflammatory Drugs?" *British Medical Journal*, June 1, 2002, pp. 1287–88.

35. Henry J. Kaiser Family Foundation, "Prescription Drug Trends: A Chartbook Update," Nov. 2001, p. 31.

36. Marcia Angell, "The Pharmaceutical Industry: To Whom Is It Accountable?" *The New England Journal of Medicine*, June 22, 2000, p. 1904.

9. THE $800 MILLION PILL

1. Joseph A. DiMasi, *Price Trends for Prescription Pharmaceuticals, 1995–1999,* Tufts Center for the Study of Drug Development, Aug. 2000. The study purported to show that me-too drugs resulted in competition. But it chose a 5-percent differential as significant. Simply by expanding the price differential to 10 percent, the number of drugs that resulted in significant price competition fell to less than half. Only five of the twenty drugs entered the market 30 percent or more below existing prices, which one would have expected from all firms intent on seizing significant market share.

2. David Noonan with Joan Raymond and Anne Belli Gesalman, "Why Drugs Cost So Much," *Newsweek*, Sept. 25, 2000, p. 22.

3. Henry J. Kaiser Family Foundation, *Prescription Drug Trends: A Chartbook Update*, Nov. 2001. See also National Institute for Health Care Management, *Prescription Drug Expenditures in 2001: Another Year of Escalating Costs*, Apr. 2002; and National Institute for Health Care Management, *Prescription Drugs and Mass Media Advertising, 2000*, Nov. 2001.

4. Henry J. Kaiser Family Foundation, *Prescription Drug Trends*.

5. Chunliu Zhan et al., "Potentially Inappropriate Medication Use in the Community-Dwelling Elderly," *Journal of the American Medical Association*, Dec. 12, 2001, pp. 2823–29.

6. Henry J. Kaiser Family Foundation, *Prescription Drug Trends*; see also Pharmaceutical Research and Manufacturers Association, "Annual Report, 2001–2002," p. 13.

7. Thomas Maeder, "The FDA Meets the Twenty-first Century," *Under-*

standing Government, http://www.understandinggovernment.org/maeder.html (accessed Mar. 25, 2003).

8. See, for instance, Chris Adams, "Doctors 'Dine n' Dash' in Style, As Drug Firms Pick Up the Tab," *Wall Street Journal*, May 14, 2001; Scott Hensley, "More Than Ads, Drug Makers Rely on Sales Representatives," *Wall Street Journal*, Mar. 14, 2002; Robert Pear, "Drug Industry Is Told to Stop Gifts to Doctors," *New York Times*, Oct. 1, 2002.

9. Harris, *The Real Voice*, p. 76.

10. Alan F. Holmer, "Innovation Is Key Mission," *USA Today*, May 31, 2002.

11. Life expectancy statistics are available on the Centers for Disease Control Web site, http://www.cdc.gov; e-mail communication from S. Jay Olshansky, Oct. 16, 2002.

12. *Runner's World*, Oct. 2002. See also National Association for Sport and Physical Education, *The Shape of the Nation Report*, Oct. 2001.

13. See Ronald Bailey, ed., *Global Warming and Other Eco-Myths: How the Environmental Movement Uses False Science to Scare Us to Death*; and Samuel S. Epstein, *The Politics of Cancer Revisited*.

14. Holmer, "Innovation Is Key Mission."

15. Joseph A. DiMasi et al., "Cost of Innovation in the Pharmaceutical Industry," *Journal of Health Economics* 10 (1991): 107–42.

16. Tufts Center for the Study of Drug Development, "Tufts Center for the Study of Drug Development Pegs Cost of New Prescription Medicine at $802 Million," press release, Nov. 30, 2001.

17. Data provided by the Division of AIDS, NIAID.

18. Government Accounting Office, "NIH Clinical Trials: Various Factors Affect Patient Participation," Report to Congressional Requesters, Sept. 1999.

19. Alice Dembner, "Critics Say Drug Trials Often a Marketing Tool," *Boston Globe*, June 25, 2002; Sheryl Gay Stolberg and Jeff Gerth, "Medicine Merchants: How Research Benefits Marketing," *New York Times*, Dec. 23, 2000.

20. Melody Petersen, "Madison Ave. Plays Growing Role in Drug Research," *New York Times*, Nov. 22, 2002; Frank Davidoff et al., "Sponsorship, Authorship and Accountability, *New England Journal of Medicine*, Sept. 13, 2001, pp. 825–27.

21. Public Citizen, "Rx R&D Myths: The Case Against the Drug Industry's R&D 'Scare Card,'" *Public Citizen Congress Watch*, Aug. 8, 2001.

22. Ernst and Young LLP, "Pharmaceutical Industry R&D Costs: Key Findings about the Public Citizen Report," Aug. 8, 2001, posted on the Pharmaceutical Research and Manufacturers Association Web site, http://www.phrma .org/mediaroom/press/releases//2001-08-11.227.pdf (accessed Oct. 15, 2003).

23. Telephone interview with Baruch Lev, Oct. 15, 2002.

24. David Willman, "'Fast-Track' Drug to Treat Diabetes Tied to 33 Deaths," *Los Angeles Times*, Dec. 6, 1998.

25. Daniel W. Sigelman, "Dangerous Medicine," *The American Prospect*, Sept. 23, 2002.

26. National Institute for Health Care Management Research and Education

Foundation, *Changing Patterns of Pharmaceutical Innovation,* May 2002; see also Melody Peterson, "New Medicines Seldom Contain Anything New, Study Finds," *New York Times,* May 29, 2002.

27. Pharmaceutical Research and Manufacturers Association, *NIHCM's Report on Pharmaceutical Innovation: Fact vs. Fiction,* a preliminary report, June 11, 2002.

28. Ibid.

29. Industry statistics from the Biotechnology Industry Organization Web site, http://www.bio.org/news/stats.asp (accessed Oct. 15, 2003).

30. Andrew Pollack, "Despite Billions for Discoveries, Pipeline for Drugs Is Far from Full," *New York Times,* Apr. 19, 2002.

31. Andrew Pollack, "Once Novel Drug Company No Longer Sets Pace," *New York Times,* Apr. 18, 2002.

32. Gardiner Harris, "Drug Firms, Stymied in the Lab, Become Marketing Machines," *Wall Street Journal,* July 6, 2000; Gardiner Harris, "Why Drug Makers Are Failing in Quest for New Blockbusters," *Wall Street Journal,* Apr. 18, 2002.

33. See Harris, "Why Drug Makers Are Failing."

34. Speech to the Association of University Technology Managers, San Diego, Feb. 28, 2002.

35. The Global Alliance for TB Drug Development, *The Economics of TB Drug Development,* Oct. 2001, p. 66.

10. THE FUTURE OF DRUG INNOVATION

1. ALLHAT officers and coordinator for the ALLHAT Collaborative Research Group, "Major Outcomes in High-Risk Hypertensive Patients Randomized to Angiotensin-Converting Enzyme Inhibitor or Calcium Channel Blocker vs. Diuretic," *Journal of the American Medical Association,* Dec. 18, 2002, pp. 2981–97. National Heart, Lung and Blood Institute, press conference, Dec. 17, 2002.

2. Edward D. Frohlich, "Treating Hypertension: What Are We to Believe?" *New England Journal of Medicine,* Feb. 13, 2003, pp. 639–41.

3. Richard Mayeux and Mary Sano, "Treatment of Alzheimer's Disease," *New England Journal of Medicine,* Nov. 25, 1999, pp. 1670–79.

4. Interview with David Blumenthal, May 30, 2000. Blumenthal, a professor at Harvard Medical School and director of the Massachusetts General Hospital Institute of Health Policy, has been tracking industry-university relations in medicine since the Carter administration.

5. Thomas M. Burton, "Left on the Shelf: Why Cheap Drugs That Appear to Halt Fatal Sepsis Go Unused," *Wall Street Journal,* May 17, 2002; Thomas M. Burton, "French Study Bolsters Steroids as Treatment for Deadly Sepsis," *Wall Street Journal,* Aug. 21, 2002.

6. Stuart H. Altman and Cindy Parks-Thomas, "Controlling Spending on Prescription Drugs," *New England Journal of Medicine,* Mar. 14, 2002, pp. 855–56.

7. Marcia Angell, "The Pharmaceutical Industry."

8. The SNP Consortium Ltd. Web site: http://snp.cshl.org/about/. In a paper prepared for a conference at Duke University in Nov. 2002 ("The Public and the Private in Biopharmaceutical Research"), intellectual property law professors Arti K. Rai and Rebecca S. Eisenberg argued that "the willingness of private firms in a patent-sensitive industry to spend money to enhance the public domain is powerful evidence that intellectual property rights in the research results threaten to create significant barriers to subsequent research and product development."

9. This point is made in several articles contained in David Korn and Stephen J. Heinig, eds., "Public versus Private Ownership of Scientific Discovery: Legal and Economic Analyses of the Implications of Human Gene Patents," *Academic Medicine*, pt. 2, Dec. 2002.

10. Scott Hensley, "Pfizer Sues to Block Viagra Rivals," *Wall Street Journal*, Oct. 23, 2002. *University of Rochester v. G. D. Searle and Co.*, U.S. District Court, Western District of New York, decided Mar. 5, 2003, http://www.nywd .uscourts.gov/decision/20030305_00cv6161_larimer.pdf (accessed Mar. 5, 2003).

11. See, for instance, the Web site of Campaign for Access to Essential Medicines on the Doctors Without Borders Web site, http://www.accessmed-msf .org/index.asp#.

12. David Perlman, "Drug Firm Seeks Cures over Cash," *San Francisco Chronicle*, Aug. 19, 2002.

13. Interview with Victoria Hale, Feb. 26, 2003.

14. Perlman, "Drug Firm Seeks Cures."

15. Interview with Carol Nacy, June 21, 2002.

16. Drews, *In Quest of Tomorrow's Medicines,* p. 234.

17. Nacy interview.

Bibliography

Arno, Peter S., and Karyn L. Feiden. *Against the Odds: The Story of AIDS Drug Development, Politics and Profits*. New York: HarperCollins Publishers, 1992.

Asbury, Carolyn H. *Orphan Drugs: Medical versus Market Value*. Lexington, Mass.: Lexington Books, 1985.

Bailey, Ronald, ed. *Global Warming and Other Eco-Myths: How the Environmental Movement Uses False Science to Scare Us to Death*. Roseville, Calif.: Forum Publishing, 2002.

Bazell, Robert. *Her-2: The Making of Herceptin, a Revolutionary Treatment for Breast Cancer*. New York: Random House, 1998.

Cohen, Jon. *Shots in the Dark: The Wayward Search for an AIDS Vaccine*. New York: W. W. Norton, 2001.

Cook-Deegan, Robert. *The Gene Wars*. New York: W. W. Norton, 1994.

Crewdson, John. *Science Fictions: A Scientific Mystery, a Massive Cover-up, and the dark Legacy of Robert Gallo*. Boston: Little, Brown, 2002.

Davies, Kevin. *Cracking the Genome*. New York: The Free Press, 2002.

Drews, Jürgen. *In Quest of Tomorrow's Medicines: An Eminent Scientist Talks about the Pharmaceutical Industry, Biotechnology, and the Future of Drug Research*. New York: Springer-Verlag, 1999.

Epstein, Samuel S. *The Politics of Cancer*. San Francisco: Sierra Club, 1978.

———. *The Politics of Cancer Revisited*. Fremont Center, N.Y.: East Ridge Press, 1998.

Epstein, Steven. *Impure Science: AIDS, Activism, and the Politics of Knowledge*. Berkeley: University of California Press, 1996

Fried, Stephen. *Bitter Pills: Inside the Hazardous World of Legal Drugs*. New York: Bantam Books, 1998.

Gallo, Robert C. *Virus Hunting: AIDS, Cancer, and the Human Retrovirus, a Story of Scientific Discovery*. New York: Basic Books, 1991.

Gambardella, Alfonso. *Science and Innovation: The U.S. Pharmaceutical Industry During the 1980s*. Cambridge, England: Cambridge University Press, 1995.

Goodman, Jordan, and Walsh, Vivien. *The Story of Taxol: Nature and Politics in the Pursuit of an Anti-Cancer Drug*. Cambridge, England: Cambridge University Press, 2001.

Grabowski, Henry G. *Health Reform and Pharmaceutical Innovation*. Washington, D.C.: AEI Press, 1994.

Greenberg, Daniel S. *Science, Money, and Politics: Political Triumph and Ethical Erosion*. Chicago: University of Chicago Press, 2001

Harris, Richard. *The Real Voice*. New York: The McMillan Company, 1964.

Johnson, Haynes, and Broder, David S. *The System: The American Way of Politics at the Breaking Point*. Boston: Little Brown and Co., 1996.

Joyce, Christopher. *Earth Goods: Medicine-Hunting in the Rainforest*. Boston: Little Brown and Co., 1994.

Kenney, Martin, *Biotechnology: The University-Industrial Complex*. New Haven, Conn.: Yale University Press, 1984.

Kluger, Richard. *Ashes to Ashes: America's Hundred-Year Cigarette War, the Public Health, and the Unabashed Triumph of Philip Morris*. New York: Vintage Books, 1997.

Kwitny, Jonathan. *Acceptable Risks*. New York: Poseidon Press, 1992.

Le Fanu, James. *The Rise and Fall of Modern Medicine*. New York: Carroll and Graf Publishers, 1999.

Lerner, Barron H. *The Breast Cancer Wars: Hope, Fear, and the Pursuit of a Cure in Twentieth-Century America*. New York: Oxford University Press, 2001.

Lewis, Sinclair. *Arrowsmith*, 1925; reprint, New York: Signet Classic, 1998.

Lewontin, Richard. *It Ain't Necessarily So: The Dream of the Human Genome and Other Illusions*. New York: New York Review Books, 2000.

Liebenau, Jonathan. *Medical Science and Medical Industry: The Formation of the American Pharmaceutical Industry*. Baltimore: Johns Hopkins University Press, 1987.

Mahoney, John Thomas. *The Merchants of Life: An Account of the American Pharmaceutical Industry*. New York: Harper, 1959.

Marsa, Linda. *Prescription for Profits: How the Pharmaceutical Industry Bankrolled the Unholy Marriage between Science and Business*. New York: Scribner, 1997.

McKelvey, Maureen. *Evolutionary Innovations: The Business of Biotechnology*. New York: Oxford University Press, 1996.

Mintz, Morton. *By Prescription Only*. Boston: Beacon Press, 1965

Moore, Thomas J. *Prescription for Disaster: The Hidden Dangers in Your Medicine Cabinet*. New York: Simon and Schuster, 1998.

Mundy, Alicia. *Dispensing with the Truth: The Victims, the Drug Companies, and the Dramatic Story Behind the Battle over Fen-phen*. New York: St. Martin's Press, 2001.

Murdock, Rick, and Fisher, David. *Patient Number One: A True Story of How One CEO Took on Cancer and Big Business in the Fight of His Life*. New York: Crown Publishers, 2000.

Office of Technology Assessment (prepared by Alan M. Garber). *Federal and Private Roles in the Development and Provision of Alglucerase Therapy for Gaucher Disease*, U.S. Government Printing Office, 1992.

Panem, Sandra. *The Interferon Crusade*. Washington, D.C.: Brookings Institution Press, 1994.

Patterson, James T. *The Dread Disease: Cancer and Modern American Culture.* Cambridge, Mass.: Harvard University Press, 1987.

Proctor, Robert N. *Cancer Wars: How Politics Shapes What We Know and Don't Know About Cancer.* New York: Basic Books, 1995

Rettig, Richard A. *Cancer Crusade.* Princeton, N.J.: Princeton University Press, 1977.

Robbins-Roth, Cynthia. *From Alchemy to IPO: The Business of Biotechnology.* Cambridge, Mass.: Perseus Publishing, 2000.

Rosenberg, Steven A., and Barry, John M. *The Transformed Cell: Unlocking the Mysteries of Cancer,* New York: G. P. Putnam's Sons, 1992.

Ryan, Frank. *The Forgotten Plague: How the Battle Against Tuberculosis Was Won and Lost.* New York: Little Brown and Co., 1992.

Schweitzer, Stuart O. *Pharmaceutical Economics and Policy.* New York: Oxford University Press, 1997.

Shilts, Randy: *And the Band Played On: Politics, People, and the AIDS Epidemic.* New York: St. Martin's Press, 1987.

Shorter, Edward. *The Health Century.* New York: Doubleday, 1987.

Silverman, Milton Morris. *Magic in a Bottle.* New York: Macmillan Co., 1948.

Silverman, Milton, and Lee, Philip R. *Pills, Profits, and Politics.* Berkeley: University of California Press, 1974.

Smith, Jane S. *Patenting the Sun: Polio and the Salk Vaccine.* New York: William Morrow and Co., 1990.

Starr, Paul. *The Social Transformation of American Medicine: The Rise of a Sovereign Profession and the Making of a Vast Industry.* New York: Basic Books, 1982.

Stokes, Donald E. *Pasteur's Quadrant: Basic Science and Technological Innovation.* Washington, D.C.: Brookings Institution Press, 1997.

Strickland, Stephen Parks. *Politics, Science, and Dread Disease: A Short History of United States Medical Research Policy.* Cambridge, Mass.: Harvard University Press, 1972.

———. *The Story of the NIH Grants Programs.* Lanham, Md.: University Press of America, 1989.

Swann, John Patrick. *Academic Scientists and the Pharmaceutical Industry: Cooperative Research in Twentieth-Century America.* Baltimore: Johns Hopkins University Press, 1988.

Waldholz, Michael. *Curing Cancer.* New York: Touchstone Books, 1999.

Weatherall, M. *In Search of a Cure.* Oxford, England: Oxford University Press, 1990.

Weinberg, Robert A. *One Renegade Cell: How Cancer Begins.* New York: Basic Books, 1999.

———. *Racing to the Beginning of the Road: The Search for the Origin of Cancer.* New York: W. H. Freeman and Co., 1998.

Werth, Barry. *The Billion-Dollar Molecule: One Company's Quest for the Perfect Drug.* New York: Simon and Schuster, 1994.

Young, James Harvey. *The Medical Messiahs: A Social History of Health Quackery in Twentieth-Century America.* Princeton: Princeton University Press, 1992.

Acknowledgments

I stumbled onto the central theme of this book while writing a cover story on drug pricing for *The American Prospect* magazine during the 2000 election campaign. Material that eventually found its way into several chapters first appeared in its pages. So I am deeply indebted to Robert Kuttner, whose wise counsel and patient editing allowed this daily news reporter to make the difficult transition to the more thoughtful, longer forms of our craft. I met Bob more than two decades ago while he was reporting his first book, and over the years his public commitment to the unfashionable idea that the public sector and public investments play a crucial role in American life has inspired my own journalism. He is an excellent editor and has become a friend, and for both, I thank him.

The book would not have been possible without the cooperation of the more than two hundred doctors, scientists, company executives, government officials, patient advocates, and patients whom I interviewed. While far too numerous to mention, many took time out from busy schedules to patiently explain their complex worlds, and I want every one of them to know that I deeply appreciated and benefited from their generosity. If I made mistakes translating their science and lives into layman's language, the fault is entirely my own.

This project received the generous support of the Kaiser Family Foundation, whose media fellowship program provided both financial and emotional sustenance during its crucial midpassage. My fellow fellows—Raney Aronson, Bob Davis, Don Finley, Andrew Julien, and Andy Miller—provided me with a virtual newsroom for talking shop and lots of good times to remember. And the director, Penny Duckham, has made the program indispensable to the field of health care journalism. I look forward to our reunions.

I received critical help at various points in the process. People who read early drafts of portions of the manuscript and provided comments include Marcia Angell, John Erickson, Don Bollinger, Joseph Weiner, and Karen Goozner. Thank you Eric Nelson for suggesting there was a book in the article. Thanks also to Lucia Fanjul for her valuable research assistance, and to Brooke Kroeger at New York University, who made my brief stay in academia more enjoyable and suggested the title for this book. And the project's early stages received financial support from Vernon Loucks, who hired me for an unrelated writing project and agreed to support my work on the initial book proposal.

Finally, I want to give thanks to my family and their unique inputs into this project. Alan and Terry are cancer survivors and constantly reminded me of the hope people bring to their thinking about the pharmaceutical industry. Robert is a patent attorney, and I hope our frequent discussions have been as useful to him as they have been to me. And my mother Estelle, now in her eighties, went through a number of medical crises in the two years leading up to the publication of this book. In addition to all the love she gave me over the past five decades, she provided an unfortunate but informative window into the world of senior citizen medical care.

The book is dedicated to my children: Rebecca and her husband Chris, Thad, and Zoe; and to my grandchild, Rachel. But my deepest thanks go to my wife Karen, who not only read the manuscript but provided a sounding board during the five years I was thinking and writing about the world of legal drugs. Without her constant support and encouragement, this book would not exist.

Index

A-77003, 119–20, 123
Aaron Diamond AIDS Research Center, 138–40, 162
Abbott Laboratories, 23–24, 119–20, 128–29; at AIDS conference in Berlin, 90; diagnostic kits, 23; Erickson and, 94, 96–97, 116, 118–21, 162; finances, 158–59; Goldwasser and, 19; government funding and, 138; history, 115–19; NCI and, 120, 121, 125, 128–30, 138; protease inhibitors and, 90, 97, 119–20, 124–25, 128, 129, 134, 137–38; Rathmann at, 23–24; ritonavir and, 152, 159
ABI Prism 3700, 63–64
"Achilles' heel of HIV," 134
acyclovir, 103
Adamson, John, 29
adrenergic blockers, 247
advertising, 233
Agenerase, 160
Agouron Pharmaceuticals, 159
AIDS: in developing countries, 244; epidemiology, 85–87, 161; in the media, 88, 91, 92, 95, 96, 107, 108, 133–38, 144, 147, 154, 156–57; public attitudes toward, 86, 87; task force to fight, 102
AIDS activism, 143
AIDS activist groups, 122
AIDS activists, 88, 114, 123, 132–33, 143, 145, 147; Merck's relations with, 132–33, 153, 154
AIDS Clinical Trials Group (ACTG), 106, 131, 133, 135, 144, 145–46, 148, 229; Abbott, ritonavir, and, 150; AIDS

activists and, 123, 145; clarithromycin and, 123; combination therapy and, 131, 134, 135, 144, 146; ddC and, 143, 144; financial incentive for companies to work with, 142; functions, 104–5; Ho and, 140; Hoth and, 88, 120, 130; Merck and, 132; origin, 104; Roche, saquinavir, and, 143, 145–46
AIDS Coalition to Unleash Power (ACT UP), 92, 122
AIDS drugs: buyers clubs, 123; combinations of, 88, 91, 130, 131, 133–38, 142, 148–50, 154, 160–61; development of, 85–86; high prices, 92, 114, 125, 127; problem of patient adherence, 161; profits from, 161; resistance to, 91, 139, 140, 148, 153, 161, 163 (see also HIV: mutations). See also specific drugs and drug classes
AIDS metaphor, 86
AIDS patients: in New York City, 112–13; surrogate markers, 144–45, 147
AIDS research: government funded, 88, 97, 102, 160, 238; money spent by private industry on, 160
AIDS test, 116
AIDS vaccines, 88, 157
AIDS virus: discovery, 94–95; sequencing of its genes, 95. See also HIV
Allegra, 221
allergy medicines, 222–24. See also antihistamines
alpha-galactosidase, 51, 53–55; patent for, 54. See also Fabry enzyme
Altman, Lawrence, 135–36
Altman, Stuart, 253

American Cancer Society (ACS), 169–70, 183; board members, 168
American Society for Clinical Oncology (ASCO), 196, 204
American Society for the Control of Cancer (ASCC), 169–71
Ames, Bruce, 180, 181
Ames test, 180
Amgen, 36–37; formation, 1–2, 22–23; Goldwasser's joining, 25, 26; Lin at, 25, 28; marketing, sales, and finances, 2–3, 28–29, 31–37; patent litigation fight with TKT, 37–38; research, 36; Vapnek as director of research, 26, 34. *See also specific products*
amino acid sequences, 26, 27, 64
amprenavir, 160
anemia. *See* erythropoietin
anesthetics, 116
angiotensin converting enzyme (ACE) inhibitors, 247, 248
antacids, 217–22
antibiotics, 106, 122–23, 211–14, 220, 232
antibodies, 139, 195, 205–6; monoclonal, 191, 193–94
antihistamines, 214, 217–18, 221, 223
Antihypertensive and Lipid-Lowering Treatment to Prevent Heart Attack Trial (ALLHAT), 248
antihypertensive drugs. *See* blood-pressure medications
antiviral drugs, market for, 161
appetite suppressants, 34
Applera. *See* Applied Biosystems
Applied Biosystems, 63, 64, 70, 74, 75. *See also* PE Biosystems
Applied Molecular Genetics. *See* Amgen
applied research, 15; funding for, 98–100. *See also under* cancer research
Aranesp, 3, 33
Argonne National Laboratory, 72–73
Ariad Pharmaceuticals, 80
arsphenamine, 93
arthritis, 35, 226–27
astimezole (Hismanal), 221, 223
Astra Pharmaceuticals, 218–22
AstraZeneca, 201, 222
atomic bomb, building, 71
Atomic Energy Commission, 71–72
Axys Pharmaceuticals, 258
AZT (azidothymidine): Barr Laboratories' license to manufacture and distribute, 123–24; clinical trials, 87–88, 103, 131, 133, 135, 144, 146, 152, 156; combined with other drugs, 88, 131, 133–36, 144–46, 151–52, 155–56;

criticism of, 104; FDA approval, 103, 104, 110; history and development, 103; patenting, 103; price, 104, 123–25; safety tests, 103; side effects and toxicity, 88, 103, 104

Baltimore, David, 178
Barney, Lawrence D., 109
Barr, David, 135
Barr Laboratories, 114
Barranger, John, 42, 44
Bayh-Dole Act (Bayh-Dole University and Small Business Patent Act), 22, 52, 109, 125, 127, 162
Beckman, Arnold, 69
Beckman Instruments, 68, 69
Berg, Paul, 127–28
Berman, Robin Ely, 45, 46
beta-blockers, 218
Bextra, 224
Bill and Melinda Gates Foundation, 192, 246, 257–58
Binder, George, 34
Biogen, 25, 27, 71, 128
biotechnology revolution, 20, 69, 183, 191, 214–15, 242–43
Bishop, Michael, 179
Black, James, 218
black fever (leishmaniasis), 244–45
Blair, Henry, 44
Blair, Tony, 62, 66
blood pressure, 95–96
blood-pressure medications, 247–49
Bobst, Elmer H., 109, 168
Boger, Joshua, 90–91, 159
Bolognesi, Dani, 103
Bowes, William, 22
Boyer, Herbert, 21, 128
Brady, Roscoe, 59; on Ceredase, 48; Genzyme and, 49–50; life history and background, 42–43; and lysosomal storage disorders, 49–50; research, 40–46
Bragman, Keith, 89, 112–14, 149
Brand, Mark, 3
breast cancer, 197
Breast Cancer Prevention Trial, 198
Bristol-Myers Squibb, 114, 124, 130, 185, 188–91, 202, 204, 238
Broder, Samuel, 102–4, 110, 120, 121, 190, 192
Burnham, Duane, 121
Burroughs Wellcome, 103, 121, 124, 125; patent suit against, 104, 114. *See also* AZT
Bush, Vannevar, 39, 98–100, 106, 107
businesses, small, 125–27

buyers clubs for AIDS drugs, 123

Calhoun, David, 51–52, 54
California Institute of Technology (Cal-Tech), 22, 25–26, 68–72
Canada, 232
cancer: diagnostic techniques, 169; dietary causes, 180, 181; environmental and toxic causes, 174–77, 180–81, 236; epidemiology, 165–66, 169; genetic factors in, 182–83 (see also oncogenes); lung, 166, 175, 201; ovarian, 187, 197; testicular, 184, 185; treatments, 167 (see also chemotherapy); viral causes, 95, 106, 177–78, 181; war on, 101, 164, 167–69, 174, 178, 185
Cancer Chemotherapy National Service Center, 173
Cancer Letter, The, 202
cancer lobby, 172
cancer research, 168; basic vs. applied/drug research, 167, 178–79; ethical guidelines, 253–54. See also cancer: war on
capillary technology, 73, 75
Carson, Rachel, 175
CD4 cells, 144, 145
celecoxib (Celebrex), 225–29, 241
Celera Genomics, 61, 63, 64, 66, 76, 77, 80–81, 258
cell reproduction, 178. See also DNA
Ceredase, 47–49; cost, 48–49; FDA approval, 46, 58
Cerezyme, 49
Cetus Corporation, 22
Chabner, Bruce, 120, 124, 128, 129, 187, 190
Chagas disease, 258
chemotherapy: drugs administered along with, 33; origin, 172, 173; targeted therapies, 2–4; for testicular cancer, 184, 185. See also National Cancer Institute (NCI): drug development program
chemotherapy drugs, 92, 124; in the media, 166, 200–201, 204; plant-derived, 185–86 (see also cancer research; specific drugs)
Childs, Starling, 170
Chinese hamster ovaries (CHO) cells, 52, 53
chloroquine, 244
Chockley, Nancy, 242
Chodakewitz, Jeffrey, 152, 155
cholesterol-lowering drugs, 238
Chow, Yung-King, 134, 135

chronic myeloid leukemia (CML), 199–201, 205
cimetidine (Tagamet), 218, 219
Cipla, 150
cisplatin, 184–85, 204
Citizen's Committee for the Conquest of Cancer, 101, 168
clarithromycin, 122–23
Claritin (loratadine), 222–23
Clark, Paul, 124
clinical trials, 28, 113–14, 237; costs, 158; recommendations regarding required, 253–54; used for marketing, 238. See also specific drugs
Clinton, Bill, 61–62, 65, 66
Clinton administration, 215
cocktail therapy. See AIDS drugs: combinations of
Coghill, Robert, 116
Cohen, Stanley, 21
Collier, Ann, 146
Collins, Francis S., 30, 61–63, 65–66, 81
"compassionate use," 113, 114, 143
competition between companies, 211. See also me-too drugs
conflicts of interest, 37, 53, 128
Conn, Doyt, 36
contract research organizations, 259
Cook-Deegan, Robert, 71
Cooperative Research and Development Agreement (CRADA), 188, 189
Corey, Lawrence, 105
Crewdson, John, 95
Crick, Francis, 20, 67, 178
cyclo-oxygenase (Cox), 224; Cox-2 and Cox-2 inhibitors, 224–28, 255
cystic fibrosis, 30, 54

Danner, Sven, 90
ddC. See zalcitabine
"dead body" trials, 114
Delaney, Martin, 150
DeLisi, Charles, 72
Democratic Party, 232
Department of Energy (DOE), 63, 67, 71–72
Depression, Great, 169, 209–10
desloratadine, 224
Desnick, Robert J., 50–54, 58, 59
developing countries, diseases in, 244–45, 257
diabetes, 179
dialysis. See kidney dialysis patients
Diamond, Aaron, 139–41. See also Aaron Diamond AIDS Research Center
Diamond, Irene, 139

Diamond v. Chakraberty, 64, 215
Dickinson, Becton, 154
didanosine (ddI), 110, 111, 114, 130, 134, 135, 144
diet, 180, 181, 236
diethylene glycol, 211
DiMasi, Joseph E., 237
diphenhydramine (Benadryl), 217
diseases, rare, 40–41, 46–48, 58
diuretics, 247–48
DNA, 20, 26; attaching dyes to chain terminators, 70; chemical method of identifying the order of bases in, 68; DNA sequencing machine, 68–74 (*see also* prototype machine); model of double helix structure, 67, 178; replication process, 68; ultra-thin capillaries for transporting fragments of, 73
Dogmagk, Gerhard, 210
Dole, Bob, 22, 59
Doll, John, 77
Dovichi, Norman, 73
Drews, Jürgen, 10, 113, 114, 148, 149, 259
Dreyer, William J., 68, 69
drotrecogin alfa (Xigris), 80, 252
drug applications: fees for new, 240; normal *vs.* priority status, 240–41
drug laws, 28
drug prescriptions: inappropriate, 233; number of, 233
drug prices, 256–60; compared with their benefits, 253; new battle over pricing, 232–35; price controls, 7, 254; reasons for high(er), 3, 234–35
drug spending: annual national, 5; runaway, 232
drugs: costs of discovering new, 3; generic *vs.* brand-name, 233–34, 249 (*see also* "new and improved" drugs); with limited or no improvement over existing drugs, 231; measuring new drugs against existing therapies, 253–54; potential new, 257
Druker, Brian, 199–201, 205
DuPont Pharmaceuticals, 91

Ehrlich, Paul, 93–94
Einhorn, Lawrence, 184
Eisenberg, Rebecca S., 79–80
elderly, 232. *See also* Medicare
Eli Lilly and Company, 66, 80, 198, 203, 252
Elion, Gertrude, 103
Embrel, 35, 36
Emini, Emilio, 106, 108, 109, 132, 134, 152–53

employers, 233–34
enantiomers, 221
Eng, Christine M., 56
entrepreneurial revolution, 20
environmental toxins, 174–77, 180–81, 236
enzyme replacement therapy, 40–41, 44–45, 55–56. *See also* Ceredase; *specific drugs*
enzymes, 2; missing, 40, 43; purification, 50. *See also* protease
epidermal growth factor (EGF), 193, 201, 202, 205
Epogen, 2; Aranesp compared with, 33; clinical trials, 28–29, 36; FDA approval, 31, 36; marketing and sales, 28–29, 36–37; price, 31; reimbursement for, 37; revenue generated by, 32
Epstein, Samuel S., 180
Erbitux, 202–5
Erickson, John, 162–63, 258; A-77003 and, 123; Abbott and, 94, 96–97, 116, 118–21, 162; background and career, 92–93; description, 92; and funding, 96–97, 118–20; HIV protease and, 96–97, 118–19; Kempf and, 119–20; meeting with NIH, 120; at NCI, 121; X-ray crystallography and, 93–94, 96, 121
erythropoietin (Epo), 14, 24, 29, 38; Abbott and, 19, 23, 24; Amgen and, 25, 26; anemia and, 28; discovery of, 13–14; Genetics Institute and, 25–27; Goldwasser and, 25–27, 250; kidney dialysis patients and, 2, 19; Lin and, 25–28; price, 14; production, 17, 19, 27, 28; Rathmann and, 24; recombinant, 24–29; research on, 17, 19, 23, 24–27. *See also* Epogen
Eschbach, Joseph, 29
esophagitis, 222
estrogen blocking. *See* tamoxifen
etanercept. *See* Embrel
European Union (EU), 58
exercise, 236
expressed sequence tags (ESTs), 65

Fabrase, 53
Fabrazyme, 56, 59
Fabry disease, 43, 49, 60; Brady and, 55; Desnick and, 50–53, 58, 59; Genzyme and, 49–50, 53–54, 56–59; NIH funding for research on, 52, 54–56; Selden and, 53–55; TKT and, 53–60
Fabry enzyme, 50; purification, production, and replacement, 50, 52 (*see also* Fabrase). *See also* alpha-galactosidase

Farber, Michael, 80, 173–74, 178–79
fast-track designation. *See* drug applications: normal *vs.* priority status
fat gene, 34
Fauci, Anthony, 120, 131, 145, 153
Federal Technology Transfer Act of 1986, 125, 127, 188
Federal Trade Commission (FTC), 212–13, 231
Fischl, Margaret, 135
Flavell, Richard, 27
Fleming, Thomas, 201–2
fluorescent tags, 70, 73
fluoxetine (Prozac), 217
folic acid, 173
Folkman, Judah, 166
food: contaminated, 211
Food and Drug Act, 211, 214
Food and Drug Administration (FDA), 28, 58–59, 135, 149; accelerated approval, 143–46, 149, 156; Antiviral Advisory Committee, 144, 152; cancer drugs approved by, 167, 201–2; Claritin and, 223–24; Cox-2 inhibitors and, 226; criticisms of, 147; and drugs for rare diseases, 58; Erbitux and, 204; guidelines for drug approval, 253, 259; history, 211; liberalization and reform, 58, 143–45, 149, 253; number of drugs approved by, 231; Orphan Drug Development office, 53; priority status, 240–41
Freire, Maria, 246
Frohlich, Edward D., 248
Furberg, Curt, 248

G. D. Searle, 160, 224, 225
Galambos, Louis, 92, 157
Gallo, Robert, 94–95, 102
Gambardella, Alfonso, 9
gastritis, 220. *See also* antacids
gastrointestinal stromal tumors (GIST), 200–201
Gates, Bill and Melinda, 192, 246, 257–58
Gaucher disease, 40–41, 43, 56, 58; Genzyme and, 44, 45, 48–50
Gaucher enzyme, 50
GenBank, 77–78
gene therapy, 54, 55
genes: activation, 54–55; diseases caused by malfunctioning, 29–30, 78–79 (*see also specific diseases*); mapping chromosomes that contain, 72; tumor suppressor, 182
gene-splicing revolution, 127
genetic engineering, 23–25, 31, 215

Genetic Engineering Technology (Genentech), 21, 24, 66, 128, 193–97, 257
genetic sequencing, 26, 27, 51, 64, 68–72; automated, 72; for commercial gain, 77; high-speed sequencing, 72. *See also* DNA: DNA sequencing machine
Genetics Institute, 25–28, 53
genome: mapping the human, 71, 78; race to complete the, 62. *See also* Human Genome Project
Genzyme: Brady and, 41, 44–46, 49–50; competition between TKT and, 57, 59; Desnick and, 53, 54; enzyme replacement therapy and, 41, 44–46, 50 (*see also* Ceredase); Fabry disease and, 49–50, 53–54; FDA and, 46, 47; finances, 48; Gaucher disease and, 44, 45, 48–50; launched by Blair, 44; NIH funding, 45, 54; Termeer and, 48–49
Genzyme test, 57
Gilbert, Walter, 25, 68, 71, 128
Gilmartin, Raymond V., 154, 155
GlaxoSmithKline, 160, 218
Gleevec (ST-571), 81, 199–201, 204–5
Global Alliance for TB Drug Development, 158, 245–46, 258
glucocerebrosidase: manufacturing, 45, 49; purifying, 44. *See also* Ceredase; enzymes; Gaucher disease
glucocerebroside, 43
Goldwasser, Eugene, 24, 37; Amgen and, 15, 25, 37; Gilbert and, 25; Jacobson and, 15–16; legal battles, 19, 37–38; life history, 13, 15–16; Miyake and, 17–18; problems funding his kidney research, 18–19, 38; rejected by Abbott Laboratories, 19; research on Epo, 18–19, 25; search for and discovery of Epo, 13–14, 16–18, 20, 71, 250
government: price controls, 7, 254 (*see also* Medicare); research funded by, 8; role in technological innovation, 98
government funding: for AIDS drugs research, 120, 121, 130 (*see also specific drugs and drug companies*)
government-funded inventions, pricing and commercialization of, 125–28
Graham, Evarts, 175
Groopman, Jerome, 167–68
Grossman, Howard, 33–34
Gurin, Samuel, 42

Hale, Victoria, 257, 258
Harrington, Mark, 145
Harris, Richard, 234

Hartwell, Jonathan, 185
Haseltine, William, 97, 243
Hassan, Fred, 243
health care advocates, 7–8
Health Care Finance Administration
  (HCFA), 37
Healy, Bernadine, 64, 123–24
heartburn, 219
Helicobacter pylori, 220
Her-2 (human-epidermal-growth-factor
  receptor-2), 193, 194, 196
Herceptin (trastuzumab), 194–97
Hewick, Rodney, 25–26
Hirsch, Jules, 35
Hismanal (astimezole), 221, 223
histamine (H2) antagonists, 218, 220
histamines and histamine blockers, 217–
  18, 221
Hitachi, 79
Hitler, Adolf, 210
HIV: biology, 89, 141; markers (see viral
  load tests); mutations, 141, 153, 161–
  62 (see also AIDS drugs: resistance to);
  rapid reproduction, 141, 142, 153. See
  also AIDS virus
HIV protease, 95, 96, 105, 111, 117, 162
Hivid. See zalcitabine
Ho, David, 92, 138–42, 155, 163
Hoffmann-La Roche, 89, 109–12, 114,
  159; ddC clinical trials, 131, 143; his-
  tory, 109; protease inhibitor program,
  111–13, 134, 137; saquinavir and,
  143, 145
Holmer, Alan F., 6–7, 234–35
Hood, Leroy, 22, 25, 26, 68–69, 72
Horovitz, Zola, 190
Horwitz, Susan, 186
Hoth, Daniel, 88, 105, 120, 124, 129,
  130, 145
Howard Hughes Medical Institute, 139
Hsu, Ming-Chu, 110–11
Huang, Henry, 70
Hueper, Wilhelm C., 174–75
Human Genome Project, 61–63, 65, 67,
  72, 77, 243; government involvement
  in, 71; Human Genome Day, 61–62, 66
Human Genome Sciences, 243
human growth hormone, 194
human-epidermal-growth-factor
  receptor-2 (Her-2), 193, 194, 196
Hybritech, 203
Hygienic Laboratory, 170
hypertensive drugs. See blood-pressure
  medications

ICI Pharmaceuticals, 197, 218
ImClone System, 202–4

immune system, 141. See also antibodies
Immunex, 35
immunotoxin therapy, 205–6
Incyte Pharmaceuticals, 75, 77
indinavir, 133, 134, 150, 152–58
inflammation, 35, 224
Institute for Genomic Research (TIGR),
  75, 76
Institute for Global Therapeutics, 258
Institute for OneWorld Health, 257–58
insulin, 66, 179
insurance companies, 7–8, 233–34, 240,
  242
Intercompany Collaboration (ICC), 150
interferon, 22, 23, 109, 183, 201
interleukin, 183
interleukin 2 (IL-2), 110
International AIDS Conference: sixth
  (San Francisco), 87–91; ninth (Berlin),
  87–91, 134
Interscience Conference on Antimicrobial
  Agents and Chemotherapy (ICAAC),
  142, 151, 156, 163
Ioannou, Yiannis, 52, 54
Iressa, 201–2

Jackson, Dudley, 170–72
Jacobson, Leon, 15–17
Jaklevic, Joseph, 74
James, John, 88
Johnson, Lyndon Baines, 101
Johnson and Johnson, 221; Ortho-
  Biotech division, 28, 33
Jordan, Craig, 197–99, 205
*Journal of the American Medical Associa-
  tion*, 175–76
Ju, Jingyue, 75

kala azar, 257
Karger, Barry, 73
Kassebaum, Nancy, 48
Kefauver, Estes, 213, 214, 234
Kempf, Dale, 96–98, 119–20, 123, 129,
  137–38
Kennedy, Edward, 168
Kennedy administration, 126
Kessler, David, 144, 145, 147, 216, 217
kidney dialysis patients, 2, 19, 29, 31–
  33. See also Fabry disease
kidney research, Goldwasser's, 18–19, 38
kidneys, 38
Kiley, Thomas D., 65
Kilgore, Harley, 99
kinase proteins, 81, 82, 182
Kineret, 35
King, Mary-Clair, 182–83
Kirin Brewery Company, 28

Klausner, Richard, 182, 192, 200
Klugman, Jack, 47
Koch, Robert, 93
Kohl, Nancy, 107
Kolata, Gina, 166
Kramer, Larry, 92
Krohn, Anthony, 111

L-661, 133
Landsberger, Frank, 53
Larimer, David, 256
Lasker, Mary, 101, 168, 176, 178
Lawrence Berkeley National Laboratory, 74
Le Fanu, James, 31
Lee, Philip R., 214
leishmaniasis (black fever), 244–45, 257
Leonard, John, 90, 128–30, 137, 138, 158
leptin, 34–35
leukemia, 173; chronic myeloid, 199–201, 205
Lev, Baruch, 240
Levinson, Arthur, 195
life expectancy, rising, 235–36
lifestyle, 236
Lin, Fu-Kuen, 24–28
lipid levels, 56–57, 59
lipids, 43
Little, Clarence Cook "Pete," 176
Long, Russell, 127
loratadine (Claritin), 222–24
lung cancer, 166, 175, 201
Lyden, Nicholas, 199–200
lymphoma, non-Hodgkin's, 205
lysosomal storage disorders, 43, 49, 50

M. D. Anderson Cancer Center, 172, 184
malaria, 244, 257
managed care, 234
marketing expenses, 230
Markowitz, Martin, 140, 148
Marshall, Barry, 220
Marshall, Garland, 97
Massachusetts Institute of Technology (MIT), 98, 99
Massengill and Company, 211
Mathies, Richard, 73–75
Maxam, Allan, 68
Mayo Clinic, 139
McCarthy, Joseph R., 213
McGowan, John, 97
McGuire, William, 187
McKinnell, Henry, 225
mechlorethamine (Mustargen), 173
media, 181; chemotherapy drugs in the,

166, 200–201, 204. *See also under* AIDS
Medicaid, 232
Medical Research Council (Britain), 68
Medicare, 4–6, 232; negotiation for reduced price of drugs, 31, 32; prescription drug benefit, 5–7, 239
Meduri, G. Umberto, 252
Megabase, 75
Memorial Hospital, 170
Memorial Sloan-Kettering Hospital, 170, 172, 173
Mendelsohn, John, 202–4
Merck, 109, 150, 154–55; commitment to combat AIDS, 105, 106, 131–32, 157, 158; Cox-2 inhibitors and, 224–28; history, 105–6; indinavir and, 133, 152–58; NNRTIs research, 132–33; omeprazole, Astra, and, 219; protease inhibitor research, 105, 106, 108–9, 133, 137; relations with AIDS activists, 132–33, 153, 154; streptomycin and, 212
Merck, George W., 10, 106
Merck 035, 155–56
Merrell Dow, 221
metabolic processes, patenting, 255
methotrexate, 35, 173
me-too drugs, 213–17, 230–32, 241, 243. *See also* allergy medicines; antacids
Metzenbaum, Howard, 48, 168
Mexico, 232
Meyers, Abbey, 48
military research and technology, 98–100
Mitsuya, Hiroaki "Mitch," 119
Miyake, Takaji, 17–18, 27–28
Molecular Dynamics, 74–75
monoclonal antibodies, 191, 193–94
Montagnier, Luc, 94–95
Moore, Francis, 179
Mt. Sinai School of Medicine, 50–54
Murad, Ferid, 117–22
Murrow, Edward R., 212
mustard gas, 172, 173
Mustargen (mechlorethamine), 173
mycobacterium avium complex (MAC), 122
Myriad Genetics, 79

Nacy, Carol, 258–60
National Breast Cancer Coalition, 196
National Cancer Act, 101, 164, 167, 178
National Cancer Institute (NCI), 120–24; Abbott and, 120, 121, 125, 128–30, 138; advisory panel, 172; and AIDS drugs, 102, 104, 110, 119, 130–31,

National Cancer Institute *(continued)* 162; and basic cancer research, 167–69, 174, 181, 182; criticisms of, 180; drug development program, 167, 168, 174; Environmental Cancer Section, 174; finances, 101, 174, 238; Gleevec and, 200; grant system, 101–3; hunt for chemotherapy drugs, 164–65, 179; origin, 171; as provider of clinical trials, 238; purpose and direction, 171–72; as research establishment focused on cancer biochemistry, 164; research on natural products, 185–91; shift in drug-hunting strategy, 191–92; tamoxifen and, 198; taxol and, 186–87; UCSD cancer center funded by, 202–3

National Cooperative Drug Development Grant (NCDDG), 97, 105

National Heart, Lung, and Blood Institute, 247

National Institute for Health Care Management, 240

National Institutes of Health (NIH), 72; AIDS and, 88; allocation of funds, 41; Brady and, 40–42; creation, 100, 170; fear of getting involved in drug pricing, 190; federal budget for, 100–101, 251; on gene patenting, 64, 65; grants, 18; licensing activity, 128; Office of Technology Transfer, 162; purpose, 251; reasonable pricing clause, 147–48, 190; technology transfer and, 127

National Institute for Allergies and Infectious Diseases (NIAID), 97, 110, 120; AIDS activists and, 145; AIDS program, 142; and approval of AIDS drugs, 144; Division of AIDS, 238; interferon and, 109; pharmaceutical assault on HIV, 104

National Kidney Foundation, 37

National Organization for Rare Disorders (NORD), 47, 48

National Science Foundation, 69, 99, 100

natural products, 124, 185–86. *See also under* National Cancer Institute: research on natural products

Navia, Manuel, 107, 108

Needleman, Philip, 224, 225

Neely, Matthew, 169

nelfinavir, 159

Neupogen, 2, 32

nevirapine, 134

"new and improved" drugs, 229, 249. *See also* drugs: generic *vs.* brand-name

New Deal, 169, 209

Nexium, 220–22

NF-KB, 80

Nissenson, Allen, 37

Nixon, Richard M., 167–69

non-nucleoside reverse transcriptase inhibitors (NNRTIs), 130, 132–34

nonprofit institutions, 139, 212, 257, 258–59

non-steroidal anti-inflammatory drugs (NSAIDs), 224–29

Norbeck, Daniel, 151

Norvir, 151

Novartis Pharma AG, 199, 200

nucleic acid molecules, 81

nucleosides, 89, 130, 149. *See also* reverse transcriptase inhibitors

obesity gene, 34

Occupational Tumors and Allied Diseases (Hueper), 175

Office of Scientific Research and Development (OSRD), 98; Committee on Medical Research, 98

Office of Technology Transfer, NIH, 162

Olshansky, Jay, 235–36

omeprazole (Prilosec), 219–22

oncogenes, 179–80, 182, 193, 202

OneWorld Health. *See* Institute for OneWorld Health

Operation Shark Fin, 220, 221

opportunity cost of capital, 237

Oracle Corp., 79

Oroszlan, Steve, 96

Orphan Drug Act, 46–48

Orphan Drug Law, 59

orphan drugs, 46–48; development, 59

Orphan Medical of Minnetonka, Minnesota, 54

ovarian cancer, 187, 197

painkillers, 115–16, 224–29

Parke-Davis, 18–19

paromomycin, 257

Parran, Thomas, 169, 171

Pastores, Gregory, 57

Patent and Trademark Office (PTO), 63, 64, 80, 212, 254–56

patent laws: recommended modifications of, 256. *See also* Bayh-Dole Act

patenting: biological/metabolic processes, 255, 256; genes, 64–67, 77, 82, 243, 255; life forms, 64, 254–55; research converted into intellectual property, 80, 215

patent(s), 22, 60, 79–80, 127; criteria for obtaining, 64; search for new drugs to replace ones coming off, 229

Patient Bill of Rights movement, 234

Patrinos, Aristides, 63

Patterson, James, 169, 172
PE Biosystems, 75. *See also* Applied
  Biosystems
PE Corporation, 76
Pearl, Laurence, 96
penicillin, 98, 211
Perelman, Ronald, 196
Perelson, Alan, 141, 142
Pernet, Andre, 123–25
Pfizer, 159, 226, 255–56
pharmaceutical firms: mergers between,
  259; outsourcing tasks, 9; revenue and
  profits, 233
Pharmaceutical Research and Manufac-
  turers Association (Pharma/PhRMA),
  26, 192, 216, 239, 242
Pharmacia, 224, 226, 227, 257
pharmacoeconomics, 253
placentas, 44, 45
platinum, 184
polio vaccine, 212
political campaign contributions to pharmaceutical industry, 6
Politics of Cancer, The (Epstein), 180
pollution, 174–77, 180–81, 236; in the
  media, 181
Praexis Pharmaceutical, 36
Prasit, Peppi, 225
Prescription Drug User Fee Act (PDUFA),
  240
price controls, 7, 254
Prilosec (omeprazole), 219–22
Procrit, 33–34
Progressive Era legislation, 211
Prontosil, 209–10
propranolol, 218
prostaglandins, 224
protease, 89. *See also* HIV protease
protease inhibitors, 88–90, 117–18, 131,
  140, 149–50, 159–63, 258; Abbott
  and, 90, 97, 119–20, 124–25, 128,
  129, 134, 137–38; cross-resistance,
  148–49, 161–62; FDA approval, 88,
  91; government-funded research on,
  90, 97; price, 125; side effects, 91. *See
  also specific drugs*
protein sequencing machines, 68–69. *See
  also* DNA: DNA sequencing machine
proteins and biotechnology, 89
proton-pump inhibitors, 219, 220, 222
proto-oncogenes. *See* oncogenes
prototype machine, 74
Prozac (fluoxetine), 217
Public Citizen/Congress Watch, 239
public health methods of disease control, 236
Public Health Service's Hygienic Laboratory, 170

public interest groups, 7–8
public opinion, 7
Pure Food and Drug Act of 1906, 211,
  214

Quincy (television show), 47
Quinn, Mary Jean, 51

raloxifene (Evista), 80, 198
randomized clinical trials (RCTs). *See*
  clinical trials
ranitidine (Zantac), 218, 219
Rathmann, George, 23–24, 26–28, 34
Reagan, Ronald, 46, 102, 181
Reagan administration, 102
recombinant DNA engineering, 21–24,
  50, 52, 82
recombinant Epo, 24–29
red blood cells. *See* erythropoietin
Reimers, Niels, 21
renin, 95, 111
renin inhibitors, 95–96, 107, 119
Replagal, 55–57, 59
research: applied (*see* applied research);
  government *vs.* private funding for,
  39–40, 237–38. *See also specific topics*
research-and-development spending, 9,
  239, 241–44, 250–51, 259; as reason
  for high prices, 234–37, 239–40, 249,
  259–60
Retrovir. *See* AZT
retroviruses, 89, 95, 178, 182
reverse transcriptase, 89, 95, 178
reverse transcriptase inhibitors, 89, 107,
  110, 130, 134
Rezulin, 241
rheumatoid arthritis, 35
Rhoads, Cornelius "Dusty," 172–73
ritonavir, 159; Abbott's license to sell,
  152; clinical trials, 138, 140, 142,
  148, 150–52, 156; combined with
  other drugs, 151–52, 155–56; effectiveness, 140, 150–51; FDA approval,
  152, 156; HIV mutations and resistance to, 140–41, 148; patenting, 138;
  price and sales, 152; problems with,
  134; synthesis, 129
RNA, 89, 178
Roberts, Noel, 111–13
Roche. *See* Hoffmann-La Roche
Rockefeller Institute for Medical
  Research, 170
Roosevelt, Franklin D., Jr., 209
Roosevelt, Franklin Delano, 39, 98, 209
Rosenberg, Barnett, 184
Rossmann, Michael, 93
Rous, Peyton, 171

Russo, Mike, 57–58
Rutgers Research Foundation, 212

Sachs, George, 218–19
Salgo, Miklos, 112–13
Salk, Jonas, 212
Salser, Winston, 22, 23
Sanger, Frederick, 20, 51, 67–68
saquinavir, 111, 148; clinical trials, 112,
 113, 133, 143, 145–46, 148, 149;
 combined with other drugs, 145–46,
 148–49, 151; effectiveness, 90, 111–
 13, 133, 134, 145–46, 149; FDA
 approval, 91, 112, 149, 150; price,
 150; reproduced by Merck, 133; resist-
 ance to, 148–49; side effects and other
 problems with, 89–90, 112, 113, 145,
 149
Schering-Plough, 222–24
Schiffmann, Raphael, 56, 59
Schlager, Seymour, 122
Schoellhorn, Robert A., 116–18, 120–21
Schuler, Jack W., 117, 118, 121
science, basic/pure: research in, 98–101,
 250 (see also under cancer research)
Scolnick, Edward M., 106–8, 118, 132,
 152, 182, 225
Searle, G. D., 160, 225
Securities and Exchange Commission
 (SEC), 55–56, 159
Seldane (terfenadine), 221, 223
Selden, Richard, 53–55
Sepracor, 221
sepsis/septic shock, 252
Sequella Foundation, 258
Sharer, Kevin, 3
Shaw, George, 138, 140, 142, 155
Shepard, Michael, 195
Sigal, Irving, 106–8
Silent Spring (Carson), 175
Silverman, Milton, 214
single-capillary machine, 75
Sinsheimer, Robert, 71
Slamon, Dennis, 193–97
Sloan-Kettering Institute, 170
Smith, Kline, and French, 218
Smith, Lloyd M., 70–71, 73
smoking, 166, 175–77
SNP Consortium, 79, 255
SNPs (single nucleotide polymorphisms),
 79, 255
Soo, Whaijen, 110–11
Special Virus Cancer Program (SVCP),
 178, 179, 181–82
Specter, Arlen, 37
Stark, Pete, 31–32, 48
statin drugs, 238

Steinberg, Wallace, 76
Stevenson-Wydler Technology Innovation
 Act, 125, 126
Stodolsky, Marvin, 72
Stokes, Donald E., 99–101
stomach acid wars, 217–20
streptococcus, 210
streptomycin, 106, 212
sulfa drugs, 209–11, 214
sulfanilamide, 210
Sullivan, Louis, 31–32
Sulston, John, 77
Supreme Court, 64, 104, 215, 254
Surgeon General, 176
surrogate markers, 144–45, 147
Swanson, Robert, 21
swelling, 35, 224
Synergen, 35

Tagamet (cimetidine), 218, 219
Takeda Chemical Industries, 117
tamoxifen, 197–98
TAP Pharmaceuticals, 117, 219
Tartikoff, Brandon, 195
tatIII and tat inhibitors, 110–11
tax deductions for research and development, 239–40
Taxol, 124, 187–91; adverse effects, 186,
 189; discovery, 174, 185–86; effectiveness, 186–87; FDA approval, 188;
 price, 124, 127, 189–90; research on,
 186–87; supply and production, 187–
 89
Taylor, Susan, 81–82
Taylor, William, 96
3TC, 155
technology-transfer policy, 127, 162;
 open-door, 126. See also Bayh-Dole
 Act; Federal Technology Transfer Act
Temin, Howard, 178
Temin, Peter, 213
terfenadine (Seldane), 221, 223
Termeer, Henri, 44, 46, 48–49
testicular cancer, 184, 185
thalidomide, 28, 214
third-world. See developing countries
Tibotec, 162–63
tiered payment plan, 233–34
TMC 114, 126, 163
tobacco industry, 176. See also smoking
Tobacco Industry Research Committee,
 176
Tobey, George, Jr., 209
tranquilizers, minor, 214
Transkaryotic Therapies (TKT), 37–38,
 53–57, 59
trihexosidase-alpha, 50

tuberculosis (TB), 158, 212, 244–46, 257, 258
Tufts University Center for the Study of Drug Development, 237, 239, 246
tumor necrosis factor (TNF), 36
tumor suppressor gene, 182
tyrosine kinase inhibitors, 199

ulcers, 220, 224, 226–28. *See also* antacids
Ullrich, Axel, 193, 195
United Nations (UN), 257
universities: discoveries made on government grants, 126, 128
University of California at San Diego (UCSD), 202–3

vaccine(s): AIDS, 88, 157; development, 258; polio, 212
Vagelos, P. Roy, 106, 108, 132, 154
Vapnek, Daniel, 26, 34, 36
Varmus, Harold, 65, 147–48, 179
Vasella, Daniel, 200–201
Venter, J. Craig, 61–66, 75, 76, 78, 80–81
Vertex Pharmaceuticals, 90–91, 108, 159–60
Viagra, 241, 256
vinblastine, 185
vincristine, 185
Vioxx, 224, 226–28, 241
Viracept. *See* nelfinavir
viral load tests, 144, 146
Vitetta, Ellen, 205–6, 250
Volwiler, Ernest H., 116

Wade, Nicholas, 76
Waksal, Harlan, 203, 204
Waksal, Samuel, 202–4

Waksman, Selman, 106, 212
Waldholz, Michael, 183
Wall Street: biotechnology revolution on, 183, 191 (*see also* biotechnology revolution); gene patents and, 66
Walpole, Arthur, 197–98
war-time research, 98–100
Watson, James, 20, 61, 67, 71, 72, 77, 177, 178
Waxman, Henry, 47, 130, 131
Weinberg, Robert A., 177
Whitcombe, Phil, 24
White, Tony, 81
Whitfield, Roy, 75
Witte, Owen, 199
Wlodawer, Alex, 108
Wolfe, M. Michael, 229
Women's Field Army, 170
World Health Organization (WHO), 257
World War II, 98
Wyden, Ron, 188–90
Wynder, Ernst L., 175

Xigris (drotrecogin alfa), 80, 252
X-ray crystallography, 108, 121, 159; commercialization, 94

Yarchoan, Robert, 91
Young, Frank, 143

zalcitabine (ddC), 113, 145; clinical trials, 112, 113, 131, 135, 143, 144, 147, 149, 151, 152; combined with other drugs, 131, 135, 145, 151, 152; companies competing to develop, 110, 149; FDA approval, 144, 147; NCI and, 110; side effects, 111
zidovudine. *See* AZT

Indexer:	Leonard Rosenbaum
Compositor:	BookMatters, Berkeley
Text:	10/13 Sabon
Display:	Akzidenz Grotesk Condensed
Printer and binder:	Maple-Vail Book Manufacturing Group